Adult Nurse Practitioner Certification Review Guide

THIRD EDITION

EDITORS

Virginia Layng Millonig, Ph.D, R.N., C.P.N.P.
President
Health Leadership Associates, Inc.
Potomac, Maryland

Sally K. Miller, M.S., C.R.N.P., C.C.R.N., A.N.P., G.N.P., A.C.N.P.
Assistant Professor
School of Nursing
Allegheny University of the Health Sciences
Philadelphia, Pennsylvania

Health Leadership Associates
Potomac, Maryland

Family Nurse Practitioner Set

(ISBN 1-878028-24-3)

by
Health Leadership Associates, Inc.

Consists of
The

Adult Nurse Practitioner Certification Review Guide

Pediatric Nurse Practitioner Certification Review Guide

Women's Health Care Nurse Practitioner Certification Review Guide

---

Health Leadership Associates
Sponsoring Editor: Virginia Layng Millonig, Ph.D., R.N.
Managing Editor: Mary A. Millonig
Production Manager: Martha M. Pounsberry
Editorial Assistants: Bridget M. Jones
                                 Cheryl C. Patterson
Cover and Design: Merrifield Graphics
Composition: Port City Press, Inc.
Design and Production: Port City Press, Inc.

Third Edition

Printed in the United States of America

Health Leadership Associates, Inc.
P.O. Box 59153
Potomac, Maryland 20859

Library of Congress Cataloging-in-Publication Data

Adult nurse practitioner certification review guide / editors,
   Virginia Layng Millonig, Sally K. Miller; contributing authors,
   Leanne C. Busby ... [et al.]. — 3rd ed.
       p. cm. — (Family nurse practitioner set)
   Includes bibliographical references and index.
   ISBN 1-878028-16-2
     1. Nurse practitioners—Examinations, questions, etc.   2. Primary nursing—Examinations,
questions, etc.   I. Millonig, Virginia
Layng.   II. Miller, Sally K.   III. Busby, Leanne C.   IV. Series.
   [DNLM: 1. Nurse Practitioners examination questions.   2. Nursing
Care examination questions.   WY   18.2A244 1999]
RT82.8.A38   1998
610.73'076—dc21
DNLM/DLC
for Library of Congress   98-30168
                                             CIP

10 9 8 7 6 5 4 3 2 1

NOTICE: The editors, authors and publisher of this book have taken care that the information and recommendations contained herein are accurate and compatible with standards generally accepted at the time of publication. However, the editors, authors and publisher cannot accept responsibility for errors or omissions or for the consequences from application of the information in this book and make no warranty, express or implied with respect to the contents of the book.

In appreciation to the authors, reviewers and nurse practitioners throughout the country who have provided suggestions and guidance in the development of the third edition of this Review Guide. And finally to those who have found this review guide not only responsible for success in the certification process, but also as an invaluable tool in the clinical setting. Your continuous input is greatly appreciated.

To my nana, Helen Miller, whose unselfish nature and caring spirit were unparalleled...and to my son Michael, who is everything.

Contributing Authors

Leanne C. Busby, M.S.N., R.N.,C.S., F.N.P.
Administrator
Vanderbilt Asthma, Sinus, Allergy Program
Adjunct Faculty
Family Health Systems
Vanderbilt University School of Nursing
Vanderbilt University Medical Center
Nashville, Tennessee

Susan Chaney, Ed.D., R.N.,C.S., F.N.P.
Professor
College of Nursing
Family Nurse Practitioner
Homeless Outreach Medical Services
Parkland Health and Hospital System
Texas Woman's University
Dallas, Texas

Sylvia Torres Fletcher, M.S., R.N.,C.S., F.N.P.
Assistant Clinical Professor
Family Nurse Practitioner
College of Nursing
Texas Woman's University
Dallas, Texas

Nancy Dickenson Hazard, M.S.N., C.P.N.P., F.A.A.N.
Executive Officer
Sigma Theta Tau International
Indianapolis, Indiana

Mary D. Knudtson, M.S.N., R.N.,C.S., F.N.P., P.N.P.
Assistant Clinical Professor
Family Medicine
Director of Family Nurse Practitioner Program
Robert Wood Johnson Executive Nurse Leadership Fellow
University of California, Irvine
Irvine, California

Debbie G. Kramer, M.S., R.N., C.S., C.R.N.P.
Gerontological\Adult Nurse Practitioner
Patient Care Manager
Baltimore Longitudinal Study of Aging
National Institute on Aging
Johns Hopkins Bayview Medical Center
VA Maryland Health Care System and EpiHealth Associates
Baltimore, Maryland

Susan B. Moskosky, M.S., R.N.C., W.H.C.N.P.
Woman's Health Nurse Practitioner
Office of Family Planning, Office of Population Affairs
U.S. Department of Health and Human Services
Washington, D.C.

Rosanne H. Pruitt, Ph.D., R.N.,C.S., F.N.P.
Associate Professor
Graduate Coordinator
School of Nursing
Clemson University
Clemson, South Carolina

Sister Maria Salerno, O.S.F., D.N.Sc., R.N.,C.S.
Associate Professor
Director Primary Care/Adult Nurse Practitioner Program
School of Nursing
The Catholic University of America
Washington, D. C.

Pamela A. Shuler, RN, D.N.Sc., R.N.,C.S., F.N.P.
Family Nurse Practitioner
Consultant and Clinician
WESTCARE Health System
Sylva, North Carolina

Madeline Turkeltaub, Ph.D., R.N.,C.S. A.N.P.
Adult Nurse Practitioner
Senior Vice President
Collingswood
Rockville, Maryland

Margaret Hadro Venzke, M.S., R.N.,C.S., F.N.P.
Instructor
Coordinator Family Nurse Practitioner Track
College of Nursing and Health Science
George Mason University
Fairfax, Virginia
Family Nurse Practitioner
Student Primary Care Clinic
Georgetown University
Washington, D.C.

Reviewers

Rosemary Goodyear, Ed.D., R.N.,C.S
Professor
Director TWU C.A.R.E.S.
College of Nursing
Texas Woman's University
Denton, Texas

Anne W. Salomone, M.S., R.N.C., C.N.M.
Woman's Health Care Nurse Practitioner
Nurse Midwife
Demis Olson Medical Group
Crystal Lake, Illinois

Bonnie Bata-Jones, M.S., R.N.,C.S., F.N.P.
Associate Education Specialist
School of Nursing
University of Minnesota
Minneapolis, Minnesota

Beth Kelsey, M.S., R.N.C., W.H.C.N.P.
Instructor
School of Nursing
Ball State University
Muncie, Indiana

Rosemary Jablonski, M.S.N., R.N.,C.S.
Adult Nurse Practitioner
Hematology, Oncology Associates, LTD
Alexandria, Virginia

Preface

The third edition of this book has been developed especially for adult and family nurse practitioners preparing to take Certification Examinations. The third edition differs from the second edition in several respects. All sections have been expanded and updated. The number of questions have been increased and the bibliographies enhanced.

The purpose of the book is twofold. This book will assist individuals engaged in self study preparation for Certification Examinations, and may be used as a reference guide in the practice setting. It is also one of three books that comprises the 'Family Nurse Practitioner Series', the others being the Pediatric Nurse Practitioner Certification Review Guide and the Women's Health Care Nurse Practitioner Certification Review Guide.

The book has been organized to provide the reader with test taking strategies first. This is followed by the chapter on health promotion. The next 13 chapters address common disorders and provide succinct summaries of definitions, etiology, signs and symptoms, physical findings, differential diagnoses, diagnostic tests\findings and management\treatment. The final chapter addresses health policy, role, trends and professional issues for the nurse practitioner in the health care industry at large.

Following each chapter are test questions, which are intended to serve as an introduction to the testing arena. In addition a bibliography is included for those who need a more in depth discussion of the subject matter in each chapter. These references can serve as additional instructional material for the reader.

Many nurses preparing for certification examinations find that reviewing an extensive body of scientific knowledge requires a very difficult search of many sources that must be synthesized to provide a review base for the examination. This publication provides a succinct, yet comprehensive review of the core material.

The editors and contributing authors are certified nurse practitioners. They have designed this book to assist potential examinees to prepare for success in the certification examination process.

It is assumed that the reader of this review guide has completed a course of study in either an adult or family nurse practitioner program. The Adult Nurse Practitioner Certification Review Guide is not intended to be a basic learning tool.

Adult Nurse Practitioner

Certification is a process that is gaining recognition both within and outside the profession. For the professional it is a means of gaining special recognition as a certified nurse practitioner which not only demonstrates a level of competency, but may also enhance professional opportunities and advancement. For the consumer, it means that a certified nurse has met certain predetermined standards set by the profession.

CONTENTS

1 **Test Taking Strategies** *Nancy A. Dickenson Hazard*
Virginia L. Millonig

2 **Health Promotion and Evaluation** *Rosanne H. Pruitt*

3 **Dermatological Disorders** *Sylvia Fletcher*
Susan Chaney

4 **Eye, Ear, Nose, and Throat Disorders** *Margaret Hadro Venzke*

5 Respiratory Disorders
Margaret Hadro Venzke

6 Cardiovascular Disorders
Sally K. Miller

7 Hematological and Oncological Disorders
Sister Maria Salerno

8   Gastrointestinal Disorders   *Sister Maria Salerno*

9   Endocrine Disorders   *Sister Maria Salerno*

10   Genitourinary and Gynecologic Disorders   *Pamela A. Shuler*
                                                                 Mary D. Knudtson

11 Pregnancy, Contraception and Menopause
Susan B. Moskosky

12 Musculoskeletal Disorders
Madeline Turkeltaub

13 Neurological Disorders
Sally K. Miller

14 Psychosocial Disorders
Sister Maria Salerno

15   Care of the Aging Adult

Debbie G.Kramer

16   Advanced Practice Trends and Issues and Health Policy

Leanne C. Busby

Test Taking Strategies and Techniques

Nancy A. Dickenson Hazard
Virginia L. Millonig

We all respond to testing situations in different ways. What separates the successful test taker from the unsuccessful one is knowing how to prepare for and take a test. Preparing yourself to be a successful test taker is as important as studying for the test. Each person needs to assess and develop individual test taking strategies and skills. The primary goal of this chapter is to assist potential examinees in knowing how to study for and take a test. Of equal importance to this study preparation is a basic understanding of how certification examinations are developed. They are based upon a universal knowledge foundation. Test items are selected from generally recognized resources available to the examinee, and specific to the type of specialty area.

STRATEGY #1 Know Yourself

When faced with an examination, do you feel threatened, experience butterflies or sweaty palms, have trouble keeping your mind focused on studying or on test questions? These common symptoms of test anxiety plague many of us, but can be used advantageously if understood and handled correctly. Over the years of test taking, each of us has developed certain testing behaviors, some of which are beneficial, while others present obstacles to successful test taking. You can take control of the test taking situation by identifying the undesirable behaviors, maintaining the desirable ones and developing skills to improve test performance.

Technique #1: From the following descriptions of test taking personalities, find yourself (Table 1). Write down those characteristics which describe you even if they are from different personality types. Carefully review the problem list associated with your test taking personality characteristics. Write down the problems which are most troublesome. Then make a list of how you can remedy these problems from the improvement strategies list. Be sure to use these strategies as you prepare for and take examinations.

STRATEGY #2 Develop Your Thinking Skills

Understanding Thought Process: In order to improve your thinking skills and subsequent test performance, it is best to understand the types of thinking as well as the techniques to enhance the thought process.

Everyone has a personal learning style, but we all must proceed through the same process to think.

Table 1

Test Taker Profile

Type	Characteristics	Pitfalls	Improvement Strategies
The Rusher	• Rushes to complete the test before the studied facts are forgotten	• Unable to read question and situation completely	• Practice progressive relaxation techniques
	• Arrives at test site early and waits anxiously	• At high risk for misreading, misinterpreting and mistakes	• Develop a study plan with sufficient time to review important content
	• Mumbles studied facts	• Difficult items heighten anxiety	• Avoid cramming and last minute studying
	• Tense body posture	• Likely to make quick, not well-thought-out guesses	• Take practice tests focusing on slowing down and reading and answering each option carefully
	• Accelerated pulse, respiration and neuromuscular excitement		• Read instructions and questions slowly
	• Answers questions rapidly and is generally one of the first to complete		
	• Experiences exhaustion once test is over		
The Turtle	• Moves slowly, methodically, deliberately through each question	• Last to finish; often does not complete the exam	• Take practice tests focusing on time spent per item
	• Repeated rereading, underlining and checking	• Has to quickly complete questions in last part of exam, increasing errors	• Place watch in front of examination paper to keep track of time
	• Takes 60 to 90 seconds per question versus an average of 45 to 60 seconds	• Has difficulty completing timed examinations	• Mark answer sheet for where one should be halfway through exam based on total number of questions and total amount of time for exam
			• Study concepts not details
			• Attempt to answer each question as you progress through the exam

Thinking occurs on six levels—the lower level of memory and comprehension and the higher levels of application, analysis, synthesis and evaluation (Sides & Korchek, 1994). Memory is the ability to recall facts. Without adequate retrieval of facts, progression through the higher levels of thinking cannot occur easily. Comprehension is the ability to understand memorized facts. To be effective,

Adult Nurse Practitioner

Type	Characteristics	Pitfalls	Improvement Strategies
The Personalizer	• Mature person who has personal knowledge and insight from life experiences	• Risk in relying on what has been learned through observation and experience since one may develop false understandings and stereotypes	• Focus on principles and standards that support nursing practice
		• Personal beliefs and experiences are frequently not the norm or standard tested	• Avoid making connections between patients in exam clinical situations and personal clinical experience
		• Has difficulty identifying expected standards measured by standardized examination	• Focus on generalities not experiences
The Squisher	• View exams as threat, rather than an expected event in education	• Procrastinates studying for exams	• Establish a plan of progressive, disciplined study
	• Preoccupied with grades and personal accomplishment	• Unable to study effectively since waits until last minute	• Use defined time frames for studying content and taking practice exams
	• Attempts to avoid responsibility and accountability associated with testing in order to reduce anxiety	• Increased anxiety over test since procrastinating study impairs ability to learn and perform	• Use relaxation techniques • Return to difficult items • Read carefully
The Philosopher	• Academically successful person who is well disciplined and structured in study habits	• Over analysis causes loss of sight of actual intent of question	• Focus on questions as they are written
	• Displays great intensity and concentration during exam	• Reads information into questions answering with own added information rather than answering the actual intent of question	• Work on self confidence and not on question. Initial response is usually correct
	• Searches questions for hidden or unintended meaning		• Avoid multiple rereadings of questions
	• Experiences anxiety over not knowing everything		• Avoid adding own information and unintended meanings
			• Practice, practice, practice with sample tests
The Second Guesser	• Answers questions twice, first as an examinee, second as an examiner	• Altering an initial response frequently results in an incorrect answer	• Reread only the few items of which one is unsure. Avoid changing initial responses

Type	Characteristics	Pitfalls	Improvement Strategies
The Lawyer	• Believes second look will allow one to find and correct errors	• Frequently changes answers because the pattern of response appears incorrect (i.e., too many ''true'' or too many correct responses)	• Take exam carefully and progressively first time, allowing little or no time for rereading • Study facts • Avoid reading into questions
	• Frequently changes initial responses (i.e., grades own test)		
	• Attempts to place words or ideas into the question (leads the witness)	• Veers from the obvious answer and provides response from own point of view	• Focus on distinguishing what patient is saying in question and not on what is read into question
	• Occurs most frequently with psychosocial or communication questions which ask for the most appropriate response	• Reads a question, jumps to a conclusion then finds a response that leads to predetermined conclusion	• Avoid formulating responses aimed at obtaining certain information
			• Choose responses that allow patient to express feelings which encourage hope, not catastrophe, those which are intended to clarify, which identify feeling tone of patient or which avoid negating or confronting patient feelings
			• Carefully read entire question before selecting a response

From: ''Making the grades as a test-taker,'' by N. Dickenson-Hazard, (1989) *Pediatric Nursing, 15,* p. 303. Adapted from: *Nurse's guide to successful test-taking* by M. B. Sides and N. B. Cailles, 1989. Philadelphia: J. B. Lippincott, Co., pp 59–70, 199–203. Copyright 1989 by A. J. Jannetti, Inc. Reprinted by permission.

comprehension skills must allow the person to translate recalled information from one context to another. Application, or the process of using information to know why something occurs, is a higher form of learning. Effective application relies on the use of understood, memorized facts to verify intended action. Analysis is the ability to use abstract or logical forms of thought to show relationships and to distinguish the cause and effect between the variables in a situation.

As related to testing situations, the thought process from memory to analysis occurs quite quickly. Some examination items are designed to test memory and comprehension while others test application and analysis. An example of a memory question is as follows:

Type 1 diabetes results from dysfunction of the:

a)   Liver
b)   *Pancreas*
c)   Adrenal glands
d)   Kidneys
e)   Pituitary gland

To answer this question correctly, the individual has to retrieve a memorized fact. Understanding the fact, knowing why it is important or analyzing what should be done in this situation is not needed. An example of a question which tests comprehension is as follows:

> You are taking a history on a 47 year-old white female during a routine health assessment visit. She reports that in the past month she has experienced increased thirst and needs to urinate frequently. She reports recurrent episodes of vaginitis and is concerned about an abrasion on her leg which will not heal. You note that her blood pressure is recorded at 150/90 and that she is overweight. You would most likely suspect which of the following?
>
> a)   Urinary tract infection
> b)   Hyperthyroidism
> c)   Type 1 diabetes mellitus
> d)   Essential hypertension
> e)   *Type 2 diabetes mellitus*

To answer this question correctly, an individual must retrieve facts about the physiology of diabetes mellitus in order to understand and differentiate the presenting symptoms.

In answering an examination question that requires a higher level of thought, an individual must be able to recall a fact, understand that fact in the context of the question, and apply this understanding to determine why one answer is correct, after analyzing possible answer choices as they relate to the situation (Sides & Korchek, 1994). An example of an application analysis question is as follows:

> A 48 year-old diabetic woman wants to enroll in a low-impact aerobics class. Her diabetes is well managed with twice daily insulin injections. Your best advice is to:
>
> a)   Increase daily doses of insulin
> b)   *Have an extra snack before exercise class*
> c)   Administer a dose of regular insulin after exercise is completed
> d)   Tell her participating in the class is not advisable

To answer this question correctly, the individual must recall physiologic facts of insulin dependent diabetes, understand what is happening in this situation, consider each option and how it applies to the patient's condition and analyze why each advice option works or doesn't work for this patient. Application/analysis questions require the examinee to use logical rationale, based on a well defined principle or fact. Problem solving ability becomes important as the examinee must think through each question option, determining its relevance and importance to the situation in the question.

Building your thinking skills: Effective memorization is the cornerstone to learning and building thinking skills (Olney, 1989). We have all experienced ''memory power outages'' at some time, due in part to trying to memorize too much, too fast, too ineffectively. Developing skills to improve memorization is important to increasing the effectiveness of your thinking and subsequent test performance.

Technique #1:   Quantity is NOT quality, so concentrate on learning important content. For example, it is important to know the various pharmacologic agents appropriate for the management of chronic obstructive pulmanary disease (COPD), not the specific dosages for each medication.

Technique #2:   Memory from repetition, or saying something over and over again to remember it, usually fades. Developing memory skills which trigger retrieval of needed facts is more useful. Such skills are as follows:

Acronyms: These are mental crutches which facilitate recall. Some are already established such as PERRLA (pupils equal, round, react to light, and accommodation), C.H.F. for (congestive heart failure), or T.I.A. for (transient ischemic attack). Developing your own acronyms can be particularly useful since they are your own word association arrangements in a singular word. Nonsense words or funny, unusual ones are often more useful since they attract your attention.

Acrostics: This mental tool arranges words into catchy phrases. The first letter of each word stands for something which is recalled as the phrase is said. Your own acrostics are most valuable in triggering recall of learned information since they are your individual situation associations. An example of an acrostic is as follows:

Sam **E**xercises **B**y **W**eight-lifting and **R**unning stands for the aspects of non-drug therapy/management for hypertension: **S**alt restriction, **E**xercise, **B**iofeedback, **W**eight reduction, and **R**elaxation techniques.

ABCs: This technique facilitates information retrieval by using the alphabet as a crutch. Each letter stands for a symptom, which when put together creates a picture of the clinical presentation of the disease. For example, the characteristics of peptic ulcer disease using the ABC technique is as follows:

    a) Antacids relieve pain
    b) Burning epigastric pain
    c) Cycle of pain two hours after eating
    d) Discomfort awakens at night
    e) Experiences weight loss
    f) Food sometimes aggravates pain

Imaging: This technique can be used in two ways. The first is to develop a nickname for a clinical problem which when said produces a mental picture. For example, "thin, barrel-chested, pink puffer" might be used to visualize a patient with emphysema who has a muscle-wasted body appearance, absent central cyanosis, hypertrophy of respiratory accessory muscles and an AP chest diameter greater than the transverse chest. A second form of imaging is to visualize a specific patient while you are trying to understand or solve a clinical problem when studying or answering a question. For example, imagine a young woman who is experiencing an acute asthma attack. You are trying to analyze the situation and place her in a position which maximizes respiratory effort. In your mind you visualize her in various positions of sidelying, angular and forward, imaging what will happen to the woman and her respiratory effort in each position.

Rhymes, music & links: The absurd is easier to remember than the most common. Rhymes, music or links can add absurdity and humor to learning and remembering (Olney, 1989). These retrieval tools are developed by the individual for specific content. For example, making up a rhyme about diabetes may be helpful in remembering the predominant female incidence, origin of disease, primary symptoms and management as illustrated by:

> There once was a woman
>   whose beta cells failed
> She grew quite thirsty
>   and her glucose levels sailed
> Her lack of insulin caused her to
>   increase her intake

And her increased urinary output
was certainly not fake
So she learned to watch her diet
and administer injections
That kept her healthy, growing
and free of complications.

Setting content to music is sometimes useful to remembering. Melodies which are repetitious jog the memory by the ups and downs of the notes and the rhythm of the music.

Links connect key words from the content by using them in a story. An example given by Olney (1989) for remembering the parts of an eye is IRIS watched a PUPIL through the LENS of a RED TIN telescope while eating CORN-EA on the cob.

Additional memory aids may also include the use of color or drawing for improving recall. Use different colored pens or paper to accentuate the material being learned. For example, highlight or make notes in blue for content about respiratory problems and in red for cardiovascular content. Drawing assists with visualizing content as well. This is particularly helpful for remembering the pathophysiology of the specific health problem.

The important thing to remember about remembering is to use good recall techniques.

Technique #3:   Improving higher level thinking skills involves exercising the application and analysis of memorized facts. Small group review is particularly useful for enhancing these high level skills. Small group interaction allows verbalization of thought processes and receipt of input about content and thought process from others (Sides & Korchek, 1994). Individuals not only hear how they think, but how others think as well. This interaction allows individuals to identify flaws in their thought process as well as to strengthen their positive points.

Taking practice tests are also helpful in developing application/analysis thinking skills. Practice tests permit the individual to analyze thinking patterns as well as the cause and effect relationships between the question and its options. The problem solving skills needed to answer application/analysis questions are tested, giving the individual more experience through practice (Dickenson-Hazard, 1990).

STRATEGY #3 Know The Content

Your ability to study is directly influenced by organization and concentration (Dickenson-Hazard, 1990). If effort is spent on both of these aspects of exam preparation, examination success can be increased.

Preparation for studying: Getting organized. Study habits are developed early in our education experiences. Some of our habits enhance learning while others do not. To increase study effectiveness, organization of study materials and time is essential. Organization decreases frustration, allows for easy resumption of study and increases concentrated study time.

Technique #1:   Create your own study space. Select a study area that is yours alone, free from distractions, comfortable and well lighted. The ventilation and room temperature should be comfortable since a cold room makes it difficult to concentrate and a warm room may make you sleepy (Burkle & Marshak, 1989). All study materials should be left in a specific study space. The basic premise of a study space is that it facilitates a mind set that you are there to study. When study is interrupted, it is best to leave study materials just as they are. Don't close books or put away notes as they will have to be relocated, wasting valuable time, when study is resumed.

Technique #2:   Define and organize the content. Secure an outline or the content parameters which are to be examined from the examining body. If outline is sketchy, develop a more detailed one for yourself using the recommended texts as a guideline. Next, identify available study resources: class notes, old exams, handouts, textbooks, review courses and books, home study programs, or study groups. For national standardized exams, such as initial licensing or certification, it is best to identify a few resources which cover the content being tested and stick to them. Attempting to review all available resources is not only mind boggling, but increases anxiety and frustration as well. Make your selections and stay with them.

Technique #3:   Conduct a content assessment. Using a simple rating scale of:

    1 = requires no review
    2 = requires minimal review
    3 = requires intensive review
    4 = start from the beginning

Read through the content outline and rate each content area (Dickenson-Hazard, 1990). Table 2 provides a sample exam content assessment. Be honest with your assessment. It is far better to recognize your content weaknesses when you can study and remedy them, rather than wishing during the exam that you had studied more. Likewise with content strengths: If you know the material, don't waste time studying it.

Technique #4:   Develop a study plan. Coordinate the content which needs to be studied with the time available (Sides & Korchek, 1994). Prioritize your study needs, starting with weak areas first. Allow for a general review at the end of the study plan. Finally, establish an overall goal for yourself; something that will motivate you when brought to mind.

Table 3 illustrates a study plan developed on the basis of the exam content assessment in Table 2. Conducting an assessment and developing a study plan should require no more than 50 minutes. It is a wise investment of time with potential payoffs of reduced study stress and exam success.

Technique #5:   Begin now and use your time wisely. The smart test taker begins the study process early (Olney, 1989). Sit down, conduct the content assessment and develop a study plan as soon as you know about the exam. DON'T PROCRASTINATE!

Getting Down To Business—The Actual Studying: There is no better way to prepare for an examination than individual study (Dickenson-Hazard, 1989). The responsibility to achieve the goal you set for this exam lies with you alone. The means you employ to achieve this goal do vary and should begin with identifying your peak study times and using techniques to maximize them.

Technique #1:   Study in short bursts. Each of us have our own biologic clock which dictates when we are at our peak during the day. If you are a morning person, you are generally active and alert early in the day, slowing down and becoming drowsy by evening. If you are an evening person, you don't completely wake up until late morning and hit your peak in the afternoon and evening. Each person generally has several peaks during the day. It is best to study during those times when your alertness is at its peak (Dickenson-Hazard, 1990).

During our concentration peaks, there are mini peaks, or bursts of alertness (Olney, 1989). These alertness ("mini") peaks occur during a concentration peak because levels of concentration are at their highest during the first part and last part of a study period. These bursts can vary from ten minutes to one hour depending on the extent of concentration. If studying is sustained for one hour there are only two mini peaks; one at the beginning and one at the end. There are eight mini peaks if that

Table 2

Sample Content Assessment

Exam Content: Gastrointestinal Health Problems of the Adult	
Category: Provided by Examining Body	*Rating: Provided by Examinee*

I. Peptic Ulcer Disease
    A. Etiology 4
    B. Pathophysiology 3
    C. Symptomatology 3
    D. Differential Diagnosis 4
    E. Diagnostic Tests 3
    F. Management/Treatment 4

II. Esophagitis
    A. Etiology 3
    B. Pathophysiology 3
    C. Symptomatology 2
    D. Differential Diagnosis 3
    E. Diagnostic Tests 2
    F. Management/Treatment 4

III. Cholecystitis
    A. Etiology 2
    B. Pathophysiology 2
    C. Symptomatology 1
    D. Differential Diagnosis 2
    E. Diagnostic Tests 4
    F. Management/Treatment 4

IV. Appendicitis
    A. Etiology 3
    B. Pathophysiology 4
    C. Symptomatology 3
    D. Differential Diagnosis 2
    E. Diagnostic Tests 3
    F. Management/Treatment 4

V. Diverticulitis
    A. Etiology 3
    B. Pathophysiology 4
    C. Symptomatology 3
    D. Differential Diagnosis 3
    E. Diagnostic Tests 2
    F. Management/Treatment 4

VI. Hepatitis
    A. Etiology 3
    B. Pathophysiology 4
    C. Symptomatology 4
    D. Differential Diagnosis 4
    E. Diagnostic Tests 2
    F. Management/Treatment 4

VII. Acute Gastroenteritis
    A. Etiology 2
    B. Pathophysiology 3
    C. Symptomatology 2
    D. Differential Diagnosis 3
    E. Diagnostic Tests 4
    F. Management/Treatment 3

VIII. Irritable Bowel Syndrome
    A. Etiology 3
    B. Pathophysiology 3
    C. Symptomatology 3
    D. Differential Diagnosis 4
    E. Diagnostic Tests 4
    F. Management/Treatment 3

Table 3

Sample Study Plan
Goal: Master Content on the Gastrointestinal Problems of the Adult Patient. Test Time Available: 2 Weeks

Objective	Activity	Date Accomplished
Master content on diverticulitis	Read Chapter 26. Take notes on chapter content according to outline	Feb. 5 & 6, 1 hour
	Review class notes combined with chapter notes	Feb. 6, 1 hour
	Review sample test questions	Feb. 6, 1 hour
Understand content on peptic ulcer disease	Read Chapter 25. Take notes on chapter content according to content outline	Feb. 7, 2 hours
	Review class notes combined with chapter notes.	Feb. 8, 1½ hours
Master content on cholecystitis	Read Chapter 24. Take notes on chapter content according to content outline	Feb. 10, 2 hours
	Review class notes combined with chapter notes	Feb. 11, ½ hours
	Review sample test questions	Feb. 12, 1½ hours
Know material on irritable bowel syndrome	Scan Chapter 27. Review class notes supplementing with text notes	Feb. 14, 2 hours
Know material on esophagitis	Scan Chapter 23. Review class notes supplementing with text notes	Feb. 15, 2 hours
Know material on hepatitis	Scan Chapter 28. Review highlights and important concepts	Feb. 16, 2 hours
Know material on appendicitis and acute gastroenteritis	Scan Chapter 29. Review highlights and important concepts	Feb. 17, 2 hours
Demonstrate understanding of all material	Review with another person	Feb. 18, 2 hours
	Review all notes	Feb. 19, 1½ hours
	Take sample test questions	Feb. 19, 1½ hours
Think positively	SMILE	ON GOING
	Take frequent breaks	
	Reward myself after each study session	
	Keep my goal in mind	

same hour is divided into four, 10-minute intervals. Hence it is more helpful to study in short bursts (Olney, 1989). More can be learned in less time.

Technique #2: Cramming can be useful. Since concentration ability is highly variable, some individuals can sustain their mini peaks for 15, 20 or even 30 minutes at a time. Pushing your concentration beyond its peak is fruitless and verges on cramming, which in general is a poor study technique. There are, however, times when cramming, a short term memory tool, is useful. Short term memory generally is at its best in the morning. A quick review or cram of content in the morning can be useful the day of the exam (Olney, 1989). Most studying, however, is best accomplished in the afternoon or evening when long term memory functions at its peak.

Technique #3: Give your brain breaks. Regular times during study to rest and absorb the content is needed by the brain. The best approach to breaks is to plan them and give yourself a conscious break (Dickenson-Hazard, 1990). This approach eliminates the "day dreaming" or "wandering thought" approach to breaks that many of us use. It is better to get up, leave the study area and do something non-study related for longer breaks. For shorter breaks of five minutes or so, leave your desk, gaze out the window or do some stretching exercises. When your brain says to give it a rest, accommodate it! You'll learn more in less stress free time.

Technique #4: Study the correct content. It is easy for all of us to become bogged down in the detail of the content we are studying. However, it is best to focus on the major concepts or the "state of the art" content. Leave the details, the suppositions and the experience at the door of your study area. Concentrate on the major textbook facts and concepts which revolve around the subject matter being tested.

Technique #5: Fit your studying to the test type. The best way to prepare for an objective test is to study facts, particularly anything printed in italics. Memory enhancing techniques are particularly useful when preparing for an objective test. If preparing for an essay test, study generalities, examples and concepts. Application techniques are helpful when studying for this type of an exam (Burkle & Marshak, 1989).

Technique #6: Use your study plan wisely. Your study plan is meant to be a guide, not a rigid schedule. You should take your time with studying. Don't rush through the content just to remain on schedule. Occasionally study plans need revision. If you take more or less time than planned, readjust the plan for the time gained or lost. The plan can guide you, but you must go at your own pace.

Technique #7: Actively study. Being an active participant in study rather than trying to absorb the printed word is also helpful. Ways to be active include taking notes on the content as you study; constructing questions and answering them; taking practice tests and discussing the content with yourself. Also, using your individual study quirks is encouraged. Some people stand, others walk around and some play background music. Whatever helps you to concentrate and study better, you should use.

Technique #8: Use study aids. While there is no substitute for individual studying, several resources, if available, are useful in facilitating learning. Review courses are an excellent means for organizing or summarizing your individual study. They generally provide the content parameters and the major concepts of the content which you need to know. Review courses also provide an opportunity to clarify not-well-understood content, as well as to review known material (Dickenson-Hazard, 1990). Study guides/certification review books and home study programs are useful for organizing study. They provide detail on the content which is important to the exam. Study groups are an excellent resource for summarizing and refining content. They provide an opportunity for thinking through your knowledge base, with the advantage of hearing another person's point of view. Each of these study aids increases understanding of content and when used correctly, increases effectiveness of knowledge application.

Technique #9: Know when to quit. It is best to stop studying when your concentration ebbs. It is unproductive and frustrating to force yourself to study. It is far better to rest or unwind, then resume at a later point in the day. Avoid studying outside your A.M. or P.M. concentration peaks and focus your study energy on your right time of day or evening.

STRATEGY #4 Become Test-wise

Most nursing examinations are composed of multiple choice questions (MCQ). This type of question requires the examinee to select the best response(s) for a specific circumstance or condition. Successful test taking is dependent not only on content knowledge but on test taking skill as well. If you are unable to impart your knowledge through the vehicle used for its conveyance, i.e., the MCQ, your test taking success is in jeopardy.

Computer based examinations are a new method of testing for some certification examinations. Eventually all of the certification paper and pencil examinations will be replaced with the computer method. Computer based testing has several advantages such as flexibility in taking the examinations at your convenience and earlier notification of test results. If the certification examination you are planning to take is computerized, the instructions will be provided both prior to the examination as well as at the time of the examination. No computer experience is required, and tutorials or introductory lessons precede the computer-based testing to familiarize you with the process.

Moreover, the strategies used to develop effective test-taking skills are applicable to both the traditional paper/pencil and computerized forms of the certification examinations (Sides & Korchek, 1994).

Technique #1: Recognize the purpose of a test question. Most test questions are developed to examine knowledge at two separate levels: memory and comprehension or application and analysis. A memory question requires the examinee to recall facts from their knowledge base while an application question requires the examinee to use and apply the knowledge. Memory questions test recall while application questions test synthesis and problem-solving skills. When taking a test, you need to be aware when you are being asked to recall a fact, and when you are being asked to use that fact.

Technique #2: Recognize the components of a test question. Multiple choice questions may include the basic components of a background statement, a stem and a list of options. The background statement presents information which facilitates the examinee in answering the question. The stem asks or states the intent of the question. The options are 3 to 5 possible responses to the question. The correct option is called the keyed response and all other options are called distractors (ABP, 1989). Knowing the components of a test question helps you sift through the information presented and focus on the question's intent (see Table 4).

Technique #3: Identify the key word(s) in a test question. Don't jump to conclusions when you read the stem. Key words are generally included in the stem of a test question, whereas key concepts or conditions appear in the background statement. You should pay particular attention to the key words in the stem and their impact on the intent of the question (See Table 5). Never "read" into a question or make assumptions beyond the information given.

Technique #4: Recognize the item types. Basically two styles of MCQs are used for examinations. One requires the examinee to select the one best answer; the other requires selection of multiple correct answers. Among the one best answer styles there are three types. The A type requires the selection of the best response among those offered. The B type requires the examinee to match the options with the appropriate statement. C type items require the examinee to compare or contrast two related conditions. The X type asks the examinee to respond either true or false to each option (ABP, 1989). Table 6 illustrates these item types. Many standardized tests such as those used for certification are composed of three to five option-A type questions.

Technique #5: Read the directions to the questions carefully. Since an examination may have several types of questions, it is imperative to read the directions carefully. If different item types are used on an exam, they are generally grouped together by type and marked clearly with directions. Be on the lookout for changing item types and be sure you understand how you are to answer before you begin reading the question.

Technique #6: Apply the basic rules of test taking. Examination candidates can avert many problems associated with test taking if they give thought to the

Table 4

Anatomy Of A Test Question

Background Statement:	A 32 year-old African-American female is being seen for a complaint of sores in the vaginal area. She has been experiencing a low-grade fever, headache and malaise over the past five days. Physical examination reveals inguinal lymphadenopathy, vaginal erythema and multiple labial and vaginal vesicular lesions.
Stem:	Which of the following causative organisms would you most likely suspect?
Options:	(A) *Herpes simplex virus 2* (B) Condylomata lata (C) Herpes simplex virus 1 (D) Treponema pallidum

Table 5

Test Question Key Words And Phrases

First	Priority	True Statements
Best	Advice	Correct Statements
Most	Approach	Contributing to
Initial	Consideration	Of the following
Important	Management	Which of the following
Major	Expectation	Each of the following
Common	Intervention	
Least	Assessment	
Except	Contraindication	
Not	Evaluation	
Greatest	Counseling	
Earliest	Facilitative	
Useful	Indicative	
Leading	Suggestive	
Significant	Appropriate	
Immediate	Accurately	
Helpful	Likely	
Closely	Characteristics	

From "Anatomy of a test question" by N. Dickenson-Hazard, 1989, *Pediatric Nursing 15*, p. 395. Copyright 1989 by A. J. Jannetti, Inc. Reprinted by permission.

mechanics of sitting down, reading the question and noting their answers. Timing yourself to avoid spending too much time on a question, returning to difficult questions, and not changing your answers are all techniques that can improve performance. Table 7 provides helpful hints for the basic rules of test-taking. Review these and apply them to the testing situation.

Technique #7   Make educated guesses. This type of guessing is the selection of an option (answer) when certainty of the correct answer is questionable. Elimination of all options except for two of them, followed by a reevaluation of these options based upon your correct knowledge base then allows you to make an educated guess.

There are some examinations that will give credit when correct answers are selected and give no credit for incorrect answers. Directions for this type of examination may state that credit will be given for correct answers, therefore all questions should be answered and you will not be penalized for guessing.

Other kinds of examinations will only give credit for correct answers, and subtract credit for incorrect answers. Directions for this type of examination will instruct you not to guess, or that there is a penalty for guessing. However, even with this kind of an examination, it is still to your advantage to make an educated guess if you can reduce your possibilities to two options and then select the best of the two. **WILD GUESSING** should be avoided since it may not be to your advantage (Nugent & Vitale, 1997).

Technique #8:   Practice, practice, practice. Taking practice tests can improve performance. While they can assist in evaluation of your knowledge, *their primary benefit is to assist you with test taking skills.* You should use them to evaluate your thinking process, your ability to read, understand and interpret questions, and your skills in completing the mechanics of the test.

Technique #9:   Be prepared for exam day. It is important to familiarize yourself with the test site, the building, the parking and travel route prior to the exam day. If you must travel, arrive early to allow time for this familiarization. It is helpful to make a list of things you need on the exam day: pencils, admission card, watch and a few pieces of hard candy as a quick energy source. On exam day allow yourself plenty of time to arrive at the site. Wear comfortable clothes and have a good breakfast that morning. The night before the exam, go to bed at a reasonable hour, and avoid excessive drinking or eating (Sides & Korchek, 1994). The idea is to arrive on time at the test site, prepared and as rested as possible.

TABLE 6

Item Type Examples

A TYPE

Directions for One Best Choice Items: This item-type requires that you indicate the one best answer from the lettered alternatives offered for each item. After you have decided on the one BEST answer, completely blacken the corresponding lettered circle on the answer sheet.

#1 A 46 year-old white female is being seen in follow-up for the treatment of migraine headaches. Your management plan would most appropriately include counseling on which of the following preventive techniques?
   a. Limiting intake of high calcium foods
   b. Encouraging additional sleep hours
   c. *Learning biofeedback techniques*
   d. Massaging posterior head and neck areas regularly
   e. Developing a rigorous exercise routine

B TYPE

Directions: Each group of questions below consists of five lettered headings followed by a list of numbered words or statements. For each numbered word or statement, select the one lettered heading that is most closely associated with it and fill in the circle beneath the corresponding letter on the answer sheet. Each lettered heading may be selected once, more than once, or not at all.

#2-#4
Medication Types::
   a. Anti-fungal
   b. Anti-protozoan
   c. Antiseptic
   d. Anti-viral
Most useful for treatment of:
   2. Trichomoniasis (B)
   3. Candidiasis (A)
   4. Bacterial vaginosis (B)

C TYPE

Directions: Each set of lettered headings below is followed by a list of numbered words or phrases. For each numbered word or phrase fill in the circle on the answer sheet under A if the item is associated with (A) only, B if the item is associated with (B) only, C if the item is associated with both (A) and (B), D if the item is associated with neither (A) nor (B).
   (A) Diabetic acidosis
   (B) Insulin shock
   (C) Both
   (D) Neither

#5 — Elevated bicarbonate level in serum (D)
#6 — The duration of the condition before proper treatment is begun may influence the prognosis (C)
#7 — Deep breathing (A)
#8 — Coma (C)
#9 — Moist skin (B)

X TYPE

Directions: Each of the questions or incomplete statements below is followed by five suggested answers or completions. For EACH lettered alternative completely blacken one lettered circle in either column T or F on the answer sheet.

Which of the following tests are useful for differentiating anemia associated with a chronic disease from iron deficiency anemia?
   a. Serum iron levels (F)
   b. Bone marrow examination (T)
   c. Reticulocyte count (F)
   d. Serum transferrin level (F)
   e. Serum ferritin level (T)

Adapted from ''Anatomy of a test question.'' by N. Dickenson-Hazard, 1989, *Pediatric Nursing 15*, p. 396. Copyright 1989 by A. J. Jannetti, Inc. Adapted by permission.

TABLE 7

Basic Rules For Test Taking

Basic Rule	*Helpful Hints*
Use time wisely and effectively	Allow no more than 1 minute per question—if you can't answer question, make an intelligent guess

Know the parts of a question
  Background statement: Informational scenario
  Stem: Specific question or intent statement
	Select the option that best completes question or solves the problem
	Relate options to question and balance against each other
	Consider all options

Read question carefully	Understand stem first, then look for answer Underline key words in background information and stem (i.e., first, best, initial, early, most, appropriate, except, least, not)
Identify intent of item based on information given	Don't assume any information not given . Don't read in or add any information not given Actively reason through question
Answer difficult questions by eliminating obviously incorrect options first	Select the best of the viable, available options using logical thought Reread stem; select strongest option Skip difficult questions and return to them later or make an educated guess
Select responses guided by principles of communication	Choose therapeutic, respectful, communication enhancing options Avoid inappropriate, punitive responses
Know the principles of nursing practice	Select options that relate to common need or the population in general Select options that are correct without exception Select options which reflect nursing judgement
Know and use test-taking principles	Avoid changing answers without good reason Attempt every question Don't rely on flaws in test construction Be systematic and use problem-solving techniques in answering questions

From ''Making the grade as a test-taker'' by N. Dickenson-Hazard, 1989. *Pediatric Nursing 15,* p. 304. Adapted from *How to take tests.* (pp 15-57) by J. Millman and W. Paul, 1969, New York: McGraw-Hill Co. and from *Nurses's guide to successful test taking.* (pp 43-53) by M. B. Sides and N. B. Cailles, 1989, Philadelphia: J. B. Lippincott Co. Copyright 1989 A. J. Jannetti, Inc. Reprinted and adapted by permission.

STRATEGY #5 Psych Yourself Up: Taking tests is stressful

While a little stress can be productive, too much can incapacitate you in your studying and test taking (Divine & Kylen, 1979). Your attitude and approach to test taking and studying can influence your outcomes. Psyching yourself up can have a positive effect and make examinations a non-anxiety laden experience (Dickenson-Hazard, 1990). The following techniques are based on the principles of successful test taking as presented by Sides & Cailles (1989). Incorporation of these techniques can improve response and performance in examination situations.

Technique #1: Adopt an ''I can'' attitude. Believing you can succeed is the key to success. Self belief inspires and gives you the power to achieve your goals. Without a success attitude, the road to your goal is much harder. We all stand an equal chance of success in this world. It is those who believe they can who achieve it. This ''I can'' attitude must permeate all your efforts in test taking from studying to improving your skills, to actually writing the test.

Technique #2:   Take control. By identifying your goal, deciding how to accomplish it and developing a plan for achieving it, you take control. Do not leave your success or failure to chance; control it through action and attitude.

Technique #3:   Think positively. Examinations are generally based on a standard which is the same for all individuals. Everyone can potentially pass. Performance is influenced not only by knowledge and skill but attitude as well. Those individuals who regard an exam as an opportunity or challenge will be more successful.

Technique #4:   Project a positive self-fulfilling prophecy. While preparing for an examination, project thoughts of the positive outcomes you will experience when you succeed. Self-talk is self-fulfilling. Expect success, not failure, of yourself.

Technique #5:   Feel good about yourself. Without feeling a sense of positive self worth, passing an examination is difficult. Recognize your professional contributions and give yourself credit for your accomplishments. Think ''I will pass,'' not ''I suppose I can.''

Technique #6:   Know yourself. Focus exam preparation and test taking on your strengths. Try to alter your weaknesses instead of becoming hung up on them. If you tend to overanalyze, study and read test questions at face value. If you're a speed demon when taking a test, slow down and read more carefully.

Technique #7:   Failure is a possibility. We all have failed at something at some point in our lives. Rather than dwelling on the failure, making excuses and believing you'll fail again, recognize your mistakes and remedy them. Failure is a time to begin again; use it as a motivator to do better. It is not the end of the world unless you allow it to be. It is best to deal with the failure and move on, otherwise it interferes with your success.

Technique #8:   Persevere, persevere, persevere! Endurance must underlie all your efforts. Call forth those reserve energies when you've had all you think you can take. Rely upon yourself and your support systems to help you maintain a sense of direction and keep your goal in the forefront.

Technique #9:   Motivation is muscle. Most individuals are motivated by fear or desire. The fear in an exam situation may be one of failure, the unknown or discovery of imperfection. Put your fear into perspective; realize you are not the only one with fear and that all have an equal opportunity for success. Develop strategies to reduce fear and use fear to your advantage by improving the imperfections. Desire is a powerful motivator and you should keep the rewards of your desire foremost in your mind. Whatever motivates you, use it to make you successful. Reward yourself during your exam preparation and once the exam has been completed. You alone hold the key to success; use what you have wisely.

Technique #10:   Overprepare. One of the best ways to reduce test anxiety is to overprepare. The more prepared you are the more confident you will be. Overpreparation requires you to study the same information over again even when you know the information. This activity will reinforce your learning and will build confidence and reduce anxiety when it comes time to take the examination.

Overpreparation can not occur unless adequate time is allowed for this process. A last minute cramming approach will not lead to an overprepared test taker. Being over prepared definitely places an individual in control and in a position of power and confidence (Nugent & Vitale, 1997).

This chapter has provided concepts, strategies and techniques for improving study and test taking skills. Your first task in improvement is to know yourself, how you study and how you take a test. You should use your strengths and remedy the weaknesses. Next you need to develop your thinking skills. Work on techniques to improve memory and reasoning. Now you need to organize your study and concentrate on using these new and used skills to be successful. Create a study space, develop a plan of action, then implement that plan during your periods of peak concentration. Before taking the exam be sure you understand the components of a test question, can identify key words and phrases and have practiced. Apply the test taking rules during the exam process. Finally, believe in yourself, your knowledge and your talent. Believing you can accomplish your goal facilitates the fact that you will.

BIBLIOGRAPHY

American Board of Pediatrics. (1989). *Developing questions and critiques.* Unpublished material.

Burke, M. M., & Walsh, M. B. (1992). *Gerontologic nursing.* St. Louis: Mosby Year Book.

Burkle, C. A., & Marshak, D. (1989). *Study program: Level 1.* Reston, VA: National Association of Secondary School Principals.

Dickenson-Hazard, N. (1989). Making the grade as a test taker. *Pediatric Nursing, 15,* 302–304.

Dickenson-Hazard, N. (1989). Anatomy of a test question. *Pediatric Nursing, 15,* 395–399.

Dickenson-Hazard, N. (1990). The psychology of successful test taking. *Pediatric Nursing, 16,* 66–67.

Dickenson-Hazard, N. (1990). Study smart. *Pediatric Nursing, 16,* 314–316.

Dickenson-Hazard, N. (1990). Study effectiveness: Are you 10 a.m. or p.m. scholar? *Pediatric Nursing, 16,* 419–420.

Dickenson-Hazard, N. (1990). Develop your thinking skills for improved test taking. *Pediatric Nursing, 16,* 480–481.

Divine, J. H., & Kylen, D. W. (1979). *How to beat test anxiety.* New York: Barrons Educational Series, Inc.

Goroll, A., May, L., & Mulley, A. (Eds.). (1988). *Primary care medicine* (2nd ed.). Philadelphia: J. B. Lippincott.

Millman, J., & Pauk, W. (1969). *How to take tests.* New York: McGraw-Hill Book Co.

Nugent, P. M., & Vitale, B. A. (1997). *Test success.* (2nd ed.). Philadelphia: F. A. Davis.

Olney, C. W. (1989). *Where there's a will, there's an A.* New Jersey: Chesterbrook Educational Publishers.

Sides, M., & Cailles, N. B. (1989). *Nurse's guide to successful test taking.* Philadelphia: J. B. Lippincott Co.

Sides, M., & Korchek, N. (1994). *Nurse's guide to successful test taking* (2nd ed.). Philadelphia: J. B. Lippincott.

Health Promotion and Evaluation

Rosanne H. Pruitt

Theoretical Aspects: Health Promotion Theories and Models

- High Level Wellness—a *continuum* that demonstrates dynamic interaction of health and environment as one moves toward high level wellness; health is dynamic with a continuous need for health promoting activity to maintain and improve one's health

- Maslow's Hierarchy of Needs (Maslow, 1954)
  1. Survival needs—food, water, sleep
  2. Safety and security—protection from physical hazards
  3. Love and belonging—affection, companionship
  4. Self-esteem—sense of self worth, recognition
  5. Self-actualization—achievement of personal potential

- Health Belief Model (Becker, 1972)—health is influenced by age, sex, race, ethnicity, and income
  1. Threats to health
     a. Perceived susceptibility
     b. Perceived seriousness of condition
  2. Outcome expectation of health action
     a. Perceived benefits of action
     b. Perceived barriers to taking action
     c. Efficacy expectations

- Self-Efficacy Theory (Bandura, 1977) explains human behavior in terms of a dynamic, reciprocal interaction between behavior, personal factors, and environmental influences—key concepts include:
  1. Personal factors which include the ability to symbolize behavior meaning, to foresee outcomes of given behavior, to learn by observing others, to self-determine and self regulate, and to reflect and analyze experience
  2. Reciprocal determinism refers to behavior as dynamic and dependent on environmental and personal constructs that influence each other simultaneously

- Health Promotion Model (Pender, 1996)—health promoting behaviors are motivated by multiple cognitive-perceptual factors such as the importance of health and perceived benefits, perceived control of health and self-efficacy, and modified by factors such as demographics and interpersonal influences

- Erikson's Stages of Psychosocial Development (Erikson, 1963)—degree of success in accomplishing developmental tasks influences the accomplishment of tasks of older adults

    1. Trust versus mistrust—trust of self and others

    2. Autonomy versus shame and doubt—self expression and cooperation with others

    3. Initiative versus guilt—focus on purposeful behavior

    4. Industry versus inferiority—belief in one's ability

    5. Identity versus role confusion—clear sense of self

    6. Intimacy versus role confusion—capacity for reciprocal love relationships

    7. Generativity versus stagnation—creativity and productivity

    8. Ego identity versus despair—acceptance of one's life as worthwhile and unique

- Health Behavior Change Models

    1. PRECEDE Model (Green & Kreuter, 1991)—involves identifying, assessing the learner=s quality of life; identifying health problems and risk factors; The acronym PRECEDE stands for Predisposing, Reinforcing and Enabling Causes in Educational Diagnosis and Evaluation: Predisposing factors (perception, knowledge, and attitudes), Reinforcing factors (significant others), and Enabling factors (environmental factors of accessibility and costs) are used to develop educational interventions for change and policies to support change

    2. Change Theory (Lewin)—advanced practice environments are dynamic; planned change involves unfreezing of current approach, implementing change, refreezing or creating, and acceptance and regular use of new approach (Cohen, 1996)

    3. Transtheoretical Model (Prochaskov & Velicir, 1997)—temporal model of behavioral change, model emerged from comparative analysis of over 300 theories

    a.   Precontemplation—no intention to take action within next six months; not ready and often resistant to health promotion change efforts; appropriate to use consciousness raising education

    b.   Contemplation—intention to take action within next six months; not ready and ambivalent toward change; appropriate to use consciousness raising education

    c.   Preparation—intends to take action within 30 days and has taken some behavioral steps in this direction; individuals at this stage should be recruited for action toward behavior change

    d.   Action—individual has changed behavior for less than six months

    e.   Maintenance—individual has changed overt behavior for more than six months; support and encouragement pf continued behavior change

- System Theories

  1. General Systems Theory (von Bertalanffy, 1968) views world in terms of sets of integrated reactions in an effort to see parts in relation to the whole—key concepts include:

    a.   System—goal directed unit with interdependent, interacting parts that also interact with environment

    b.   Boundaries regulate exchange of energy, information, and matter between systems; may be open or closed depending on interaction with surrounding environment

    c.   Input, output, and feedback loop provide for an exchange of energy, information, and matter

  2. Neuman's Systems Model (Neuman, 1995)—uses a systems format and includes levels of prevention as well as multiple dimensions of health promotion (physical, psychological, spiritual, and social); health promotion efforts are used to strengthen line barriers of defense

Related Concepts

- Levels of prevention from public health science are used by most authorities when differentiating health promotion activities from other interventions. *Healthy People 2000* and other federal documents use a broader interpretation including health protection, with specific screenings and safety factors which are also included in this chapter

    1. Primary prevention includes measures to promote optimum health prior to the onset of any problems—health promotion, care intended to minimize risk factors and subsequent disease e.g., promoting a healthy diet, exercise, stress management, safety, avoiding harmful substances

    2. Secondary prevention focuses on early identification and treatment of existing health problems, e.g., screening for disease, pap smear, mamogram

    3. Tertiary Prevention is care intended to improve the course of a disease; the rehabilitation and restoration to health, e.g., cardiac rehabilitation

- Cultural influence must be considered with any health encounter. Cultural beliefs of disease causation influence health practices e.g., magic or evil spirits (Latino); violation of a natural law (American Indian); imbalance between "hot" or "cold" forces (Asian, Latino). Varied beliefs affect the acceptance of practices such as handwashing and immunizations. There are differences between and among cultural groups. Certain beliefs are common among cultural groups (Clark, 1996)

    1. Native Americans—harmony with nature and supernatural forces are important factors in health beliefs; social networking is also important; note taking is often considered taboo; silence is a sign of respect

    2. Hispanic American—extended family is important in decision making; illness may be related to imbalance of hot and cold; sustaining eye contact is considered rude (mal ojo); higher risk of vitamin A, iron and calcium deficiency due to dietary habits

    3. Asian Americans—naturalistic beliefs are common; saying no is considered rude and is avoided; eye contact may be avoided out of respect; a need to balance hot and cold through food and medication is prevalent; use of acupuncture therapy is widespread

4. African-Americans—diverse group with beliefs that include "health is harmony with nature" and "life is a process, not a state;" maternal grandmother is often important in decision making

Lifestyle/Health Behaviors

- Stress Management: Stress is an imbalance between environmental demands and one's individual and social resources required to cope with those demands

    1. Types of stressors

        a. Major life events—discrete events that disrupt normal functioning (e.g., marriage, divorce, death of family member)

        b. Daily hassles—minor daily events perceived as frustrating

        c. Chronic strains—challenges, hardships, and problems

        d. Cataclysmic events—sudden disasters that require major adaptive responses (e.g., natural disasters)

        e. Ambient stressors—continuous and often unchanging conditions in physical environment, such as chronic pollution or noise

    2. Theoretical basis of stress

        a. General Adaptation Syndrome—Selye's (1974) continuum demonstrates how small amounts of stress are motivating and improve the quality of life (eustress or good stress), however beyond a certain point the stress becomes psychologically and physically debilitating (distress)

        b. Physical indicators of stress

            (1) Gastrointestinal symptoms—upset stomach, change of appetite

            (2) Headache, muscle tension, elevated blood pressure (BP)

            (3) Restlessness

            (4) Cold, sweaty palms

        c. Emotional indicators of stress

            (1) Irritability, emotional outbursts, crying

            (2) Depression, withdrawal

        (3)   Hostility, tendency to blame others

        (4)   Anxiety, suspiciousness

  d. Behavioral indicators of stress

        (1)   Lethargy, loss of interest

        (2)   Poor concentration, forgetfulness

        (3)   Decreased productivity, absenteeism

        (4)   Sleep disturbance

  e. Related terminology—Karoshi (Japanese) death by overwork; associated with long hours and stressful working conditions

3. Stress management intervention techniques

  a. Stress reduction techniques

        (1)   Time management—determine goals and priorities, set time priorities, and learn to say no to nongoal related activities

        (2)   Time blocking—set aside time to adapt to change and incorporate it into daily routine

        (3)   Change avoidance—during periods of high life change, avoid unnecessary change to prevent need to make multiple adjustments simultaneously

        (4)   Habituation—incorporate routine into daily activities during stressful situation (e.g., park in same place to avoid having to look for car upon return)

        (5)   Environmental modification—identify experiences and/or personalities that are abrasive or stress producing and minimize contact as much as possible

        (6)   Involvement with activities of interest—doing something for others and helping with activities of interest to decrease focus on self

  b. Behavioral aspects to build stress resistance

        (1)   Increase self esteem—focus on own strengths and attributes

        (2)   Increase assertiveness—substitute positive assertive behavior for negative passive actions

        (3)   Meditation/prayer (includes Zen and yoga)

  c.   Counter-conditioning to lower stress response

        (1)   Autogenic training repetition of autogenic suggestions such as ''my arms and legs are heavy''

        (2)   Imagery—image visualization used to relax, or assist with past frightening experiences

        (3)   Tension-relaxation exercises—tense muscles for 8 to 10 seconds, then relax; longer training sessions are usually required initially to enhance benefits (may be contraindicated in severe heart disease or hypertension)

        (4)   Biofeedback—awareness and control to influence response that is not ordinarily under voluntary control

           (a)   Electromyography—measures the amount of electrical discharge in muscle fibers (usually forearm and forehead)

           (b)   Skin temperature feedback—peripheral temperature measurement by vasomotor control found in bio-dots, mood rings, etc.

        (5)   Exercise—produces physiological changes that counteract effects of stress

  d.   Contraindications for stress management

        (1)   Severe depression

        (2)   Hallucinations or delusions

        (3)   Temporary hypotensive or hypoglycemic states

        (4)   Severe pain

- Social Support: Supportive relationships (Friedman, 1998)

  1.   Four types of supporting behaviors

    a.   Emotional support—provision of empathy, love, trust and caring (strongest, most consistent relationship to positive health status)

    b.   Instrumental support, such as direct assistance or services

    c.   Informational support such as advice, suggestions and information for problem solving

      d. Appraisal support or provision of information useful for self-evaluation purposes (feedback, affirmation)

  2. Related research

      a. Research evidence suggests that quality of supportive relationships rather than quantity is a better predictor of health—relationships are thought to provide buffering effects to protect people from the negative consequences of stressful situations

      b. The importance of social support has been demonstrated in multiple studies related to recovery from illness, disaster, success with weight loss and other positive life changes; support groups can provide encouragement for those without a strong positive social network (Pender, 1996)

- Nutrition

  1. Healthy diet guidelines

      a. Eat a variety of foods, more fruit, vegetables, whole grains, poultry and fish (herbs/spices can enhance diminished taste associated with normal aging)

      b. Calorie breakdown—55 to 60% carbohydrates, < 30% fat with remainder protein (.8 to 1.0 g/kg)

      c. Limit total fat to less than 30% of total calories and saturated fat to less than 10% of total calories

      d. Limit cholesterol intake to 300 mg/day

      e. Use sugar, salt and sodium in moderation

      f. The food guide pyramid (U.S. Department of Agriculture) includes the following daily recommendations

         (1) Bread, cereal, rice—6 to 11 servings

         (2) Vegetable and fruit groups—3 to 5 servings

         (3) Milk, yogurt, and cheese—2 to 3 servings

         (4) Meat, poultry, fish, dry beans, eggs, and nuts—2 to 3 servings

         (5) Oils, sweets, and fats used sparingly

Table 1:

Recommended Calcium Intakes

	Amount mg/day
Young Adults (11–24 years) Pregnant/Lactating Women	1,300–1,500
Women, 25–29 years (premenopausal) Women, 50–64 years (postmenopausal,taking estrogen Men, 25–64 years	1,000
Men and women, 65+ years Women, 50-64 years (postmenopausal, not taking estrogen)	1,500

Food sources of calcium: Yogurt, milk, cheese, calcium fortified juices and cereal, turnip and mustard greens, collards, kale, broccoli, sardines and salmon with bones

    g.   Multivitamins with folic acid (0.4mg/day) are recommended for all women of childbearing age

    h.   Vitamin D is needed for proper calcium absorption—200 to 800 IU/day

    i.   Calcium (NIH Consensus Panel, 1994), See Table 1

2.   Assessment for weight loss

    a.   Symptoms indicative of underlying pathology (associated with and/or aggravated by excessive weight)

        (1)   Polyuria/polyphagia/polydipsia (diabetes)

        (2)   Joint pain or marked swelling (osteoarthritis or gout)

        (3)   Angina/palpitations/dyspnea (cardiovascular disease)

        (4)   Edema/cold intolerance (hypothyroidism)

        (5)   Recent weight gain with edema, pruritus (renal disease)

    b.   Contraindications for weight loss

        (1)   Pregnancy

        (2)   Chemotherapy due to already compromised nutritional status and potential impact on therapy

Table 2

Body Mass Formula

1. To convert weight to kilograms, divide pounds(without clothes) by 2.2
2. To convert to meters, divide height in inches(without shoes) by 39.4, then square it
3. Divide weight in kilograms (#1) by meters squared (#2)

Table 3

Body Mass Index Chart

Weight				Height(feet/inches)				
(lbs)	5'0	5'2"	5'4"	5'6"	5'8"	5'10"	6'0"	6'2"
125	24	23	22	20	19	18	17	16
130	25	24	22	21	20	19	18	17
135	26	25	23	22	21	19	18	17
140	27	26	24	23	21	20	19	18
145	28	27	25	23	22	21	20	19
150	29	27	26	24	23	22	20	19
155	30	28	27	25	24	22	21	20
160	31	29	28	26	24	23	22	21
165	32	30	28	27	25	24	22	21
170	33	31	29	28	26	24	23	22
175	34	32	30	28	27	25	24	23
180	35	33	31	29	27	26	25	23
185	36	34	32	30	28	27	25	24
190	37	35	33	31	29	27	26	24
195	38	36	34	32	30	28	27	25
200	39	37	34	32	30	29	27	26
205	40	38	35	33	31	29	28	26
210	41	38	36	34	32	30	29	27
215	42	39	37	35	33	31	29	28
220	43	40	38	36	34	32	30	28
225	44	41	39	36	34	32	31	29
230	45	42	40	37	35	33	31	30

	BMI
Overweight	25-29.9
Obese	30 and above

NHLBI June 17, 1998

3. Body mass determinations—useful in determining both under-and-over nutrition or weight-for-frame-size calculate the body mass using the body mass formula in Table 2 or the body mass index chart in Table 3

4. Guidelines for healthy weight loss should include:

   a. A diet deficient in calories, not nutrients, with a focus on diet composition/preparation methods

b. A balanced diet (food guide pyramid); should not depend on vitamins, weight loss pills, prepared liquids, "fad diets"

c. A diet that supplies all essential vitamins and minerals

d. Adequate fiber for proper GI functioning

e. Adequate fluid for renal functioning

f. Enough fat to supply essential fatty acid linoleic acid

g. Consumption of a variety of highly nutritious foods

h. A goal of up to 3 lbs/wk (gradual) weight loss

i. A focus on regular meals, avoiding snacks and modifying bad eating habits

5. Weight control strategies

a. Regular physical activity (increases caloric use, aids and sustains weight loss, preserves lean body mass and metabolism (Keller, Oveland, & Hudson, 1997)

b. Social support by family, friends, colleagues, and support groups

c. Focus on internal motivation for loss (e.g., control, personal goals, self-monitoring) and positive health benefits

d. Smaller, more frequent meals to maintain blood sugar levels and avoid feelings of hunger

e. Control home environment (e.g., limit eating to one room, sit down at table without watching television)

f. Control eating environment (e.g., avoid serving bowls at the table, use smaller plates and glasses, and eat slowly)

g. Limit snacks (e.g., keep low calorie snacks available, ready to eat)

h. Control work environment (e.g., eat away from your desk, store food away from work area, and take exercise breaks)

i. Use a shopping list, do not shop when hungry

j. Food diary (thoughts and feelings regarding eating patterns for two weeks) to guide intervention strategies

6. Health effects of severe dieting (metabolic response to starvation)

    a.   Lower metabolic rate

    b.   Hypertension as a result of norepinephrine release

    c.   Overcompensation, gain beyond pre-diet weight

    d.   Loss of fat and protein, regain fat

    e.   Fat cells multiply as protective response against starvation

7.   Weight loss prognostic factors

    a.   Stability of present weight—number of years at present weight

    b.   Motivation to change, conditions making weight loss a high priority

    c.   Realistic expectations

8.   Nutritional risk factors for older adults—three or more factors indicate a moderate nutritional risk (U.S. Dept. of Health and Human Services, 1994)

    a.   Presence of illness or condition affecting amount and kind of food eaten or dental/mouth problems which make eating difficult

    b.   Eats < 2 meals/day, few fruits, vegetables or dairy products

    c.   Inadequate finances for food

    d.   Physically unable to shop, cook or feed self

    e.   Three or more drinks of beer, wine or liquor daily

    f.   Unintentional loss or gain of 10 pounds in past 6 months

    g.   Three or more different medications taken daily

- Exercise: Any exercise performed regularly for a total of 30 minutes a day is beneficial, if sedentary, a gradual increase is recommended; added benefit may be derived from further increases (NIH Consensus panel, 1996)

1.   Physical fitness

    a.   Psychological benefits

        (1)   Increased alertness

        (2)   Improved self esteem, feeling better

        (3)   Decreased depression

(4) Lower stress

b. Physical benefits

(1) Heart—increases efficiency, lowers heart rate, lowers BP, increases oxygen capacity

(2) Decreases LDL, increases HDL

(3) Muscles—improves strength and endurance

(4) Improves flexibility

(5) Increases BMR during and after exercise

(6) Weight loss of fat, not muscle

(7) Body composition—lowers fat percentage

(8) Anti-aging effect

c. Components of effective exercise

(1) Performed most, but preferably all days of the week

(2) Enjoyable for participant

(3) Rhythmic movement with alternating relaxation and contraction of large muscle groups

(4) Moderate intensity for at least 30 minutes; talk test—one should be able to talk with some labored breathing during exercise

d. Components of an exercise plan

(1) Warm up (increases blood flow, loosens and strengthens muscles), e.g., brisk walk and deep breathing

(2) Stretch (maintains and increases flexibility), e.g., stretch slowly and hold position several seconds to point of tightness, not pain; do not bounce

(3) Endurance—select a variety of activities to work different muscle groups; start slow and build up gradually

(4) Cool down period allows body temperature and heart rate to decrease slowly, prevents pooling of blood in extremities and decreases muscle soreness, e.g., walk, deep breathe and loosely shake extremities

e. Exercise counseling

    (1)   Exercises to avoid

        (a)   Bouncing with stretch (strains involved joints)

        (b)   Sit-ups with legs straight or double leg lifts (strains lower back)

        (c)   Duck walk (bent knee walk) (stresses knees)

        (d)   Toe touching (stresses hamstrings)

        (e)   Leg splits and leg thrusts in kneeling position (stresses legs and groin area and also creates potential hip strain)

    (2)   Exercise self-care

        (a)   Appropriate clothing with layers in winter

        (b)   Caps for cold weather and summer heat

        (c)   Appropriate footwear, snug socks

        (d)   Plenty of fluids before, during and after exercise

        (e)   Alternate exercise program during weather extremes, e.g., stationary bike, treadmills, steppers etc

    (3)   Tolerance barometer—refers to potentially dangerous physical symptoms or early signs of injury

        (a)   Breathlessness (inability to talk while exercising)

        (b)   Excessive fatigue—fatigue for more than one hour after exercise

        (c)   Chest discomfort, dizziness, faintness, exertional dyspnea, nausea or vomiting

        (d)   Stiffness in joints with slight loss of motion

        (e)   Swelling and localized pain

f. Exercise prescription components:

    (1)   Specify duration, intensity, and frequency

    (2)   Progression of physical activity—gradual onset, increasing in intensity/duration, e.g., begin walking, then gradually replace with jogging

    (3)   Individualized to client capabilities

      (4)   Client motivation, goals, and interest (motivators)—adolescent females—weight control, improved appearance; adolescent males—increased skills, strength, competition; women—weight control, appearance, stress reduction; men—pleasure, fun, and challenge abilities (Jones, 1997)

      (5)   Based on available time, equipment, and facilities

      (6)   Refer individuals with abnormal exercise stress tests (bicycle ergometer or treadmill), chronic/recent heart or lung pathology, or any positive cardiac risk factors to the appropriate health care provider

  g. Physical fitness evaluation

      (1)   Cardiorespiratory endurance or aerobic fitness is usually measured by performance on 1.5 mile run, step test (5 minute pulse-recovery step test), bicycle ergometer test or swimming test

      (2)   Skinfold test or other determination of body fat composition

      (3)   Back flexibility of back—hyperextension, sit/reach test

      (4)   Muscle strength—tested by determining maximum amount of weight that can be lifted comfortably, a single time, by four different muscle groups; test is usually conducted following completion of approximately six weeks of training

      (5)   Muscle endurance—determined by push-ups (shoulder, arm and chest muscle endurance) and bent knee sit-ups (abdominals)

      (6)   Leg power—tested by height of vertical jump from squat position

  h. Nutrition for athletic performance

      (1)   Drink 17 ounces of fluid approximately 2 hours prior to exercise to promote hydration; allow time for excretion of excess ingested fluid; drink approximately two cups of fluid for every pound of weight loss during extended athletic activities

      (2)   Maintain well balanced diet—adequate carbohydrates to

optimize respiratory metabolism, adequate protein to preserve lean body mass, adequate minerals to maximize oxygen delivery, and calcium to develop high density bones (Kenney, 1996)

- Safety and Environment

    1. General

        a. Fire safety (smoke alarms, fire extinguishers)

        b. Home safety (secure locks on doors and windows)

        c. Automobile (use of safety belts, harnesses, defensive driving)

        d. Helmets (bikes, motorcycles, roller blades)

        e. Personal safety (avoid risk-taking behaviors; always be on the defensive, especially women)

    2. Safety for aging adult

        a. Home safety

            (1) Adequate lighting especially around stairs; light switches near doorways and accessible from bed

            (2) Home should be surveyed for risk factors that may create walking hazards (loose rugs, furniture placement, electrical cords); traffic lanes in each room free of hazards

            (3) Nightlight or flashlight by bed is recommended to avoid falls or disorientation in the dark

            (4) Avoid housekeeping hazards by cleaning up spills as they occur and avoiding clutter on floors/stairways

            (5) Bathroom—non-slip mat in tub/shower, secure ''grab bar''

            (6) Stairwell—secure handrail, steps in good repair

        b. Personal safety

            (1) Avoid dangers of hypothermia with adequate heat and caloric intake

            (2) Set up daily surveillance system with others

            (3) Assess ability to take medications correctly

    c. Physical deficit concerns

        (1) Gait and balance problems

            (a) Slippery or irregular surfaces

            (b) Clutter or obstructions

            (c) Stairs, steep or without rails

            (d) Lack of space to maneuver assistive device (e.g., walker)

            (e) Bathtub without rail or slip guards

        (2) Decreased vision

            (a) Inadequate lighting

            (b) Poorly marked stairs

        (3) Decreased sensitivity to pain/heat

            (a) Hot water bottle/heating pad

            (b) Hot bath water

        (4) Potential driving/traffic hazards

            (a) Decreased visual acuity and hearing

            (b) Decreased reaction time

            (c) Difficulty moving head (arthritis)

            (d) Ambulation too slow for traffic signals

3. Four categories of environmental hazards

    a. Biological (e.g., viruses, microorganisms)

    b. Chemical (e.g., lead, asbestos)

    c. Physical (e.g., natural disasters)

    d. Sociological and psychological hazards (e.g., overcrowding, lack of resources)

4. Components of an environmental assessment

    a. Home hazards—fire safety, pest control, inadequate heat or toilet facilities

    b. Work-site hazards and protection—noise, inhalants, lifting, hazardous materials; related exposures

   c. Neighborhood hazards—noise, air/water pollution, inadequate police protection, overcrowding or isolation from neighbors

   d. Community hazards—lack of availability of grocery stores, drugstores, public transportation

Health Evaluation Across the Lifespan

- Health History: Important in identifying risk behaviors and need for health education

  1. Demographics and biographical data

  2. History of present illness

    a. Symptom analysis

      (1) Location and radiation

      (2) Quality or character

      (3) Quantity, frequency, intensity, duration, effect on daily activities

      (4) Gradual, abrupt onset, course, length of time, pattern

      (5) Setting

      (6) Aggravating and alleviating factors

      (7) Associated symptom/manifestations

    b. Reason for seeking health care or chief complaint—signs/symptoms and duration; preferably in client's own words

  3. Past medical history (Swartz, 1994)

    a. General state of health (client's perception)

    b. Past illnesses (hospitalizations)

    c. Past injuries, surgery (dates, treatment, and follow-up)

    d. Emotional health (past problems including assistance, history of domestic violence)

    e. Sexual health (obstetric and contraceptive history, number of partners, sexual preference, sexual problems, disease prevention efforts)

    f. Food or drug allergies (specify reaction and treatment, if any)

    g. Medications (prescription and over the counter)

    h. Immunizations (type and date)

    i. Sleep patterns (approximate hours, difficulties)

    j. Last examinations (physical, dental, vision, hearing, radiography, electrocardiogram (ECG), cancer screenings)

4. Personal habits

    a. Tobacco use—cigarettes, pipe, cigars, smokeless; record number of cigarettes per day, number of use years, if stopped, how long ago; approach adolescents with declarative statements related to drugs at school, drugs in common use at school, drugs used by friends, and by individuals; inquire about tobacco use in terms of number of packs smoked daily

    b. Alcohol and drug use (type, amount)

    c. Use of caffeine (coffee, colas, etc.)

    d. Diet (24 hour intake, including nutritional supplements)

    e. Exercise (type, frequency)

    f. Leisure activities (type, frequency)

    g. Sports (type, frequency)

    h. Additional questions may be required regarding sports participation, especially contact sports that may include:

        (1) Have you ever been dizzy or passed out during or after exercise?

        (2) Have you had a seizure, concussion or been unconscious?

        (3) Are you able to run $\frac{1}{2}$ mile or more?

        (4) Are you missing a kidney?

        (5) Have you ever had a heart murmur, high blood pressure or heart abnormality?

5. Psychosocial history

    a. Living situation at present

    b. Education—for adolescents ask, if in school, grades, positive or negative attitudes toward school

    c. Religious beliefs in relation to health and treatment

      d. Positive or negative perspective of the future

      e. Perception of ''typical day''

      f. Stress, stress management

      g. Depression or anxiety, suicide ideation (adolescents and young adults require direct questioning, e.g., have you ever thought of killing yourself)

      h. Support systems

6. Family history: Include age, health status or cause of death of parents, siblings, children in a genogram, (diabetes, heart disease, cancer, hypertension, lung disease, alcoholism, blood disorders, birth defects and any other illnesses that seem to run in the family)

7. Occupational and environmental history

      a. Type of work, former occupation(s)

      b. Hazardous exposures at home or work

      c. Military service, wartime employment, if any

      d. Location of home, length of time

      e. Home location adjacent to factories, shipyards, or other potentially hazardous facilities

      f. Hobbies, potential exposures

8. Adolescent interviewing guidelines

      a. Adolescent is primary historian, interviewed alone

      b. Explain ground rules—unless serious problem emerges threatening life or health, interview is confidential

      c. Home, Education, Activities, Drugs, Sex, Suicide (HEADSS) interview format is widely suggested—see age related anticipatory guidance

- Risk Factor Identification: Virtually every disease, condition has risk factors; select conditions are presented related to prevalence, in addition to protective factors.

  1. Research over the past 20 years has identified factors associated with physical health and longer healthier life. (Pender, 1996)

      a. Exercise—regular, (see exercise, this chapter)

  b. Non-smoker, recently extended to smoke-free environment

  c. Seven to eight hours of sleep

  d. Moderate or no alcohol

  e. Regular and moderate eating (including breakfast)

  f. Weight control

  g. Ample exercise, good nutrition and healthy lifestyle to slow aging process

2. Cardiac risk factors:

  a. Age—male 45+, female 55+ or premature menopause without estrogen replacement therapy

  b. Family history of premature heart disease, myocardial infarction or death of father/first degree male relative < 55, mother/female relative < 65

  c. Cigarette smoking

  d. Hypertension $\geq$ 140/90 mm Hg, or on anti-hypertensive medication

  e. Low HDL cholesterol < 35mg/dL, (> 60 mg/dL negative risk)

  f. LDL > 160mg/dL (< 130 mL negative risk)

  g. Diabetes mellitus

3. Obesity (20% above desirable weight)—mortality rates increase with weights 10% above desirable weights; obesity is associated with multiple attendant health risks (Clinical Preventive Services, 1997)

  a. Three times more prevalent in hypertensives and type 2 diabetes

  b. Increased risk of high cholesterol and coronary artery disease

  c. Increased risk of cancer (colon, rectal, prostate, gallbladder, biliary tract, breast, cervical, endometrial, and ovarian)

  d. Abdominal adiposity associated with increased risk of stroke and death from all causes

4. Suicide risk factors

    a. Family history of psychiatric disorders (especially depression or suicide)

    b. Previous suicide attempts

    c. Family violence (verbal, physical or sexual abuse)

    d. Family instability (frequent separation from, or loss of loved one)

    e. Alcohol or substance abuse

    f. Availability and accessibility of firearms in the home

- Age Related Health Monitoring (if asymptomatic)—Specific health screenings are part of secondary prevention, see Table 4

  1. Screening guidelines

    a. Generalized screening indicated for diseases of high prevalence in the population and diseases with profound morbidity/mortality if not diagnosed

    b. Screening tests must be reliable with acceptable technical process; must include appropriate follow-up

    c. Test should be sensitive (true positive, those with disease screen positive) and specific (true negative, those without disease screen negative)

  2. Adolescence (12 to 19 years of age)—American Medical Association (AMA) recommends three visit intervals 11 to 14 years, 15 to 17 years, and 18 to 21 years unless more frequent examinations are indicated (Elster & Kuznets, 1994)

    a. Complete physical examination including:

      (1) Height/weight (use anthropometric chart)

        (a) Screen for eating disorders if indicated

        (b) Assess perception of food, weight

      (2) Complete skin examination

      (3) Assessment for gingivitis, caries, and malalignment

      (4) Assessment for signs of abuse or neglect

      (5) Hearing assessment (if exposed to excessive noise), and vision

Table 4

Adult Screening Guidelines (U.S. Preventive Services Task Force, 1996, American Cancer Society, 1994)

Service	Who Needs	Frequency*	Risk Factors
Blood Pressure	All Adults	Every 2 years	male, blk, fam hx
Cholesterol	All Adults	Every 5 years	Male, tob, htn, fam hx
Dental	All Adults	Annual	
ECG	Adults 40+	Annual (only with cardiac risk factors)	
Pap Smear	Women 18+	Annual recommended every 3 years after two normal exams for women without risk factorscm**	
Self-Breast Exam	All Women	Monthly	
Breast exam	Women 40+	Annual	
Mammogram	Women 50+	Annual	
Colorectal screen (fecal occult or sigmoid)	Adults 50+	Annual	
Prostate Ca	Men 50+	Controversy	blk, fam hx
Glaucoma screen	Adults 40+	Annual	***
Hearing	Only w/excessive noise exposure		
Chest x-ray	Not recommended		
Thyroid palpation	Adults 20 to 39	Every 3 years	
	Adults 40+	Annual	
Urinalysis	Controversy		Yes, w/sx, preg., dm.
Hgb/Hct	Controversy		Yes, w/sx, pregnancy
Health ed/prom. (nutrition, exercise, stress management, substance abuse, safety, safe sex and cancer prevention)	All Adults	Every encounter	

*Increased frequency in the presence of risk factors
**Risk factors for cervical cancer—history of STD, multiple partners, tobacco use(tob), first intercourse before age 18
***Risk factors for glaucoma—myopia, diabetes mellitus(dm), family history (fam hx), African-American(blk) > 40
The term controversy indicates that the U.S. Task Force recommends against routine screening.
Adopted from the U.S. Preventative Task Force *Guide to Clinical Preventive Services*, 1996 and American Cancer Society, 1994. Consult full reports for details

b. Blood pressure (BP) every two years, normal systolic 110 to 135 mm Hg, diastolic 60 to 85; refer BP > 140/90

c. Tuberculin skin test (PPD) every two years with any exposure or if at risk

d. Female

    (1) Teach self-breast examination (SBE)

    (2) Determine Tanner stage (Hay, Groothuis, Hayward, Levin (1995)

        (a) Tanner Stages usual sequence of pubertal events —**T**elarche (breast development), **P**ubarche (growth of axillary and pubic hair), **A**drenarche (increased secretion of adrenal androgens), **G**rowth spurt and **M**enarche (first menstrual period) (TPAGM)

        (b) Stage I—growth spurt (height and weight) average age for girls 10 years

        (c) Stage II—breast bud, sparse pubic hair

        (d) Stage III–IV—breast development

        (e) Stage V—mature stage

    (3) If sexually active or 18 years old—Papanicolaou (pap) smear

e. Male

    (1) Teach self-testicular examination (STE)

    (2) Determine Tanner stage

        (a) Stage I—growth spurt (height and weight) average age for boys 12.5 years

        (b) Stage II—sparse pubic hair

        (c) Stage III–IV—male organ enlargement

        (d) Stage V—mature stage

f. If high risk, counseling and test for human immunodeficiency virus (HIV) and VDRL; assess knowledge of contraceptives and protective barriers

g. Immunization

    (1) Tetanus-diptheria booster (Td)

(2) Others if needed; see Immunization Guidelines this chapter

h. Remain alert for depressive symptoms, any suicide risk factors

i. Dental checkup with cleaning annually

3. Young adult (20 to 39 years of age) (see Table 4)

a. Complete physical examination (age 20, then every 5 to 6 years

b. BP every 2 years; normal systolic 110 to 135 mm Hg, diastolic 60 to 85 mm Hg

c. Total cholesterol every 5 years with additional tests if total cholesterol exceeds 200 mg/dL

d. Female

(1) SBE monthly

(2) Pap and pelvic examination every 3 years , GC and chlamydia tests

(3) Clinical breast examination (by health professional) every 3 years

e. Male—STE monthly

f. PPD if exposed to tuberculosis

g. Immunizations—Td every ten years

h. Self-skin examination

i. Dental checkup with cleaning annually

4. Middle-aged adult (40 to 59 years of age) (see Table 4)

a. Complete physical examination (every 5 to 6 years)

b. B.P. every 2 years; normal systolic 110 to 135 mm Hg, diastolic 60 to 85 mm Hg

c. Total cholesterol every 5 years with additional tests if total cholesterol exceeds 200 mg/dL

d. ECG, age 40+ with cardiac risk factors

e. Female

(1) SBE monthly

      (2) Clinical breast exam yearly (performed by a health professional)

      (3) Mammogram annually age 50 years

      (4) Pap and pelvic examination every 3 years

  f. Male—STE monthly

  g. Colorectal screen (fecal occult or sigmoidoscopy)—age 50 annually

  h. Glaucoma screen, annually

  i. Dental examination with cleaning every 6 to 12 months

  j. Cancer screening yearly

  k. Immunizations—tetanus every 10 years

5. Elderly adult (60 + years of age) (see Table 4)

  a. Complete physical examination every 2 years with laboratory assessments

  b. BP every 2 years, normal systolic 110 to 135mm Hg, diastolic 60 to 85mm Hg

  c. Total cholesterol every 5 years with additional tests if total cholesterol exceeds 200 mg/dL

  d. ECG annually with cardiac risk factors

  e. Female

      (1) SBE monthly

      (2) Annual mammogram

      (3) Pap and pelvic examination every 3 years

  f. Male—STE monthly

  g. Colorectal screen (fecal occult or sigmoidoscopy) age 50—annually

  h. Glaucoma screen—annually

  i. Dental examination with cleaning every 6 to 12 months

  j. Immunizations—tetanus every 10 years, pneumococcal vaccine once, and annual influenza vaccine

- Age Related Anticipatory Guidance (Allender, 1998)
  1. Adolescence (12 to 19 years of age)
     a. Leading causes of death—motor vehicle accidents (MVA), suicide, other accidents, homicide, malignancy, cardiovascular disease, congenital disease
     b. Normal growth and development
        (1) Physical changes with puberty
        (2) Need for increased self responsibilities for own health—nutrition, exercise, adequate sleep and safety habits
     c. Nutrition
        (1) Variety of foods, including breakfast
        (2) Nutritious snacks, limit sweets and fast food
     d. Skin care/skin protection
     e. Dental care (brushing and flossing)
        (1) Fluoride supplementation
        (2) Dental visits with cleaning every 6 to 12 months
     f. Injury prevention
        (1) Athletics, safety helmets, pads, mouthguards
        (2) Safety belts
        (3) Firearm safety
        (4) Defensive driving, driver education
        (5) Violent behavior/gangs
     g. Physical activity
        (1) Need for regular physical activity
        (2) Encourage team activities, peer interaction
        (3) Encourage participation in after school and/or church activities
     h. Substance abuse
        (1) Tobacco use avoidance or cessation emphasizing

unattractive cosmetic effects (stained teeth and finger-nails, foul smelling breath and clothes) and athletic con-sequences (decreased endurance, shortness of breath)

    (2)   Smokeless tobacco is not safer, can be addicting/life-threatening

    (3)   Alcohol and other drugs

  i. Sexuality

    (1)   Dating

    (2)   Responsible sexual behaviors, abstinence, contraception

    (3)   Risks, sexually transmitted diseases, unwanted preg-nancy

2. Young adult (20 to 39 years of age)

  a. Leading causes of death—motor vehicle accidents, homicide, suicide, injuries, heart disease, AIDS

  b. Nutrition and exercise

    (1)   Weight management with changing basal metabolic rate

    (2)   Selection of exercise program

  c. Dental care

  d. Sexuality

    (1)   Family planning, contraception

    (2)   Sexually transmitted diseases

  e. Cancer warning signs/skin protection

  f. Substance use/abuse

    (1)   Tobacco cessation/primary prevention

    (2)   Alcohol and other drugs

  g. Injury prevention

    (1)   Athletics

    (2)   Safety belts/safety helmets

    (3)   Firearm safety

    (4)   Defensive driving

        (5)   Violent behavior

    h. Lifestyle choices

        (1)   Family and parenting skills

        (2)   Stress management

    i. Safety and environmental health

  3. Middle aged adult (40 to 59 years of age)

    a. Leading causes of death—heart disease, accidents, lung cancer, cerebrovascular disease, breast and colorectal cancer, obstructive lung disease

    b. Nutrition and exercise

        (1)   Weight management with changing basal metabolic rate

        (2)   Selection of exercise program

    c. Dental care

    d. Sexuality

        (1)   Menopause

        (2)   Sexual changes due to aging

        (3)   Sexually transmitted diseases

    e. Cancer warning signs/skin protection

    f. Substance use/abuse

        (1)   Tobacco cessation/primary prevention

        (2)   Alcohol and other drugs

    g. Injury prevention

        (1)   Athletics

        (2)   Safety belts/safety helmets

        (3)   Firearm safety

        (4)   Defensive driving

        (5)   Violent behavior

    h. Midlife changes

        (1)   Empty nest syndrome, grandparenting

      (2)   Planning for retirement

      (3)   Stress management

   i. Safety and environmental health

4. Elderly adult (age 60+ years of age)

   a. Leading causes of death—heart disease, cerebrovascular disease, obstructive lung disease, pneumonia and/or influenza, lung and colorectal cancer

   b. Nutrition and exercise

      (1)   Weight management with changing basal metabolic rate

      (2)   Selection of exercise program

   c. Dental care

   d. Sexuality

      (1)   Sexual changes due to aging

      (2)   Sexually transmitted diseases

   e. Cancer warning signs/skin protection

   f. Substance use/abuse

      (1)   Tobacco cessation/primary prevention

      (2)   Alcohol and other drugs

   g. Injury prevention

      (1)   Athletics

      (2)   Safety belts/safety helmets

      (3)   Firearm safety

      (4)   Defensive driving

      (5)   Violent behavior

   h. Life changes

      (1)   Retirement

      (2)   Loss of spouse, friends

      (3)   Physical changes (vision, hearing, reaction time, alterations of bowel and bladder habits)

> i. Safety and environmental health
>
> > (a) Home safety
> >
> > (b) Personal safety

- Immunization Guidelines (Centers for Disease Control and Prevention (CDC) (1996)

  1. Tetanus-diptheria vaccine (Td)—primary series is recommended if not completed during childhood with two doses at least four weeks apart and a third dose 6 to 12 months after the second; Td booster is recommended every 10 years

  2. Measles-Mumps-Rubella vaccine (MMR)—recommended for adolescents who have not received two doses at or after 12 months of age; second dose is now given routinely as part of preschool immunizations or at age 12 to 14, or prior to post secondary education or military service; adults without documentation of disease or immunization need only one dose; adults born prior to 1956 are considered immune due to prevalence of diseases before that time

  3. Varicella vaccine—recommended for individuals who have never had chicken pox; adolescents and adults need two doses 4 to 8 weeks apart

  4. Influenza vaccine—recommended annually for adults and children with chronic disorders of the pulmonary and cardiovascular systems including asthma, diabetes and renal disease, persons 65 years of age or older and persons with any chronic health condition

     a. Groups that can transmit influenza to high risk persons should be immunized (e.g., health care workers and household members)

     b. Optimal time for immunization (mid-October through mid-November)

     c. Contraindications—history of anaphylactic hypersensitivity to eggs or other components; refer to physician for appropriate therapy and possible allergy evaluation

  5. Pneumococcal vaccine—recommended for any person over two years of age who is at increased risk of complications due to chronic illness (e.g., heart or lung disease and diabetes, alcoholism, Hodgkin's disease, cirrhosis, sickle cell disease) and individuals who work or live with high risk individuals); anyone over age 65

and persons without a spleen; revaccination after six or more years is recommended for those at highest risk of antibody decline, e.g., renal disease or organ transplant

6. Hepatitis B vaccine (HBV)—three dose regimen recommended for all individuals who are or will be at increased risk of infection; the second dose is given one month after the first with a third dose six months later; categories include health care workers, individuals at high risk of exposure to blood and blood products, and individuals at increased risk of exposure due to sexual practices; the timing and need for periodic boosters is determined by serologic testing; recommended for all young adults who were not previously immunized

7. Hepatitis A vaccine (HAV)—two to three doses recommended for individuals working in or traveling to countries with high levels of HAV infection; men who have sex with men, parenteral drug use, persons exposed to non-human primates, persons with chronic liver disease; adolescents up to eighteen require three doses, the first two doses one month apart and the third dose 6 to 12 months later; adults (>18) require two doses 6 to 12 months apart

8. Polio—inactivated poliovirus vaccine-enhanced potency (IVP-e) is indicated for unimmunized adults who are traveling outside the U.S. and healthcare workers; partially immunized or unimmunized adults with close contact with children receiving OPV; the second dose is given one month after the first with a third dose six months later

9. Catch up schedule, contraindications and precautions

   a. For individuals with uncertain immunization histories (lacking documentation):

      (1) First visit—Td, IPV, MMR, HBV; HAV, varicella, influenza, pneumococcccal are optional depending upon risk factors

      (2) Second visit (4 to 6 weeks after first visit)—Td, IPV, HBV, with second dose of HAV, varicella, if given initially

      (3) Third visit (6 months after second visit)—Td, IPV, HBV, with third dose of HAV for adolescents

   b. Contraindications

      (1) Anaphylactic reaction to known component:

               (a)   MMR (eggs)

               (b)   Hepatitis (Bakers yeast)

          (2)   Moderate to severe illness (fever > 100.4°F)

          (3)   Immunocompromised individuals (no live virus)

     c.   Precaution with MMR—delay pregnancy for 3 months following immunization

  10.   Immunization schedule synopsis for adolescents and adults with documentation of immunizations during childhood

     a.   Adolescents and adults

          (1)   Hepatitis B Series

          (2)   Td Booster, repeat every 10 years

          (3)   Varicella, if needed, two doses 4 to 8 weeks apart

          (4)   MMR if born after 1956

     b.   Adults over 65, chronic disease (heart, lung or diabetes; those who work or live with high risk individuals)

          (1)   Influenza vaccine each fall

          (2)   Pneumococcal vaccine

Resources

Agency for Health Care Policy and Research (AHCPR)
(800) 358-9295
FAX (301) 594-2800
http://www.ahcpr.gov/
AHCPR Publications Clearinghouse
P.O. Box 8547,
Silver Spring, MD 20907
Automated instructions available 24 hours/day
(Pocket guide on smoking cessation, etc.)

American Association for Retired Persons
(202) 872-4700
1909 K Street N.W. Fifth Floor
Washington, D. C. 20049
Services for age 50 and older include lobby for senior citizens, mail-order pharmacy, bimonthly magazine, support group for widowed persons.

Calcium Information Center
(800) 321-2681
Affiliate of Clinical Nutrition Research of the Oregon Health Sciences University and Cornell University

National Cancer Institute Cancer Information Service
(800) 4-CANCER (800) 422-6237
http://wwwicic.nci.nih.gov/
Bldg 31 Room 10A16,
9000 Rockville Pike,
Bethesda, MD 20892
(Pamphlets on breast examination, pap smear, colorectal screening)

National Heart, Lung and Blood Information Center, (NHLBI)
(800) 575-WELL (800) 575-9355
or (301) 251-1222
Fax (301) 251-1223
http://www.nih.gov/
P.O. Box 30105,
Bethesda, MD 20824-0105

National Education Program Resources NIH Pub. No.:
   92-2725 *Churches as an avenue to high blood pressure control*
   95-3045 *Recommendations regarding public screening for measuring blood cholesterol*
   94-3648 *Stay young at heart kit*
   95-3802 *The sports guide: Guide for cardiovascular risk reduction projects at sporting events*

National Institute on Aging Information Officer
(800) 622-2225
Building 31, Room 5C-35
9000 Rockville Pike
Bethesda, MD 20205
Self-care and Self-help groups for the elderly (Directory)

National Institutes of Health Consensus Conference.
(800) NIH-OMAR
Fax (301) 480-5144
http://text.nlm.nih.gov
Statement printouts available free of charge by phone

Office of Disease Prevention and Health Promotion
(800) 336-4797
http://www.os.dhhs.gov:81//PPIP/
Putting Prevention into Practice
Government Printing Office.
National Health Information Center.
P.O. Box 1133,
Washington, DC 20012-1133

President's Council on Physical Fitness and Sports
(202) 272-3421
U.S. Consumer Product Safety Commission
Washington DC 20207
Pamphlet "Safety for older consumers: Home safety check list"

Additional internet resources for Health Promotion:
American College of Nurse Practitioners http://www.nurse.org/acnp
American Dietetic Asociation http://www.eatright.com
American Health Line http://www.apn.com/info/am   health/
American Red Cross http://www.redcross.com
American Nurses Association http://www.nursingworld.org
American Journal of Nursing http://www.ajn.org
Centers for Disease Control and Prevention
http://www.cdc.gov
(888) 232-3299
International traveler's immunization hot line (404)332-4559

Food and Drug Administration http://www.fda.gov/fdahomepage.html
Food Insight
Current topics in food safety and nutrition
http://ificinfo.health.org

Health Canada http://www.hwc.ca/
Health Care Financing Administration (Medicare/Medicaid) http://
www.os.dhhs.gov/

Healthgate http://www.healthgate.com
Healthy People 2000 http://odphp.osophs.dhhs.gov/pubs/hp2000
Healthy People 2000: Citizens Chart the Course http://www.nap.edu/read-
ingroom

Modern Healthcare http://modernhealthcare.com
National Health Information Center http://nhic-nt.health.org
New England Medical Journal On-line http://www.nejm.org. /Jhome.htm

NOAH http://www.noah.cuny.edu
Nursing and Health Care Resources on the Net http://www.shef.ad.uk/nhcon/
National Institutes of Safety and Health http://www.cdc.gov/niosh.htm
National Library of Medicine http://www.nlm.nih.gov/
Safety Checklist for the Elderly http://www.usc.edu/go/hmap/library/safe-
ty.html
U.S. Department of Health and Human Services http://www.os.dhhs.
World Health Organization http://www.who.ch/

Check the telephone directory for local chapters of:
American Cancer Society National Headquarters
(800) 227-2345
1599 Clifton Road NE
Atlanta, GA 30329

American Heart Association
(800) AHA-USA1 (800) 242-8721
http://www.amhrt.org/index.html
7320 Greenville Avenue
Dallas TX 75231

American Lung Association
(212) 315-8700 (800) LUNG-USA
1740 Broadway
P.O. Box 596
New York, NY 10019

Questions
Select the best answer

1. Using the Health Belief Model, determine which of the following individuals would be most motivated for behavior change?

    a. 42-year-old married female with excess weight for over 20 years
    b. 16-year-old female with poorly controlled sugar levels and poor dietary habits consistent with her friends
    c. 50-year-old male with recent myocardial infarction, whose prognosis is good with positive changes in diet and weight loss
    d. 40-year-old who reports spouse wants him to lose weight

2. Which of the following activities would prepare an individual planning retirement to successfully resolve the final developmental tasks proposed by Erickson?

    a. Plan to simultaneously complete any community obligations
    b. Become involved with community activities
    c. Plan several extended trips early in retirement while able
    d. Avoid any commitments initially, wait for opportunities to present themselves

3. Screening for breast cancer is which level of prevention?

    a. Primary
    b. Secondary
    c. Tertiary
    d. Preliminary

4. Client (age 70) comes into your clinic the first week of November for health screening. Her last immunization, a Td (tetanus) was ten years ago. Which immunization will you recommend?

    a. Td, influenza and pneumococcal vaccine
    b. Influenza and pneumococcal vaccine and schedule Td within three months.
    c. Td and influenza
    d. Td only

5. A temporary certificate for school attendance is given following initial immunizations for a 14-year-old boy. When should the adolescent return for more immunizations?

    a. Six months
    b. Four to six weeks
    c. One year
    d. Four months

6. Female, age 19 will be entering college in January. She is not pregnant. Without evidence of recent immunization, she should receive which of the following today?

    a. Second MMR, Td and polio boosters
    b. Hemophilus influenzae (HIB) and a tetanus booster
    c. Second MMR and Td
    d. Immunization for rubella, tetanus, and influenza

7. Joe, age 15, has just moved to your community and is staying in a temporary foster home. He has no record of any immunizations. Which of the following does Joe need today?

    a. MMR, Td, and varicella
    b. IPV, MMR, HBV and Td
    c. Td only
    d. MMR and Td

8. According to research, which type of social support has the strongest relationship with health status?

    a. Emotional
    b. Instrumental
    c. Informational
    d. Appraisal

9. According to research, how much sleep is associated with a longer healthier life?

    a. 5–6 hours
    b. 6–7 hours
    c. 7–8 hours
    d. 8–9 hours

10. Josh, age 32, is ready to start exercising and wants to jog. Guidelines should include which of the following?

    a. Jog one mile initially, then add distance daily until goal is reached.
    b. Jog at least once a week for 30 minutes to condition your heart and lungs.

c. Begin with brisk walking and gradually replace with jogging.

d. Warm up exercises before or after jogging.

11. Several cups of coffee immediately prior to the clinic visit would likely elevate which of the following?

a. Heart rate

b. Respiratory rate

c. Cholesterol

d. Blood sugar

12. Jim asks why cooling down is necessary for an exercise plan?

a. Allows body temperature and heart rate to decrease slowly

b. Loosens and strengthens muscles

c. Maintains and increases flexibility

d. Sustains heart rate for longer period of time

13. According to the Transtheoretical Model, intervention at which level is most likely to result in behavior change?

a. Maintenance

b. Contemplation

c. Precontemplation

d. Preparation

14. Which stress management technique would be most appropriate for a newly diagnosed diabetic?

a. Change avoidance

b. Habituation

c. Time blocking

d. Imagery

15. According to the U.S. Preventive Services Task Force Recommendations, a woman age 21 needs which of the following annually?

a. Blood pressure and cholesterol

b. Clinical breast exam

c. Pap and pelvic

d. Dental screen

16. Your female client age 49, has had a normal baseline mammogram. She asks when she should get her next mammogram:

    a. Annually beginning next year at age 50
    b. Every other year from age 50 to 59, then yearly
    c. Every three years until you are age 60
    d. Every 5 years for the rest of your life

17. Which of the following individuals has a body mass index at the desirable level?

    a. Male, 6 feet 2 inches, 200 pounds (BMI 26)
    b. Female, 5 feet 6 inches, 125 pounds (BMI 20)
    c. Female, 5 feet 10 inches, 160 pounds (BMI 23)
    d. Male, 5 feet 10 inches, 145 pounds (BMI 21)

Answers

1. c
2. b
3. b
4. a
5. b
6. c
7. b
8. a
9. c
10. c
11. a
12. a
13. d
14. c
15. d
16. a
17. c

11/17 64%

Bibliography

Allender, M. (1998). Adolescent. In C. Edelman & C. Mandle (Eds.). *Health promotion throughout the lifespan* (4th ed.). Baltimore: Mosby.

American Cancer Society. (1994). *Summary of the American Cancer Society recommendations for the early detection of cancer in asymptomatic people.* Atlanta, Georgia, GA: American Cancer Society.

Bandura, A. (1986). *Social foundations of thought and action.* Englewood Cliffs, NJ: Prentice-Hall.

Becker, M. (1972). The health belief model and personal health behavior. *Health Education Monographs 2,* 326-7.

Centers for Disease Control and Prevention. (1996). Immunization of adolescents: Recommendations of the Advisory Committee on Immunization Practices, the American Academy of Pediatrics, the American Academy of Family Physicians, and the American Medical Association. *Morbidity and mortality weekly report. 45* (RR-13) November 22 Atlanta, GA: CDC.

Cohen, E. (1996). *Nurse case management in the 21st Century.* St. Louis: Mosby.

Clark, M. (1996). *Nursing in the community* (2nd ed.). Norwalk, CT: Appleton & Lange.

Clinical Preventive Services. (1997). *Clinician's handbook of preventive services: Put prevention into practice.* Waldorf, MD: American Nurses Publishing.

Elster, A., & Kuznets, N. (1994). AMA guidelines for adolescent and preventive services (GAPS). Baltimore: Williams & Wilkins.

Erikson, E. (1963). *Childhood and society* (2nd ed.). NY: Norton.

Friedman, M. (1998). *Family nursing: Research, theory, and practice* (4th ed.). Stanford, CT: Appleton & Lange.

Green, L., & Kreuer, M. (1991). *Health promotion planning: An educational and environmental approach* (2nd ed.). Mountain View, CA: Mayfield.

Hay, W., Groothuis, J., Hayward, A., & Levin, M. (1995). *Current pediatric diagnosis & treatment.* Norwalk, CT: Appleton & Lange.

Jones, K., & Jones, J. (1997). Physical activity & exercise. *Clinician Reviews, 7*(3) 81–102.

Keller,C., Oveland, D., & Hudson, S. (1997). Strategies for weight control success in adults. *Nurse Practitioner, 22*(3), 33–54.

Kenney, W. (1996). *American college of sports medicine fitness book.* Champaign, IL: Human Kinetics.

Maslow, A. (1954). *Motivation and personality.* New York: Harper & Row.

Neuman, B. (1995). *The Neuman systems model.* Norwalk, CT: Appleton & Lange.

Pender, N. (1996). *Health promotion in nursing practice* (3rd ed.). Norwalk, CT: Appleton & Lange.

Prochaska, J., & Velicir, W. (1997). The transtheoretical model of health behavior change. *American Journal of Health Promotion,* 12(1).

Public Health Service. (1990). *Healthy people 2000.* Publication No. (PHS) 91-50212. Washington, DC: Department of Health and Human Services.

U.S. Department of Health and Human Services. (1994). *Clinical handbook of preventive services: Put prevention into practice.* Waldorf, MD: American Nurses Publishing.

Selye, H. (1974). *Stress without distress.* NY: J. B. Lippincott.

Swartz, M. (1994). *Textbook of physical diagnosis.* Philadelphia: W. B. Saunders.

von Bertalanffy (1968). *General systems theory.* New York: George Braziller.

$\dfrac{20}{26}$ 77%

Dermatological Disorders

Sylvia Fletcher
Susan Chaney

Acne Vulgaris

- Definition: Self limited disorders characterized by development of open comedones (white heads) and closed comedones (black heads) due to an increase in sebum release by the sebaceous gland after puberty; if further inflammation is present, pustules, cysts, and nodules on erythematous bases may be present

- Etiology/Incidence
  1. Four primary pathogenic factors
     a. *Propionibacterium acnes*
     b. Increased sebum production
     c. Abnormal follicular keratinization
     d. Chemotactic factors
  2. Factors that predispose to comedone formation
     a. Cosmetics and hair products
     b. Coal tar and insoluble oils
     c. Corticosteroids (topical and systemic), oral contraceptives
  3. Contributing host factors
     a. Heredity
     b. Environment
     c. Stress
  4. May occur as a result of polycystic ovarian disease
  5. May be worse in fall and winter seasons
  6. Seen primarily in adolescents and young adults; may persist to fifth decade
  7. More common in males than females

- Signs and Symptoms
  1. Lesions are nonpruritic, may be tender
  2. Females may notice an increase in symptoms prior to menses

- Differential Diagnosis
  1. Acne rosacea

2. Eosinophilic folliculitis (seen in HIV patient)

3. Drug induced folliculitis

4. Pyogenic folliculitis

- Physical Findings

  1. Morphology

     a. Closed comedones "white heads" are papular lesions found in hair follicles due to blockage of sebum and keratinous materials

     b. Open comedones, "black heads", dilated follicular orifice with easily expressed darkened oily debris

     c. Inflamed comedones, pustules, cysts, and nodules

  2. Distribution

     a. Forehead

     b. Cheek, nose, and chin

     c. Chest, upper arms, back, and buttocks

- Diagnostic Tests/Findings: Culture for causative agent rarely necessary

- Management/Treatment

  1. Reduce bacterial population on skin

     a. Mild skin cleansing twice daily

     b. Benzoyl peroxide 2.5% to 10%—apply 1 to 2 times daily

     c. Topical erythromycin, clindamycin, tetracycline, minocycline, or meclocycline once daily for moderate papulopustular lesions

     d. For widespread distribution on chest and back

        (1) Erythromycin 250 mg 1 to 4 times daily

        (2) Tetracycline 250 mg 1 to 4 times daily (teratogenic with females)

        (3) Females—oral contraceptives with high estrogen component

  2. Prevent development of comedone with comedolytic agent

     a. Retinoic acid cream 0.025% applied nightly

      b.   Caution patient about photosensitivity

      c.   Apply benzoyl peroxide in a.m. if used concurrently

  3. Severe nodulocystic acne may requires aggressive treatment to decrease sebum production—13-cis-retinoic acid 0.5 to 2.0 mg/kg/day for 16 to 20 weeks

      a.   Teratogenic—use with extreme caution in child bearing females

      b.   Multiple systemic side effects

      c.   Monitor liver function tests (LFT), CBC, triglyceride levels

  4. Patient education

      a.   Noticeable improvement may not be apparent for six weeks

      b.   Reassure patient, advise on stress reduction

      c.   Skin care including mild skin cleansing twice daily; advise patient to not squeeze or pick lesions

Alopecia

- Definition: The complete or partial loss of hair from areas where it normally is present; may be total, diffuse, patchy, or localized

- Etiology/Incidence

  1. Hair loss involving hair matrix or follicle destruction due to chemical, physical agents, or both, and by infectious or immunologically mediated inflammation; may also result from a slowing of hair growth due to metabolic diseases

  2. Cicatricial alopecia—scarring

      a.   Hair cannot regrow due to follicle loss

      b.   Caused by *Lichen planopilaris,* severe fungal or bacterial infections, physical trauma

      c.   Other causes include severe cases of herpes zoster, chronic lupus erythematosus, or excessive ionizing radiation

      d.   Permanent and irreversible

  3. Noncicatricial alopecia—nonscarring alopecia

      a.   95% of alopecia seen in primary care

      b. Most common is male or female baldness which is genetic or developmental

      c. Other causes include secondary syphilis, systemic lupus erythematosus, pituitary insufficiency, or iron deficiency anemia

- Signs and Symptoms

    1. Usually the client is symptom free, but verbalizes distress over hair loss

    2. Hair loss resulting from physical agents or infectious disease such as tinea capitis may cause pain or pruritus

- Differential Diagnosis

    1. Tinea capitis

    2. Lichen planus

    3. Folliculitis

    4. Lupus erythematosus

    5. Dermatomyositis

- Physical Findings

    1. Genetic pattern baldness of

      a. Males—frontotemporal hairline recession with various amounts of hair loss at scalp vertex

      b. Females—diffuse or vertex hair loss

    2. Traumatic alopecia findings are patchy hair loss and breakage of hairs

    3. Infectious alopecia—patches of partial hair loss

    4. Alopecia areata (immunologic)—smooth, salmon-colored patches

- Diagnostic Tests

    1. Usually a clinical diagnosis

    2. Hair pull test of 10 or 20 grouped hairs; if over 40% of shafts are removed, disease is more advanced

    3. KOH preparation—negative for fungus

    4. Wood's light—nonfluorescence rules out fungal infections

    5. Refer for scalp biopsy for uncertain cases

6. Hair count of actual hairs lost daily; over 100 would be considered abnormal

- Management/Treatment

    1. Treatment of genetic alopecia

        a. Topical minoxidil 1 mL of 2% b.i.d.

        b. Best results with baldness under 5 years, under age 50, and smaller diameters of alopecia

    2. Refer clients with scarring alopecia for surgical hair transplants.

    3. For premenopausal women, order serum testosterone, DHEAS, iron, TIBC, TSH, CBC to reveal other causes of hair loss

    4. For diffuse hair loss in women, spironolactone 25 mg orally daily

    5. Topical estrogen may be of some value for baldness in women

    6. Refer alopecia areata clients for intralesional corticosteroids

    7. Patient education

        a. About 40% of clients have moderate hair growth within one year

        b. Treatment with minoxidil must be continued indefinitely

        c. Discontinuation of treatment will result in regression to pre-treatment levels of baldness within 2 to 3 months

        d. Side effects of minoxidil are minimal; some clients may experience dryness or pruritus

Bacterial Infections/Pyodermas

- Definitions:

    1. Impetigo—contagious and autoinoculable bacterial infection of skin; the two types are small vesicle and bullous

    2. Folliculitis—infection surrounding hair follicle caused by occlusion of ostium

    3. Furunculosis—deep-seated, autoinoculable infection involving entire hair follicle and adjacent subcutaneous tissue

    4. Carbuncle—several furuncles developing in adjoining hair follicles and coalescing to form deep mass with multiple drainage points

5. Hidradenitis suppurativa—chronic suppurative disease of the apocrine gland-bearing areas of the skin

6. Cellulitis—spreading infection of epidermis, subcutaneous tissue, and superficial lymphatic system

- Etiology/Incidence

    1. Impetigo

        a. Most frequent causative organisms—*Staphylococcus aureus* (*S. aureus*), group A beta hemolytic *Streptococcus pyogenes* (GAS)

        b. Seen primarily in children, bullous in children and young adults

        c. Predisposing factors

            (1) Humid, warm climate

            (2) Pre-existing skin disease, especially atopic

            (3) Prior antibiotic therapy

            (4) Poor hygiene, crowded living conditions,

            (5) Chronic staph carrier (nose, axilla, perineum, bowel)

    2. Folliculitis, furunculosis, carbuncule

        a. Most frequent causative organism—*S. aureus*

        b. Predisposing factors

            (1) Chronic staph carrier (nose, axilla, perineum, bowel

            (2) Diabetes

            (3) Obesity

            (4) Poor hygiene

    3. Hidradenitis suppurativa

        a. Variety of pathogens—most commonly staphylococcus, streptococcus, *E. coli*

        b. Males—anogenital involvement; females axillary involvement

        c. Predisposing factors

            (1) Obesity

        (2)   Seen in all races, most severe in African-Americans

        (3)   Family history of nodulocystic acne, hidradenitis suppurativa

4. Cellulitis

   a. Most frequent causative organisms *S. aureus*. and GAS

   b. Less common—*H. influenzae*, group B streptococci (GBS), pneumococci

   c. Diabetic/immunocompromised—*E. coli, Proteus mirabilis, Acinetobacter, Enterobacter, Pseudomonas aeruginosa*

   d. Predisposing factors:

        (1)   Multiple dermatoses—tinea, inflammatory, bullous, ulceration, pyodermas

        (2)   Trauma

        (3)   Surgical wounds

        (4)   Infections

   e. Risk factors

        (1)   Immunocompromised, cancer, and diabetes

        (2)   Alcohol and drug abuse

- Signs and Symptoms
  1. Localized pain, redness, swelling, or heat
  2. More severe infections—malaise, fever, chills, e.g., cellulitis
- Differential Diagnosis
  1. Contact dermatitis
  2. Allergic dermatitis
  3. Fungal dermatitis
  4. Herpes dermatitis
- Physical Findings
  1. Severe infections
     a. Regional lymphadenopathy
     b. Fever

    c.   Skin tracking

2.   Morphology

    a.   Impetigo—small vesicle caused by sreptococcus

        (1)   Small red macules that progress to water filled vesicles

        (2)   Ruptured vesicles leave characteristic honey-colored crusted area

    b.   Bullous impetigo caused by *Staphylococcus aureus*

        (1)   Large flaccid blister

        (2)   Cloudy to purulent contents

    c.   Folliculitis, furuncle, carbuncle,

        (1)   Abscess—tender, fluctuant nodule

        (2)   Furuncle—firm, tender nodule with central necrotic plug

        (3)   Carbuncle—multiple abscess/furnuncles with sieve like openings draining purulent material

    d.   Hidradenitis suppurativa

        (1)   Initial—inflamed nodule/abscess with serous/purulent drainage and sinus tracks; closed, black, comedones when active nodules are absent

        (2)   Late phase—fibrous "bridge" scarring and contractures

    e.   Cellulitis

        (1)   Bright red plateau, sharply demarcated from surrounding skin.

        (2)   Lymphangitis (red streaking from the area of cellulitis toward proximal lymph nodes) may be present

3.   Distribution

    a.   Impetigo—anywhere

    b.   Folliculitis, furuncle, carbuncle

        (1)   Hair bearing area—beard, axilla, occipital scalp, back of neck

        (2)   Any non-weight bearing area, buttock, upper trunk, puncture wound site

    c. Hidradenitis suppurativa

        (1) Axilla

        (2) Inguinal area

        (3) Anogenital area

        (4) Buttocks, scalp

    d. Cellulitis

        (1) Any area where normal lymphatic drainage has been disrupted

        (2) Recent venous and lymphatic surgical sites

        (3) Previous cellulitis sites

        (4) Cheek or cheek bone and lower extremities

- Diagnostic Tests/Findings

    1. Gram's stain—positive for cocci

    2. Culture and sensitivity of exudate especially on immuno-compromised patient

    3. KOH—negative

    4. Wood's lamp—no fluorescence

    5. Tzanck test—negative

- Management/Treatment

    1. Impetigo

        a. Prevention

            (1) Wash with benzoyl peroxide soap

            (2) Evaluate family members; highly contagious

        b. Gently wash lesion to remove crust

        c. Small area not involving the face

            (1) Mupirocin applied q.i.d. for 10 days

            (2) Effective against GAS and methicillin-resistant *S. aureus* (MRSA)

        d. GAS—small vesicular impetigo

      (1)   Erythromycin 250 mg q.i.d. for 10 days

      (2)   Cephalexin 250 to 500 mg q.i.d. for 10 days

  e. S. aureus—bullous impetigo

      (1)   Dicloxacillin 250mg q.i.d. for 10 days

      (2)   Cephalexin 250 mg q.i.d. for 10 days

      (3)   Erythromycin (as ethylsuccinate) 400 to 800 mg q.i.d. for 10 days

2. Folliculitis, furuncle, carbuncle and hidradenitis suppurativa

  a. Mild folliculitis

      (1)   Benzoyl peroxide 5% b.i.d. for 10 days

      (2)   Erythromycin 2% solution b.i.d. for 10 days

  b. Moderate infection

      (1)   Warm moist compresses to promote spontaneous drainage

      (2)   Incision and drainage (I & D) usually required

      (3)   Culture recurrent abscesses

      (4)   Dicloxacillin 250mg q.i.d. for 10 days

      (5)   Cephalexin 250 mg q.i.d. for 10 days

  c. Hidradenitis suppurativa—additional measures to reduce inflammation

      (1)   Intralesional triamcinalone 3 to 5 mg/mL diluted with lidocaine prior to I & D

      (2)   Prednisone 70 mg tapered over 14 days

3. Cellulitis

  a. Facial involvement—consult with physician for possible inpatient management

  b. I & D may be required

  c. Antibiotic should be selected based upon suspected pathogen

      (1)   Penicillin V Potassium 250 to 500 mg q.i.d. for 10 days (*S. aureus*, GAS)

　　　　(2)　Amoxicillin/clavulanate 500 mg t.i.d. for 10 days (*S. aureus*)

　　　　(3)　Erythromycin 250 mg q.i.d. for 10 days (GBS)

　　d.　Rest, immobilization, elevation, moist heat, analgesia

　　e.　Re-evaluate in 48 hours

Dermatitis

- Definition: Group of inflammatory pruritic skin diseases that have different etiologies but share common symptoms and clinical manifestations

　1.　Atopic dermatitis—acute, subacute, but usually chronic, pruritic inflammation of the epidermis and dermis; term often used synonymously with eczema, IgE dermatitis

　2.　Contact dermatitis—acute or chronic inflammatory reactions to substances that come in contact with the skin

　3.　Stasis dermatitis—inflammatory response to extravasated blood in dermis and subcutaneous tissue resulting from stasis

　4.　Seborrheic dermatitis—chronic dermatosis characterized by redness and scaling reaction where sebaceous glands are most active

- Etiology/Incidence

　1.　Atopic dermatitis

　　a.　Thought to have genetic basis; often seen as part of an "atopy" triad; dermatitis, asthma and allergic rhinitis

　　b.　Two-thirds of patients have personal or family history of respiratory atopy

　　c.　Seen in all populations and geographic locations

　　d.　More common in males than in females

　　e.　Highest incidence in childhood, usually resolves by third decade

　　f.　More prevalent in urban areas and developed countries

　　g.　Exacerbated by allergies, skin dehydration, emotional stress, hormonal changes, and infection

　2.　Contact dermatitis

　　a.　Irritant contact dermatitis

(1) More common than allergic contact dermatitis

(2) Most irritants used daily in work and home environments

(3) Accounts for high percentage of work-related skin disorders

    (a) Low-caustic irritants—soapy water, cleansers, rubbing alcohol, kerosene

    (b) High-caustic irritants—bleach, strong acids, alkalis

(4) Higher incidence in those with compromised skin integrity

b. Allergic contact dermatitis

(1) Delayed (type IV) cell-mediated hypersensitivity to a substance

    (a) Substance (antigen) binds with epidermal protein

    (b) Antigen-protein complex presented to T-helper cells causing release of mediators

    (c) T-helper cell expansion occurs in regional lymph nodes producing T-effector lymphocytes

    (d) T-effector lymphocytes circulate in bloodstream and produce the epidermal response

    (e) Entire process occurs in 5 to 21 days

    (f) Re-exposure—dermatologic response in 12 to 48 hours

(2) Most common sensitizer in U.S. is oleoresin of Rhus family of plants—poison oak, ivy, and sumac

(3) Other common sensitizers are nickel in jewelry, fragrances, and preservatives in topical preparations

3. Stasis dermatitis

  a. Occurs as a result of chronic venous insufficiency

  b. Complicated by low grade tissue ischemia associated with stasis at capillary level

  c. History of varicosities, thrombophlebitis, or postphlebitic syndrome

      d.   Often complicated by allergic contact dermatitis and chronic infection

   4. Seborrheic dermatitis

      a.   Etiology unknown, thought to have a genetic basis

      b.   Overgrowth of naturally occurring yeast, *Pityrosporum ovale*

      c.   Often begins in early adulthood, aggravated by stress

      d.   Can be an early cutaneous sign of HIV infection

      e.   Often severe in patients with chronic neurological diseases

      f.   Seen in patients with severe acne

      g.   More common in males

- Signs and Symptoms: Pruritic scaly rash
- Differential Diagnosis

   1. Scabies

   2. Tinea

   3. Atopic/eczema dermatitis

   4. Contact dermatitis

   5. Nummular dermatitis

   6. Psoriasis

   7. Cellulitis (stasis dermatitis)

- Physical Findings

   1. Common clinical findings for all types of dermatitis

      a.   Initial stage—erythema, papules, microvesicles, and excoriation

      b.   Chronic stage—lichenification

   2. Atopic dermatitis

      a.   Papules, erythema, excoriations and lichenification

      b.   Pustules represent secondary infections with staphylococci

      c.   Distribution—flexural areas of neck, antecubital fossae, and popliteal fossae

    d. Other locations—face, wrist, and forearm

3. Irritant contact dermatitis

    a. Mild irritants—erythema, chapped skin, dryness, and fissuring

    b. Severe cases—edema, serous oozing, tender, crusting, scaling

    c. Painful bullae may develop with potent irritant

    d. Distribution—hands most common, also face and eyes

4. Allergic contact dermatitis

    a. Erythema, edema, papules, vesicles, serous oozing, crusting, scaling

    b. Distribution—corresponds to exposed area

    c. Lesions outline site of irritant, often linear pattern with plant exposure

5. Stasis dermatitis

    a. Early stage—mottled pigmentation and slight erythema

    b. Evidence of varicosities, ankle edema

    c. Mild tenderness with deep palpation; pulses normal

    d. Chronic stage—subcutaneous tissue becomes thick, fibrous

    e. Distribution—lower legs

6. Seborrheic dermatitis

    a. Ill defined, greasy yellow scales overlying erythematous patches

    b. Distribution—scalp, within external ear, postauricular area, eyebrows, nasolabial folds, central chest, and at times axilla, groin, submammary folds

- Diagnostic Tests/Findings

1. Serum IgE—levels elevated in patients with atopy

2. KOH—negative for spores/hyphae

3. Skins scrapings—negative for burrows

- Management/Treatment

1. Three goals of therapy

a. Treatment of inflamed skin

b. Control of pruritus

c. Control of exacerbating factors

2. Treatment of inflamed skin

a. Mild disease—low-potency steroid cream

   (1) Hydrocortisone 1% cream 2 to 4 times daily

   (2) Triamcinolone acetonide 0.025% cream 2 to 4 times daily

b. Severe disease—medium potency steroid cream

   (1) Triamcinolone acetonide 0.5% cream 2 to 3 times daily

   (2) Desoximetasone 0.05% cream 2 times daily

c. Topical corticosteroid with occlusion may be helpful

   (1) Treat area with steroid cream and cover with plastic wrap

   (2) Leave on overnight and remove cover in morning

d. Acute flares may require short term ''burst'' oral glucocorticoids

   (1) Prednisone 70 mg tapered over 14 days

   (2) Solu-medrol

e. Ultraviolet light therapy and oral glucocorticoids for most severe cases

f. Wet to dry compresses with water or aluminum acetate (Burow's solution) to dry vesicular lesions

g. Bullous lesions—may be drained; do not remove top thin skin

3. Control of pruritus

a. Antihistamines, sedating H blockers

   (1) Hydroxyzine 25 mg t.i.d./q.i.d. prn

   (2) Diphenhydramine 25 to 50 mg every 4 to 6 hours prn

   (3) Doxepin 10 to 25 mg b.i.d./t.i.d. prn

b. Tepid bathes to cool and hydrate skin

    c. Mild soaps

    d. Emollients

    e. Control of exacerbating factors

        (1) Treat secondary bacterial infections

        (2) Maintain good hydration and integrity of skin

        (3) Gently towel dry skin, no brisk rubbing

        (4) Continued use of emollients to prevent skin drying

        (5) Wear gloves to avoid contact irritants

        (6) Identify and avoid offending irritants

        (7) Stasis dermatitis—special measures

           (a) Elevate legs; support stockings

           (b) Exercise daily to help reduce venous pressure and edema

        (8) Seborrheic dermatitis—special measures

           (a) Daily use of shampoos containing tar, sulfur, salicylic acid, or selenium

           (b) Ketoconazole 2% cream and shampoo is an alternative to topical steroids

        (9) Educate patient on stress reduction to avoid exacerbation

        (10) Follow-up in 1 to 2 weeks

Fungal and Yeast Infections

- Definitions:
  1. Tinea (dermatophytosis)—fungal infection of skin, nails, and hair; characteristic lesions varies by site
  2. Tinea (pityriasis)versicolor—chronic, asymptomatic, scaly dermatitis
  3. Candidiasis—yeast-like fungal infection of skin and mucous membrane
- Etiology/Incidence
  1. Tinea

      a.   Causative organisms—*Trichophyton, Microsporum,* and *Epidermophyton*

      b.   Transmitted by fomites, animals (pets), and to a lesser extent, soil

  2. Tinea versicolor

      a.   Causative organism—nondermatophyte fungus *Pityrosporum orbiculare;* normal inhabitant of skin

      b.   Most common in young adults when sebum production high

  3. Candidiasis

      a.   Causative organism usually *Candida albicans;* normal saprophytic inhabitant of GI tract; overgrowth often due to antibiotic use

      b.   Occurs in intertriginous, moist, cutaneous areas

  4. Contributing factors

      a.   Warm moist environments for fungal infections

      b.   Obesity

      c.   Altered immunity

         (1) HIV

         (2) Diabetes

         (3) Pregnancy

         (4) Inhaled or oral steroids

      d.   Oral contraceptives

      e.   Antibiotic therapy

- Signs and Symptoms (depends upon area of involvement)

  1. Mild pruritus

  2. Inflamed, tender rash

  3. Thickened nails

  4. Hair loss

- Differential Diagnosis

  1. Seborrheic dermatitis

2. Psoriasis

3. Alopecia

4. Atopic dermatitis

5. Contact dermatitis

6. Pityriasis rosea

7. Bacterial infection

- Physical Findings

    1. Morphology

        a. Tinea (dermatophytosis)—characteristic lesion varies by site

            (1) Tinea capitis—well defined or irregular, diffuse areas of scaling and hair loss on scalp

            (2) Tinea corporis—annular appearance (ringworm), deep inflammatory nodules, or granulomas

            (3) Tinea cruris—sharply demarcated, erythematous scaly patches

            (4) Tinea pedis—erythema/edema, scaling, and occasional vesiculation; fissured toe webs

            (5) Tinea unguium—opacified thickened nails with subungal debris

            (6) Immunocompromised patient—may see abscess or granulomas

        b. Tinea (pityriasis) versicolor—oval scaly hyper or hypopigmented macules

        c. Candidiasis

            (1) Skin (intertrigo)—erythematous macerated areas with satellite pustules

            (2) Mucous membranes—white friable patches on mucous membranes

    2. Distribution

        a. Tinea

            (1) Capitis—scalp

    (2) Corporis—non-hair-bearing skin

    (3) Cruris—(males) groin and upper thigh sparing scrotum

    (4) Pedis—feet, usually between 4th and 5th toes

    (5) Unguium—nails, usually 1st and 2nd toenails

  b. Tinea versicolor

    (1) "Shawl like" back, chest, and shoulders

    (2) Less common—groin, thigh, genitalia

  c. Candidiasis

    (1) Body folds—axillae, submammary, groin, intergluteal, webspaces of fingers and toes

    (2) Oral and vaginal mucous membranes

- Diagnostic Test/Findings

  1. Wood's lamp (T. versicolor)—golden fluorescence

  2. KOH—positive for hyphae, pseudohyphae, and/or spores

  3. Fungal culture—may be useful for inflammatory T. corporis and T. capitis

- Management/Treatment

  1. Tinea

    a. Scalp

      (1) Selenium sulfide shampoo 2.5% twice weekly for two weeks

      (2) Oral antifungals

        (a) Terbinafine 250 mg daily 4 to 6 weeks, (most effective)

        (b) Itraconazole 100 mg b.i.d. 4 to 6 weeks

        (c) Ketoconozole 200 to 400 mg daily for 4 to 6 weeks

        (d) Griseofulvin

      (3) Advise hair regrowth will be slow

    b. Body

          (1)   Multiple topical imidazoles and triazoles taken b.i.d. until 1 to 2 weeks after clinical clearing, e.g., clotrimazole 1% cream b.i.d.

          (2)   Terbinafine 1% cream b.i.d. 1 to 2 weeks after clinical clearing

          (3)   Griseofulvin

          (4)   If topical antifungals fail, use oral agents (see T. capitis)

          (5)   Avoid occlusive footwear for tinea pedis

   c.   Nails

          (1)   Terbinafine 250 mg daily (most effective)

              (a)   Fingernails—six weeks

              (b)   Toenails—12 weeks

          (2)   Poor results with topical agents; usually reserved for maintenance after successful systemic treatment

   d.   Follow up in two weeks to re-evaluate treatment

2.   Tinea versicolor

   a.   Selenium sulfide lotion 2.5%—apply at bedtime, rinse in morning

   b.   Clotrimazole 1% cream b.i.d. for four weeks

   c.   Ketoconozole 200 mg daily for one week

          (1)   Cure rate 90%

          (2)   No shower for 12 to 18 hours after treatment

   d.   Recurrence common as organism is normal inhabitant of skin

   e.   Sulfur-salicylic acid soap or shampoo on a continuing basis may be effective prophylaxsis

3.   Candidiasis

   a.   Nystatin cream or powder b.i.d. 2 to 4 weeks

   b.   Ketoconazole cream daily for 2 to 4 weeks

   c.   Fluconazole 150 mg orally once

      d.   Dry intertriginous area—wet Burow's compresses 3 to 4 times daily

      e.   Rule out HIV or diabetes in patients with multiple recurrences

Papulosquamous Disorders

- Definition: Group of disorders with unique scales due to abnormal keratinization process; these lesions are sharply delineated, distinguishing them from scaling lesions of eczematous diseases

  1. Psoriasis vulgaris—genetically determined, chronic, epidermal proliferate disease of unpredictable course

  2. Pityriasis rosea—self-limited mild, inflammatory skin disease lasting 3 to 8 weeks

- Etiology/Incidence

  1. Psoriasis

     a. Genetic predisposition, although not totally understood

     b. Affects 2% of population in U.S., Caucasians > African-Americans

     c. Type 1, early onset, occurring in 2nd decade

     d. Type 2, late onset, occurring in 6th to 8th decades

     e. Approximately 5% of patients will develop psoriatic arthritis affecting primarily distal interphalangeal (DIP) joints

     f. Abrupt onset seen with early HIV infection

     g. Trigger factors

        (1) Physical trauma

        (2) Infection

        (3) Stress

        (4) Drugs—corticosteroids, lithium, antimalarial, interferon, beta-blockers

  2. Pityriasis rosea

     a. Etiology unknown; viral cause suspected

     b. Seen primarily in the spring and fall seasons

     c. Patients frequently report recent upper respiratory infection

    d. 50% more common in females

- Signs and Symptoms
  1. Psoriasis
     a. Frequently asymptomatic
     b. Severe pruritus in body fold eruptions
     c. Chronic, recurring
  2. Pityriasis rosea
     a. Mild pruritus
     b. Initial lesion precedes general eruption by one to two weeks
     c. Self-limiting—heals without scarring in four to eight weeks

- Differential Diagnosis
  1. Psoriasis
     a. Seborrheic dermatitis
     b. Candidiasis
     c. Intertrigo
     d. Onychomycosis
     e. Reiter's syndrome
  2. Pityriasis rosea
     a. Syphilis
     b. Tinea infections
     c. Seborrheic dermatitis

- Physical Findings
  1. Psoriasis
     a. Cutaneous lesions reveal four prominent features:
        (1) Sharply demarcated lesions with clear-cut borders
        (2) Erythematous plaque base
        (3) Overlapping silvery scales
        (4) Auspitz sign—removal of scales results in small blood droplets

      b.   Fingers/nails

          (1) Stippling or pitting of nail plate

          (2) Yellow or brown-red staining of oncholytic patches with accumulation of yellow debris under nails

          (3) Swelling, redness and scaling of paronychial margins

  2. Pityriasis rosea—classic disease pattern

      a.   A single lesion termed "herald patch" precedes generalized eruption by 7 to 10 days

      b.   "Herald patch" is found usually on neck or lower trunk; oval, slightly erythematous, rose or fawn-colored

      c.   Oval patches seen in general eruption have an unusual fine, white scale located near the border of the plaques, forming a collarette

      d.   Lesions follow skin cleavage lines in a "Christmas tree" pattern

- Diagnostic Tests/Findings

  1. Psoriasis

      a.   Diagnosis generally based on clinical presentation

      b.   Biopsy rarely needed

      c.   KOH—negative for spores/hyphae

  2. Pityriasis rosea

      a.   Diagnosis generally based on clinical presentation

      b.   KOH—negative for spores/hyphae

      c.   Throat culture or rapid strep test—negative for scarlatina

      d.   RPR—negative for syphilis

- Management/Treatment

  1. Psoriasis—limited disease (< 30% body surface affected)

      a.   Initial approach—scalp

          (1) Tar-based shampoo daily for two to three weeks

          (2) High potency topical steroid lotion twice daily for two to three weeks

b. Initial approach—face

    (1) Low potency topical steriod cream twice daily for two to three weeks

    (2) Calcipotriene ointment 0.005% twice daily for several weeks

c. Initial apporach—trunk and extremities

    (1) High potency topical steroid cream twice daily for two to three weeks

    (2) Occulsion therapy—thin duoderm or tegaderm for five to seven days, then replace until resolved

d. A variety of regimens with alternative tar, steroids, and occlusion therapy are utilized in cases unresponsive to initial treatment

e. Topical steroids rarely produce a lasting remission

f. Topical steroids may not be used in body folds

g. Resistant cases may require treatment with therapies described in next section (psoriasis—generalized)

2. Psoriasis—generalized (> 30% body surface affected)

a. Goeckerman regimen—phototherapy ultraviolet B radiation (UVB) used in combination with topical coal tar

b. Ingram regimen—phototherapy ultraviolet B radiation (UVB) used in combination with anthralin 0.1% to 0.5% applied daily

c. Psoralen and ultra violet light type A (PUVA)—combines psoralens (methoxsalen or trioxsalen) with long wave ultraviolet light therapy

3. Pityriasis rosea

a. Treatment often not necessary

b. Topical corticosteroids and antihistamines for control of pruritus

4. Patient education—family issues, emotional support, decrease stress, National Psoriasis Foundation

5. HIV test in suspected or high risk population

Scabies

- Definition: Common highly pruritic transmissable ectoparasite infection
- Etiology/Incidence
    1. Caused by itch mite *Sarcoptes scabiei*
    2. Adult female mite burrows into skin shortly after contact; lives for 4 to 6 weeks
    3. Incubation period four weeks from initial contact; generalized hypersensitivity eruption 1 to 2 weeks later
    4. Transmitted primarily by person to person or sexual contact
    5. Transmission via clothing, bedding less common—mite cannot survive more than one day without host
    6. May affect entire families
    7. Frequently seen in institutionalized persons, such as homeless shelters, nursing homes, correctional facilities
- Signs and Symptoms
    1. Pruritus always present; most intense when individual is in bed or after a hot shower
    2. Pruritus frequently less intense in the HIV client
- Differential Diagnosis
    1. Atopic dermatitis
    2. Contact or irritant dermatitis
    3. Urticaria
    4. Pediculosis
- Physical Findings
    1. Burrows, small pruritic vesicles, or wavy dark lines a few millimeters to 1 cm in length with papule at open end
    2. May be difficult to visualize since client scratching destroys burrows
    3. Lesions are believed to be due to a hypersensitivity reaction to the excreta deposited by mite

4. Generalized excoriations surrounding vesicles and pustules on fingers, palms, wrists, elbows, axillae, feet, nipples in females, scrotum or penis in males, buttocks

5. Usually spares the head and neck, except in the elderly or patients with AIDS—in the client with HIV, hyperkeratotic plaques may be located on any area of the body

- Diagnostic Tests/Findings: Microscopic examination of skin scraping in oil immersion—presence of mite, eggs, or fecal pellets

- Management/Treatment

    1. Treatment of choice is 5% permethrin cream applied to all areas of the body from the neck down; left on for 8 to 14 hours, and then removed with soap and water

    2. Alternative is 1% lindane (no longer the drug of choice)

        a. Lotion or cream applied from neck down to all areas of the body and removed with soap and water after eight hours

        b. Not recommended for pregnant or lactating women, patients with extensive dermatitis, nor infants

    3. Alternative is 10% crotamiton cream applied to the body from the neck down for two consecutive nights and then removed with soap and water 48 hours after the last application

    4. All household members and sexual contacts should be evaluated and treated if necessary to prevent reinfection

    5. For persistent pruritus, triamcinolone 0.1% cream to affected areas b.i.d.

    6. Secondary pyoderma is generally due to staphylococcus; treat with topical mupirocin or oral erythromycin

    7. Patient education

        a. Launder all bedding and clothing in hot water and on hot dryer cycle

        b. Place clothing that cannot be laundered in plastic storage bags for at least four days— mites will not survive off the host longer than four days

        c. Advise client that pruritus may continue for several weeks

Skin Cancer

- Definition:

  1. Basal cell carcinoma (BCC)—slow growing locally destructive carcinoma of basal cell layer of epidermis; limited potential for metastasis

  2. Squamous cell carcinoma (SCC)—malignant, nodular, tumor arising from squamous cells in epithelium; hyperkeratotic growth

  3. Malignant melanoma (MM)—cancer that arises in melanocytes; accounts for 5% of all skin cancers; two most common types are superficial spreading melanoma (SSM) and nodular melanoma (NM)

  4. Kaposi's sarcoma (KS)—multisystem vascular neoplasm characterized by mucocutaneous and violet lesions and edema; involves nearly all body organs

- Etiology/Incidence

  1. Basal cell carcinoma

     a. Cause is multifactorial; cumulative sunlight exposure (UVB) is most significant factor

     b. Primarily affects fair-skinned persons with tendency to sunburn easily

     c. Most common form of human cancer

     d. Over 400,000 new cases in U.S. per year; mostly persons in 4th decade

     d. Additional risk factors

        (1) Extensive sun exposure as a youth

        (2) History of treatment with x-ray for facial acne

  2. Squamous cell carcinoma

     a. Causal/contributing factors

        (1) UVB light

        (2) Human papillomaviruses have also been implicated

        (3) Immunocompromise

        (4) Chemical carcinogens—topical nitrogen mustard; oral

PUVA (psoralens with UVA [used to treat psoriasis]); industrial carcinogens

    (5) Increased risk of oral and lip SCC in cigarette and cigar smokers

  b. Mainly seen on sun-damaged areas of fair-skinned persons, but can appear anywhere on the body

  c. Also found in brown and black-skinned person

  d. Frequency of metastasis is by location; SCC of the cutaneous tissue has an overall metastatic rate of 3% to 4%; invasive SCC arising from chronic osteomyelitis sinus tracts, burn scars, and sites of radiation dermatitis have metastatic rates of 31%, 20%, and 18% respectively

3. Malignant melanoma

  a. All causes not known

  b. Brief, intense exposure to long-wave ultra-violet radiation contributes to development

  c. Predisposing/risk factors:

    (1) Presence of precursor lesions, e.g., Clark's dysplastic melanocytic nevus, congenital melanocytic nevus

    (2) Family history of melanoma

    (3) Fair complexion; red or blonde hair; freckles; tendency to sunburn easily

    (4) Excessive sun exposure

  d. Peak age distribution 30 to 50 years

  e. Slightly more common in men

  f. Incidence has increased 300% in 40 years

4. Kaposi's sarcoma

  a. Human herpesvirus 8 present in all forms

  b. Epidemic clusters in U.S. predominantly found in HIV infected individuals—incidence has decreased from 40% to 18% of HIV population

  c. Occurs when $CD4^+$ count < 500

d. Non-HIV related forms are less common but do occur

(1) African-endemic—accounts for 8% to 12% of malignancies in Zaire

(2) Classic (European)—occurs predominantly in elderly white males, rarely fatal

(3) Iatrogenic immunosuppressive drug associated—occurs infrequently in patients on immunosuppressive or cytotoxic chemotherapy, resolves when drug withdrawn

- Signs and Symptoms
  1. BCC/SCC—painless sore that will not heal
  2. Malignant melanoma—6 signs ABCDEE
     a. **A**symmetry in shape
     b. **B**order is irregular
     c. **C**olor is mottled
     d. **D**iameter is usually large > 6.0 mm
     e. **E**levation is almost always present
     f. **E**nlargement or a history of an increase in size is perhaps the most important sign
  3. Kaposi's sarcoma—small reddish-purple to brown lesion
- Differential Diagnosis
  1. BCC/SCC
     a. Seborrheic keratosis
     b. Malignant melanoma
     c. Actinic keratosis
     d. Psoriasis
     e. Nummular eczema
  2. Malignant melanoma
     a. Melanoma in situ
     b. Solar lentigo
     c. Dysplastic melanocytic nevus with marked atypia

    d. Recurring melanocyte nevus

    e. Hemangioma

    f. Pyogenic granuloma

    g. Pigmented BCC

3. Kaposi's sarcoma

    a. Sclerosing hemangioma

    b. Ecchymosis

    c. Stasis dermatitis

- Physical Findings

1. Basal cell carcinoma

    a. Most commonly found on face and head

    b. Papular, nodular, ulcerated, sclerosing pigmented lesions

    c. Pearly appearance with telangiectatic vessels is most diagnostic

    d. Lesions may have a central crust or erosion

    e. Slow growing—may reach 1 to 2 cm diameter after several years

2. Squamous cell carcinoma

    a. In situ (Bowen's Disease)

        (1) Erythematous plaque, slightly raised, sharp borders with little infiltration

        (2) Presents most commonly on mouth and lower lip

    b. Invasive squamous cell carcinoma

        (1) Highly differentiated SCC

            (a) Keratinization within or on surface of tumor

            (b) Firm or hard upon palpation

        (2) Poorly differentiated SCC

            (a) Shows no sign of keratinization

            (b) Fleshy, granulomatous; soft on palpation

3. Malignant melanoma

   a. SSM

      (1) Pigment variation of dark brown, black, pink, or gray; starts as flattened papule, progressing to plaques, and then nodules.

      (2) Asymmetrical to 12 mm (early), to 25 mm (late)

      (3) Isolated single lesions found primarily on sun exposed areas—back, legs, anterior chest (males)

      (4) Regional lymphadenopathy (later stages)

   b. NM

      (1) Dark blue, black uniformly elevated ''blueberry-like'' nodule ranging in size from 1 to 3 cm; oval or round with smooth sharply defined borders

      (2) Distribution and regional lymphadenopathy same as SSM

4. Kaposi's sarcoma

   a. Red, purple or dark color palpable plaques or nodules on cutaneous or mucosal surfaces

   b. Lymph node involvement in 50% of patient's with HIV associated KS

   c. May also involve the lung, gastrointestinal tract, or urogenital system

- Diagnostic Tests/Findings—total excisional biopsy with narrow margins for SSM and NM

- Management/Treatment

   1. Basal cell carcinoma

      a. Electrodesiccation and curretage (ED&C)—most common

      b. Excision—for more aggressive tumors and high-risk locations referral to oncology for therapy

         (1) Radiotherapy with 4000-5000 rads in 6 to 10 doses (cure 95%)

         (2) Mohs surgery—removal of tumor; 98% cure rate

2. Squamous cell carcinoma

    a. Referral to oncologist for therapy

    b. Surgical excision is preferred treatment

    c. Other treatment options include:

        (1) Mohs surgery

        (2) Electrodesiccation and curettage with radiation

        (3) Intralesional chemotherapy

    d. Follow up for recurrence or metastasis

3. Malignant melanoma

    a. Refer to oncologist for therapy

        (1) Initial excision to establish histologic diagnosis

        (2) Re-excision of the area with adequate margins—margins range from 0.5 to 3.0 cm based upon depth of invasion

        (3) Elective lymph node dissection controversial

    b. Close follow up for evidence of recurrence of metastasis

4. Kaposi's sarcoma

    a. Referral for cryotherapy, radiation or laser surgey—treatment depends upon underlying condition and location of sarcoma

    b. Supportive care, counseling for HIV infected patients

Viral Dermatoses

- Definitions

    1. Herpes simplex I (HS-I) ("fever blister")—recurrent cutaneous viral infection characterized by single or multiple clusters of small vesicles on an erythematous base; lesions appear on the lips, in the mouth or pharynx

    2. Herpes (varicella) zoster ("shingles")—an acute CNS cutaneous viral infection characterized by vesicular eruptions and neurologic pain; involves primarily the dorsal root ganglia

    3. Warts—common contagious epithelial tumors; usually benign

- Etiology/Incidence

1. Herpes Simplex (HS-I)

   a. Caused by herpes simplex virus (HSV-I)

   b. Usually follows a minor infection, trauma, stress or sun exposure

   c. 90% of adults have serologic evidence of virus

   d. Prolonged incubation period 2 to 18 months

2. Herpes (varicella) zoster

   a. Reactivation of varicella zoster virus (VZV) in chickenpox

   b. Proposed that VZV is dormant in dorsal root ganglia

   c. May occur at any age, but most common after age 50

   d. May precede marked immunosuppresion in patients with HIV or Hodgkin's disease

   e. Post-transplant patients on immunosuppression medication are also at risk

3. Warts

   a. Caused by over 60 human papillomaviruses (HPV)

   b. Squamous cell carcinoma associated with HPV infections in anogenital region

   c. Common in young adults, but uncommon in the aged

- Signs and Symptoms

   1. HS-I

      a. Small vesicles appear after a short prodrome of tingling, burning, or itching

      b. Vesicles dry to a yellow crust within a few days

   2. Herpes zoster

      a. Pain along nerve root precedes eruption by 48 hours

      b. Characteristic crops of vesicles then appear

   3. Warts—generally asymptomatic

- Differential Diagnosis

   1. HS-I

    a. Contact dermatitis

    b. Pyoderma

    c. Chickenpox (VZV)

    d. Chancroid syphilis

2. Herpes zoster (local lesion and pre-eruptive pain)

    a. Contact dermatitis

    b. Herpes simplex

    c. Migraine

    d. Myocardial infarction

    e. Acute abdomen

3. Wart

    a. Squamous cell carcinoma

    b. Hypertrophic actinic keratosis

    c. Molloscum contagiosum

    d. Seborrheic keratosis

- Physical Findings

1. Regional lymphadenopathy may be seen with herpetic diseases

2. HS-I

    a. Small grouped vesicles on an erythematous base that progress to a crusted erosion

    b. Duration 5 to 7 days

    c. Distribution lips, mouth, pharynx

3. Herpes zoster

    a. May present 3 to 4 days prior to pain and vesicular eruptions with prodrome of chills, fever, malaise

    b. Painful unilateral vesicular eruptions within a dermatome

    c. Duration 2 to 3 weeks

    d. Distribution—face and trunk

    e. Regional lymph glands may be tender or edematous

      f.   Complication of post-herpetic neuralgia involving trigeminal region

  4. Warts

      a.   Common wart (verrucae vulgaris)

          (1)   Solitary flesh-colored papule with scaly irregular surface 2 to 10 mm in diameter

          (2)   Appear most often on fingers, around nail plate, elbows, knees

      b.   Flat wart (verruca plantaris)

          (1)   Groups of smooth flat-topped, flesh-colored lesions

          (2)   Distribution—face and extremities

      c.   Plantar warts

          (1)   Endophytic (growing inward) with thick keratin surface

          (2)   Common on sole of foot

          (3)   May be exquisitely painful

- Diagnostic Tests/Findings

  1. HS-I and zoster

      a.   Direct immunofluorescent antibody (ELISA)—positive

      b.   Tzanck smear—multinucleated cells (least sensitive)

      c.   Viral culture—positive (not highly sensitive)

      d.   Consider testing for HIV or Hodgkin's if recurrence of herpes

  2. Warts

      a.   Acetic acid 5%—lesions turn white

      b.   Biopsy—rule out squamous cell carcinoma

- Management/Treatment

  1. HS-I

      a.   Immunocompetent patient

          (1)   Initial episode—acyclovir 200 mg four times day for 7 to 10 days

          (2)   Recurrent episodes—acyclovir not effective

            (3)   Topical acyclovir not recommended

    b.   Immunosuppressed patient

        (1)   Initial episode—acyclovir 400 mg 4 times/day for 7 to 10 days

        (2)   Localized external lesion

            (a)   Topical acyclovir 5% 4 to 6 times/day

            (b)   Limit use to this group of patients due to development of resistant HS-1 viral strain

        (3)   To prevent reactivation (i.e., immediate post-transplant)—acyclovir 400 mg 3 to 5 times/day

    c.   Caution family—virus may remain on fomites for several hours

  2.   Herpes zoster

    a.   Immunocompetent

        (1)   Acyclovir 800 mg five times/day for seven days started within 48 to 72 hours

        (2)   Good hydration essential

        (3)   Nerve block for analgesia may be necessary

        (4)   Monitor renal function in patient with renal disease

    b.   Immunosuppressed

        (1)   Consult with physician

        (2)   Goal of therapy is to prevent life threatening viral spread

        (3)   IV acyclovir 12.5 mg/kg/dose every eight hours for seven days

        (4)   Try to wean patients from immunosuppression treatment

    c.   Post-zoster neuralgia

        (1)   Regional nerve blockade

        (2)   Narcotic and nonnarcotic analgesia

        (3)   Amitriptyline 25 mg t.i.d. (if no response to conventional pain therapy)

    d. Warts

        (1) Most are unresponsive to all therapeutic modalities

        (2) Most will resolve spontaneously in 1 to 2 years

        (3) Multiple keratolytic agents—salicylic acid or salicylic acid and lactic acid combination

        (4) Tretinoin—good for facial lesions

        (5) Liquid nitrogen every two weeks for several weeks

        (6) Carbon dioxide laser excision

Questions
Select the best answer.

1. Mrs. Trevino is a 35-year-old patient with patchy hair loss as a result of chronic systemic lupus erythematosus. You have determined that she has scarring or cicatrical alopecia. The most effective treatment you can offer is:

    a. Topical minoxidil
    b. Intralesional corticosteroids
    c. Topical estrogen
    d. Referral to dermatologist

2. Mr. Johnson is a 45-year-old patient with diabetes who is homeless. He presents with tender fluctulant nodules on the skin around his beard. He has been previously treated with benzoyl peroxide 5% with minimal response. You order warm moist compresses and:

    a. Dicloxacillin 250 mg q.i.d. for 10 days
    b. Trimethoprim/sulfamethoxazole every day for 5 days
    c. Acyclovir topical
    d. Clotrimazole 1% b.i.d. for 10 days

3. Mr. Johnson returns to your office with his friend. His friend presents with multiple abscesses and "boils" on the back of his neck that have coalesced and developed sieve-like openings draining pus. Your diagnosis is:

    a. Scabies
    b. Folliculitis
    c. Carbuncle
    d. Contact dermatitis

4. To reduce inflammation in a hidradentitis suppurativa lesion, immediately prior to incision and drainage you would:

    a. Apply cold packs to axilla
    b. Order solu-medrol dosepak
    c. Apply tretinoin topically
    d. Inject intralesional triamcinlone 3 to 5 mg/mL diluted with lidocaine

5. The most common sensitizer in the U.S. responsible for allergic contact dermatitis is:

    a. Oleoresin
    b. Tinea

   c. Rubbing alcohol

   d. Bleach

6. Mrs. Waterman is a 64-year-old with a history of varicosities and a single episode of thrombophlebitis. On inspection of both lower extremities you note mottled pigmentation, erythema, varicosities, and ankle edema. Your initial impression is:

   a. Cellulitis

   b. Stasis dermatitis

   c. Atopic dermatitis

   d. Contact dermatitis

7. The most effective antifungal agent used in the treatment of tinea capitis is:

   a. Terbinafine orally

   b. Clotrimazole 1% cream

   c. Ketoconozole orally

   d. Nystatin cream

8. Janet is a 22-year-old white female who presents for evaluation of lesions on the palm of her right hand. The lesions consist of silvery scales on an erythematous base and are isolated by a sharply demarcated border. You remove the scales and minute drops of blood appear giving a positive Auspitz sign. Your diagnosis is:

   a. Pityriasis rosae

   b. Squamous cell carcinoma

   c. Psoriasis

   d. Eczema

9. Common mode(s) of transmission of scabies include:

   a. Moist fomites

   b. Person to person

   c. Household pets

   d. Soil

10. A 24-year-old presents to clinic with a 5 cm purple, palpable plaque on the upper right posterior chest. He admits to unprotected homosexual activity for the past 10 years. On further exam you note axillary and inguinal lymphadenopathy. You suspect this patient may have:

   a. Squamous cell carcinoma

    b. Malignant melanoma

    c. Basal cell carcinoma

    d. Kaposi's sarcoma

11. Initial laboratory evaluation(s) for this patient should include:

    a. HIV antibody screening

    b. Complete blood count

    c. GC/chlamydia cultures

    d. Liver function tests

12. The common wart, *Verrucae vulgaris,* is characterized as:

    a. Solitary flesh colored papule with scaly irregular surface

    b. Group of flat-topped flesh colored papules

    c. Thick, endophylitic papules or plaques

    d. Papular, nodular, ulcerated sclerosing pigmented lesion.

13. Joan is a 15-year-old with multiple closed comedones, and a few pustules on her face and upper back. She has been on tretinoin for her face but is distressed at the progression of acne to her back. You would prescribe:

    a. 13-cis-retinoic acid (Accutane)

    b. Erythromycin 250 mg q.i.d. for 10 days

    c. Benzoyl peroxide cleansing soap

    d. Amoxil 250 mg t.i.d. for 10 days

14. Janice is an 18 year old who presents to your clinic with a scaly, pruritic rash on the dorsal aspect of her toes. This rash has occurred each winter for the past eight years. Her family history is unremarkable except for her father who has asthma. The most likely diagnosis is:

    a. Psoriasis

    b. Candidiasis

    c. Contact dermatitis

    d. Atopic dermatitis

15. Overgrowth of *Pityrosporum obiculare* in the young adult results in:

    a. Tinea corporis

    b. Tinea versicolor

    c. Tinea capitis

    d. Tinea pedis

16. A 30-year-old male presents with multiple, scattered, discrete vesicular lesions on the right leg for 5 days. There are honey-colored "stuck-on" crusts and erosions in some of these lesions. The culture yields *Staphylococcus aureus*. The most likely diagnosis is:

    a. Herpes simplex
    b. Herpes zoster
    c. Stasis dermatitis
    d. Impetigo

17. A 19-year-old female presents with small grouped vesicles on an erythematous base on her lower lip. The lesion is painful. She has had this before and it has always gone away in a week or so. You suspect herpes simplex 1. You would confirm your diagnosis with which of the following laboratory test?

    a. Direct immunofluorescent antibody (ELISA)
    b. KOH test
    c. Culture and sensitivity
    d. Wood's lamp

18. Mr. Smith, age 46, presents to the FNP with fever, malaise, and a painful, linear vesicular rash on just one side of his trunk. The most likely diagnosis is

    a. Tinea corporis
    b. Carbuncle
    c. Herpes simplex
    d. Herpes zoster

19. Mr. Thompson has chronic eczema. He presents with pruritic, dry, leathery patches with accentuated skin markings on his forearm. The most appropriate treatment is:

    a. Amoxicillin orally
    b. Clotrimazole 1% cream
    c. Triamcinolone acetonide 0.5% cream
    d. UVB with coal tar

20. Melissa, age 22, presents to the FNP's office with a slightly pruritic red rash on her trunk and breast following the line of skin cleavage giving a "Christmas tree" configuration. She states that the rash started as a single red patch on her abdomen. Medical history is unremarkable, except for a recent upper respiratory infection. Your initial diagnosis is:

    a. Tinea versicolor

b. Folliculitis

c. Pityriasis rosea

d. Seborrheic dermatitis

21. Mr. Kirk is a 45-year-old African American who presents with a sore on his lip that will not heal. Medical history includes psoriasis treated with oral PUVA. Upon inspection you note an erythematous plaque, slightly raised with sharp borders and no sign of infiltration or telangiectatic vessels. You make a referral to the dermatologist for further evaluation of what you suspect is:

   a. Basal cell carcinoma

   b. Squamous cell carcinoma

   c. Kaposi's sarcoma

   d. Psoriasis refractory to treatment

22. Mrs. Summers presents to the FNP with a complaint of red rash and large blister after wearing a new prosthetic leg for three days. This prosthesis has a new polyurethane material she did not have with her old prosthesis. She is a below the right knee amputee secondary to an accident as a child. Upon inspection you note a tender, erythematous, scaly, maculopapular rash. It is warm and edematous with a large bullous lesion on the posterior popliteal fossae. Your initial diagnosis is:

   a. Eczema

   b. Severe irritant contact dermatitis

   c. Herpes zoster

   d. Carbuncle

23. Your management of Mrs. Summers includes oral glucocorticoids steroids, UVB (sunlight exposure) and:

   a. Reducing bullae with sterile needle and syringe

   b. Leaving bullae alone and let rupture spontaneously

   c. Advising continued use of new prosthesis

   d. Removing top of bullae and applying high potency steroid cream

24. The following medication has no severe teratogenic properties and is safe for use in the sexually active young female with acne:

   a. Erythromycin

   b. Tretinoin

   c. Accutane

   d. Tetracycline

25. Mrs. Lopez is a 45-year-old who presents with a tender, mildly pruritic rash under both breasts and on her abdomen. She is a diabetic with poor control due to poor medication compliance and is at 160% ideal body weight (IBW). Upon inspection you note moist erythematous macerated areas with satellite pustules under both breasts and under abdominal peniculous. Your initial impression is:

    a. Candidiasis intertrigo
    b. Tinea corporis
    c. Herpes zoster
    d. Pityriasis rosea

26. Along with better control of Mrs. Lopez's diabetes and continued effort at weight modification, you would prescribe the following:

    a. Nystatin cream or powder
    b. Selenium sulfide lotion 2.5%
    c. Terbinifine 1% cream
    d. Hydrocortisone 1% cream

Answers

1. d	10. d	19. c
2. a	11. a	20. c
3. c	12. a	21. b
4. d	13. b	22. b
5. a	14. d	23. a
6. b	15. b	24. a
7. a	16. d	25. a
8. c	17. a	26. a
9. b	18. d	

Bibliography

Fauci, A. S., Isselbacher, K. J., Braunwald, E., Wilson, J. D., Martin, J. B., & Kasper, D. L. (Eds.). (1998). *Harrison's principles of internal medicine* (14th ed.). New York:McGraw Hill.

Fenstermacher, K., & Hudson, B. T. (1997). *Practice guidelines for family nurse practitioners.* Philadelphia: W. B. Saunders.

Fitzpatrick, T. B., Johnson, R. A., Wolff, K., Polano, M. K., & Suurmond, D. (1997). *Color atlas and synopsis of clinical dermatology common and serious diseases* (3rd ed.). New York: McGraw-Hill.

Hurst, J. W. (1996). *Medicine for the practicing physician* (4th ed.). Stamford, CT: Appleton & Lange.

Lesh, D. (1996). "Dermatophytosis." *Journal of the American Academy of Nurse Practitioners,* (6)8, 289-292.

Noble, J., Greene, H. L., Levinson, W., Modest, G. A., & Young, M. J. (Eds.). (1996). *Textbook of primary care medicine* (2nd ed.). St. Louis: Mosby.

Mengel, M. B., & Schwiebert, L. P. (1996). *Ambulatory medicine.* Stamford, CT: Appleton & Lange.

Stobo, J. D., Hellmann, D. B., Ladenson, P. W., Petty, B. G., & Traill, T. A. (1996). *The principles and practice of medicine* (23rd ed.). Stamford, CT: Appleton & Lange.

Tierney, L. M., McPhee, S. J., Papadakis, M. A. (Eds.). (1998). *Current medial diagnosis and treatment* (37th ed.). Stamford, CT: Appleton & Lange.

Wasson, J. (1997). *The common symptom guide. New York: McGraw-Hill.*

Eye, Ear, Nose, and Throat Disorders

Margaret Hadro Venzke

Conjunctivitis

- Definition: Inflammation of palpebral and/or bulbar conjunctiva; classic description "red eye" or "pink eye"
- Etiology/Incidence
    1. Bacterial
        a. *Staphylococcus aureus*
        b. *Streptococcus pneumoniae*
        c. *Haemophilus influenzae*
        d. *Neisseria gonorrhoeae*
        e. Proteus species
    2. Viral
        a. Adenoviruses (most common)
            (1) Adenopharyngeal conjunctivitis (APC)—"swimming pool"
            (2) Epidemic keratoconjunctivitis (EKC)—highly contagious, corneal involvement
        b. Herpes simplex
        c. Herpes zoster
    3. Allergic
        a. Seasonal allergies—pollen, grass, trees
        b. Hypersensitivity
        c. Chemical irritants
    4. Chlamydia/trachoma
    5. Other
        a. Trauma
        b. Contact lens wearer—more susceptible than general population
        c. Foreign body
        d. Drug induced—preservative in eye drops, antimicrobials
        e. Systemic illness

            (1)   Measles

            (2)   Varicella

            (3)   Rocky Mountain spotted fever

            (4)   Reiter's syndrome

     f.   Contaminated contact lens solution

     g.   Mascara/eyeliner, makeup

  6. Mode of transmission—direct contact with contagion or allergen

  7. Most common eye disease in primary care; usually benign, self-limiting disorder

- Signs and Symptoms

  1. Mild to moderate redness and irritation

  2. No acute change in visual acuity

  3. Absence of photophobia

  4. Mild discomfort/pain, often associated with itching, burning sensation or excessive tearing

  5. Watery to purulent discharge

  6. Bacterial conjunctivitis

     a.   Mucopurulent discharge (profuse exudate suggests *Neisseria gonorrhoeae*)

     b.   Thick purulent crust of material on eyelids after night's sleep

     c.   Unilateral (initially)

     d.   Self limiting—10 to 14 days without treatment, resolves in 2 to 4 days with treatment

  7. Viral conjunctivitis

     a.   Redness, general discomfort, profuse watery discharge

     b.   Preauricular adenopathy common

     c.   Association with upper respiratory illness, fever, pharyngitis

     d.   Bilateral presentation

     e.   Symptoms last 2 to 3 weeks (contagious, viral shedding in tears for approximately 2 weeks)

Table 1

	Conjunctivitis	Iritis	Acute Glaucoma
Pain	mild	moderate	severe
Vision	normal	slightly blurred	blurred
Discharge	mucopurulent	clear	clear
Cornea	clear	clear	cloudy
Pupil	normal	small irregular	oval dilated
Light Response	normal	poor	poor
Conjunctival injection	diffuse toward fornices	circumcorneal	corneal/ conjunctival hyperemia

    8. Allergic

        a. Moderate to severe bilateral itching

        b. Clear to stringy mucoid discharge

        c. Chronic hypersensitivity—vernal conjunctivitis associated with corneal ulceration

    9. Chlamydial conjunctivitis

        a. More often unilateral than bilateral

        b. Moderate exudate

        c. Enlarged, tender preauricular nodes

        d. Symptoms persist 3 to 9 months without treatment

- Differential Diagnosis

    1. Urgent ophthalmic conditions—prompt referral to avoid compromised eyesight. See Table 1

        a. Acute uveitis/iritis

        b. Acute glaucoma

        c. Corneal trauma/infection

        d. Orbital cellulitis

- Physical Findings

    1. Injected conjunctiva

    2. Discharge (see signs and symptoms)

3. Cornea—clear

4. Pupillary response—equal and reactive to light

5. Visual acuity (Snellen)—no acute change

6. Preauricular adenopathy—often viral etiology

- Diagnostic Tests/Findings

    1. Fluorescein uptake staining—dye uptake suggests corneal involvement

    2. Culture—only if chronic problem or gonococcal conjunctivitis suspected

    3. Gram stain of discharge/scrapings—rarely done unless gonococcal conjunctivitis suspected

- Management/Treatment

    1. Pharmacologic

        a. Bacterial conjunctivitis

            (1) Sodium sulfacetamide 10% ophthalmic solution, one to two drops every 4 hours while awake or q.i.d. for 5 to 7 days

            (2) Bacitracin/polymyxin ophthalmic ointment, apply thin layer in lower conjunctival sac b.i.d. for 7 days

            (3) Erythromycin ophthalmic ointment, apply thin layer in lower conjunctival sac q.i.d. for 5 to 7 days

        b. Gonococcal conjunctivitis—refer to ophthalmologist

            (1) Topical antibiotics—erythromycin

            (2) Intravenous (IV) antibiotics

                (a) Ceftriaxone

                (b) Aqueous penicillin

        c. Chlamydia conjunctivitis

            (1) Doxycycline 100 mg orally b.i.d. for 21 days

            (2) Erythromycin 250 mg 6 times/day for 21 days

        d. Viral conjunctivitis

            (1) Self-limiting

(2) Topical antibiotics—to prevent secondary bacterial infection

(3) Corticosteroids contraindicated

e. Allergic conjunctivitis

(1) Topical vasoconstrictors/antihistamines

(a) Naphazoline HCL/pheniramine maleate—1 to 2 drops q.i.d.

(b) Oral antihistamines

(c) Allergen avoidance

2. General measures

a. Cool/warm compresses

b. Frequent gentle eye wash to remove discharge

c. Artificial tears

d. Strict handwashing

e. Use separate towels; avoid handshaking

f. Contact lens care—clean contacts, use new solutions, avoid "homemade" tap water solutions

g. Avoid eye cosmetics during infection; change eye products frequently

h. Refer if no improvement in 48 hours or if vision is impaired

Blepharitis

- Definition: Inflammation of eyelid margins and eyelashes
- Etiology/Incidence

1. Commonly affects elderly persons

2. Associated with seborrheic dermatitis and acne rosacea

3. Often a chronic condition

4. Seborrheic blepharitis

a. Erythematous lid margins

b. Dry flakes, oily secretions

    c. Cosmetics and chemicals aggravate the condition

  5. Staphylococcal (ulcerative) blepharitis

    a. Acute/chronic inflammation of glands of lid margins

    b. *Staphylococcus aureus* and *Staphylococcus epidermidis* are causative organisms

    c. Mild ulceration of lid margin

    d. Loss of lashes

  6. Mixed blepharitis—most common (seborrheic with secondary staphylococcal infection)

  7. Infestation of eyelashes with lice

- Signs and Symptoms

  1. Gritty, burning sensation

  2. Crusted material on eyelids upon awakening

  3. Redness

  4. Swelling of lid margins

  5. Dry or greasy scales on lashes

  6. Mild conjunctival irritation and erythema

- Differential Diagnosis

  1. Conjunctivitis

  2. Chronic chalazia

  3. Sebaceous cell carcinoma (rare)

  4. Keratitis

- Physical Findings

  1. Erythematous eyelid margins

  2. Scaly lesions on lashes

  3. Sclera—white

  4. Conjunctivae—usually clear

  5. Masses on lids/lid margins (palpate with gloves)

  6. Preauricular adenopathy

7. Visual acuity (no change)

- Diagnostic Tests/Findings—none usually indicated
- Management/Treatment
    1. Warm water compresses
    2. Eyelid margin scrubs 2 to 4 times a day
        a. Use washcloth or cotton tip applicator, moisten with dilute solution of water and baby shampoo or commercial lid cleaner
        b. Rinse well
    3. Antibiotic ointment q.i.d. to lid margins for 7 days (erythromycin, sulfacetamide sodium)
    4. Systemic antibiotics for severe infection—doxycycline 100 mg b.i.d. for 6 weeks
    5. Co-existing seborrhea of face/scalp—treat with selenium sulfide shampoo
    6. Maintain hygiene (lid washes) to prevent recurrence of seborrheic and mixed blepharitis
    7. Infestation of lice
        a. 1% permethrin creme rinse, following shampoo of head, which kills both lice and eggs; requires one application whereas others require more than one
        b. Apply thick petrolatum to eyelashes b.i.d.
        c. Remove nits from lashes and hair

Foreign Body in Eye

- Description: Object or debris in eye causing irritation
- Etiology/Incidence
    1. Most common ocular injury in primary care
    2. Foreign body (FOB) often lodges in conjunctiva or cornea
- Signs and Symptoms
    1. Unilateral, acute onset
    2. Sensation of "something in my eye"

3. Photophobia

4. Redness

5. Mild pain

6. Mild decrease in visual acuity

- Differential Diagnosis

   1. Intraocular foreign body (penetrates eye globe)

   2. Corneal laceration

   3. Corneal abrasion

   4. "Contact lens wearer" keratitis

- Physical Findings

   1. Diagnosis based on physical findings

   2. Visual acuity may be normal

   3. Cornea—examine under magnification and bright light, FOB may show up as a dark speck

   4. Ring-shaped orange stain—embedded iron or steel body

   5. Observe for laceration, hyphema, irregular pupil or absent red reflex—immediate ophthalmic referral

   6. Conjunctiva—instruct patient to look down, grasp lashes, evert eyelid, inspect upper eye and lid

- Diagnostic Tests/Findings—fluorescein stain highlights presence of foreign body and corneal abrasion

- Management/Treatment

   1. Remove simple (non-penetrating) foreign body with moistened cotton applicator with water or sterile normal saline; re-evaluate visual acuity

   2. Irrigation of eye—use only for chemical splash to eyes

   3. Antibiotic ophthalmic ointment

   4. Eye pad

   5. Follow-up in 24 hours to evaluate

   6. Patient education:

        a.   Caution—no rubbing of eye

        b.   Advise protective eye wear

   7. Refer

        a.   Intraocular foreign body

        b.   Change in visual acuity

        c.   Acute ocular pain

        d.   Large corneal abrasion

Corneal Abrasion

- Definition: Disruption in the epithelial surface of the cornea by mechanical or chemical factors
- Etiology/Incidence
  1. Common eye injury
  2. Direct trauma to eye; most commonly a scratch from contact lens, fingernail or piece of paper
  3. Chemical splash
- Signs and Symptoms
  1. Unilateral severe eye pain
  2. Redness
  3. Tearing
  4. Photophobia
  5. Scratchy sensation that worsens with blinking
  6. Decreased visual acuity
  7. Difficulty keeping eye open
- Differential Diagnosis
  1. Keratitis (viral, bacterial, or acanthamoeba)
  2. Foreign body
  3. Corneal laceration
- Physical Findings
  1. Document visual acuity—often decreased

2. Visualization of corneal lesion following fluorescein stain illuminated with cobalt blue light

- Diagnostic Tests/Findings: Fluorescein dye—abraded or ulcerated areas will become stained and fluorese yellow-green color

- Management/Treatment

    1. Antibiotic ointment or sulfonamide drops to affected eye

    2. May use pressure patch to decrease movement of eye

    3. Oral analgesics or short acting cycloplegic agent for pain relief

    4. Follow-up eye evaluation in 24 hours to assess healing—refer immediately if no improvement

    5. Topical antibiotics q.i.d. for 24 to 48 hours

    6. Avoid topical anesthetic drops; retard healing

    7. Topical steroids contraindicated; retard healing and increase risk of infection

    8. If chemical or thermal injury to eye, refer immediately to ophthalmology

Glaucoma

- Definition: Increased intraocular eye pressure resulting in atrophy of optic nerve, loss of visual fields and acuity

- Etiology/Incidence

    1. Inadequate drainage of aqueous fluid in the anterior chamber of the eye

    2. Most common type is chronic open angle (wide angle)

    3. Chronic open angle glaucoma

        a. Accounts for 90% of all cases

        b. Predominately seen over age 40

        c. Blacks are affected more frequently

        d. Positive family history

        e. Diabetes mellitus is a risk factor

    4. Primary angle closure (closed angle or narrow angle)

      a. Positive family history

      b. African-Americans and Asians more affected than Caucasians

      c. Predominately age 55 to 75 years

      d. Females more than males

      e. Less common than "open angle" but more severe in presentation

      f. May be precipitated by stress, anxiety, darkness, increased fluid intake or medications

5. Congenital glaucoma (developmental) in young children

6. Approximately 0.5% of total population

- Signs and Symptoms

  1. Chronic open angle glaucoma—obstruction to aqueous outflow

     a. Asymptomatic at onset

     b. Mid-peripheral vision affected in early stages

     c. Frequent change of glasses

     d. Central vision loss is a late sign

     e. Gradual, painless visual loss and ultimate blindness

  2. Primary angle closure—mechanical obstruction of flow of aqueous humor; iris may obstruct the trabecular meshwork at canal of Schlemm resulting in elevated intraocular pressure

     a. Acute ocular pain

     b. Nausea, vomiting

     c. Photophobia

     d. Blurred vision

     e. Halos around lights at night

     f. Unilateral frontal headache

     g. Tearing

     h. Erythema

- Differential Diagnosis

  1. Uveitis

2. Conjunctivitis

3. Ocular trauma

4. Neurological disease

- Physical Findings

    1. Visual acuity—decreased

    2. Cornea is clear

    3. Change in peripheral vision as measured by direct confrontation

    4. Chronic open angle glaucoma

        a. Cupping of optic disc

        b. Normal or elevated intraocular pressure (IOP)

    5. Primary angle closure

        a. Lid edema

        b. Injected conjunctiva

        c. Fixed mid-dilated pupil

        d. Shallow anterior chamber, often cloudy

- Diagnostic Tests/Findings

    1. Tonometry (normal range 10 to 20 mm Hg)

    2. Pressure reading 20 mm Hg or greater requires further evaluation

    3. U.S. Preventive Task Force recommends glaucoma testing after age 65, no consensus on frequency of screening

- Management/Treatment

    1. Refer all patients with

        a. Elevated IOP

        b. Decreased visual acuity

        c. Visual field loss

    2. Goal of therapy to stabilize IOP to prevent optic nerve damage and visual loss

    3. Pharmacological—chronic open angle glaucoma

       a. Parasympathomimetics—topical miotics (pilocarpine) facilitates aqueous outflow

       b. Beta blockers decrease aqueous (timolol, betaxolol) production

       c. Carbonic anhydrase inhibitors (acetazolamide)—reduces aqueous production

       d. Hyperosmotics—reduces formation of fluid (mannitol)

  4. Pharmacological—primary angle closure

       a. Emergency treatment with IV acetazolamide, mannitol and oral glycerol

       b. Maintenance therapy with additional miotic agents and corticosteriods

  5. Laser and surgical intervention may be indicated after maximizing medication therapy

  6. General measures

       a. Encourage frequent follow-up with ophthalmology

       b. Monitor side effects of medications

       c. Avoid over the counter cold preparations that may exacerbate glaucoma

Cataracts

- Definition: Clouding/opacity of crystalline lens, causing disruption of visual acuity
- Etiology/Incidence

  1. Single largest cause of blindness

  2. 90% of cataracts due to aging process (senile cataract)

  3. Congenital cataract (rubella)

  4. Systemic disease (diabetes and thyroid)

  5. Drug induced, especially steroid use

  6. Ocular trauma

  7. Chronic uveitis

  8. Ultraviolet B light exposure

- Signs and Symptoms
    1. Painless
    2. Cloudy, fuzzy, blurred vision
    3. Change in refractive error
    4. Glare associated with bright lights (night driving)
    5. Alteration in color perception
    6. Unilateral or bilateral development
- Differential Diagnosis
    1. Senile macular degeneration (loss of central vision)
    2. Retinal detachment
    3. Diabetic retinopathy
    4. Ocular tumor
- Physical Findings
    1. Lens opacity
    2. Disruption of red reflex
    3. Visual acuity decreased
    4. Reduced color discrimination
- Diagnostic Tests/Findings—refer to ophthalmology
- Management/Treatment
    1. Refer to ophthalmologist
    2. Surgical intervention—lens implant is preferred treatment
    3. Follow-up post operatively to observe for hemorrhage or infection
    4. Non-surgical treatment—frequent changes in glasses, bifocals, or contacts
    5. Optimize the environment of the inoperable patient with increased light sources, decreased glare, reorganize living space to prevent accidents/falls
    6. Prevention with protective eyewear to filter ultraviolet B exposure

Impaired Vision

- Definition: Decreased/blurred visual acuity
- Etiology/Incidence
    1. Associated with lens opacity, damage to photoreceptor cells, damage to optic nerve, visual cortex or refractory error
    2. Legal blindness—20/200 or less in best eye with correction
    3. Presbyopia—loss of accommodative capacity of lens with age; inability to focus on objects at normal reading distance
- Signs and Symptoms
    1. Decreased vision
        a. Sudden or gradual
        b. Unilateral or bilateral
    2. Pain
    3. Floaters
    4. Peripheral vision loss
    5. Association with systemic symptoms
- Differential Diagnosis
    1. Refractive error
    2. Cataract
    3. Macular degeneration
    4. Glaucoma
    5. Retinal vascular occlusion/detachment
    6. Temporal arteritis
    7. Optic neuritis—often first sign of multiple sclerosis
    8. Cerebrovascular accident (CVA) or tumor
- Physical Findings—vary according to etiology
    1. Decreased visual acuity
    2. Unilateral visual loss, often seen in retinal detachment, temporal arteritis, or optic neuritis

3. Conjunctiva—clear or injected (glaucoma)

4. Cornea—clear or cloudy (cataracts)

5. Visual field deficit—associated with glaucoma, cerebrovascular disease, or tumor

6. Pupils—small, irregular size, with poor response to light, common in iritis or glaucoma

7. Extraocular movements—nystagmus associated with neurological disease

8. Funduscopic examination may reveal

   a. Absent red reflex (cataracts)

   b. Hemorrhages, exudates (diabetes)

   c. Optic disc swelling/cupping (glaucoma, papilledema)

- Diagnostic Tests

  1. Tonometry

  2. Slit lamp

- Management/Treatment—based upon cause of visual loss

  1. Refer to ophthalmologist

     a. Sudden loss of vision—requires emergency consultation

     b. Abnormal physical examination findings

     c. Complaints of flashing lights

     d. Visual loss associated with systemic disease

     e. Diabetics

  2. Prevention

     a. Visual disorders in the elderly often lead to trauma from falls and motor vechicle accidents

     b. U.S. Preventive Task Force recommends screening for glaucoma after age 65; no consensus on routine visual acuity screening

Acute Otitis Media

- Definition: Inflammation of middle ear

- Etiology/Incidence
  1. Eustachian tube dysfunction (ETD) or obstruction secondary to viral nasal pharyngitis—major pathogenic factors causing ineffective drainage of middle ear
  2. Bacterial pathogens
     a. *Streptococcus pneumoniae* (most common)
     b. *Haemophilus influenzae*
     c. *Moraxella* (branhamella) *catarrhalis*
     d. Occasional streptococcus or *Staphylococcus aureus*
  3. More frequent in young children (under age 7) than adults
  4. Risk factors include:
     a. Recent URI
     b. Congenital disorders—cleft palate, Down syndrome
     c. Active or passive smoking
     d. Native American/Eskimo heritage
     e. Family history of otitis media
- Signs and Symptoms
  1. Earache
  2. Fever
  3. Hearing loss (conductive)
  4. Otorrhea (if perforated eardrum)
  5. Intense pain, followed by popping sound; acute relief indicative of perforated tympanic membrane (T.M.)
  6. Vertigo
- Differential Diagnosis
  1. Otitis externa
  2. Referred pain from jaw/teeth
  3. Dental abscess
  4. Mastoiditis

5. Ear canal furuncle

- Physical Findings

    1. May see bulging tympanic membrane

    2. Distorted light reflex/obscured landmarks

    3. Pneumatic otoscopy may show decreased T.M. mobility

    4. Erythema—inconsistent finding

    5. Bullae may form on T.M.—associated with *Mycoplasma pneumoniae* organism

    6. Preauricular or cervical adenopathy

- Diagnostic Tests/Findings

    1. Usually no tests ordered

    2. Needle aspiration of middle ear fluid for culture—only in immunosuppressed patients and severe mastoiditis

    3. Tympanometry—for recurrent infections; indicator of fluid posterior to T.M.

    4. CBC with differential—if patient appears toxic; elevated WBC count

- Management/Treatment

    1. Antibiotics

        a. Amoxicillin 250 to 500 mg orally t.i.d. for 10 days

            (1) Advantage—inexpensive

            (2) Disadvantage—ineffective against Beta lactamase producing pathogens

            (3) Avoid in those with penicillin allergy

        b. Trimethoprim/sulfamethoxazole (TMP/SMX)—(160 mg TMP/800 mg SMX) every 12 hours for 10 days

        c. For recurrent otitis media with resistant pathogens:

            (1) Amoxicillin clavulanate

            (2) Cephalosporins—such as cefixime, cefaclor

2. If perforation is present, combined therapy of oral antibiotic and topical cortisporin otic suspension—4 drops in each ear t.i.d. or q.i.d. for 10 days

3. Pain management

    a. Acetaminophen

    b. Codeine

    c. Topical local anesthetic otic solution—pain reliever

4. Refer/consult with MD or otolaryngologist

    a. No response to treatment after 48 to 72 hours

    b. Persistent hearing loss after adequate treatment

    c. Complications

        (1) Mastoiditis

        (2) Facial nerve palsy

        (3) Chronic perforation

        (4) Recurrent infections

    d. Surgical procedures—myringotomy, tympanostomy tubes for recurrent infection

Serous Otitis Media

- Definition: Effusion in middle ear (also known as chronic otitis media with effusion)

- Etiology/Incidence

    1. Patency of eustachian tube is impaired; prevents equalization of pressure

    2. Associated with:

        a. Subacute infection

        b. Allergic manifestations

        c. Barotrauma

        d. Deviated septum

        e. Hypertrophic adenoids

        f. Benign or malignant neoplasms

3. More common in children than adults

- Signs and Symptoms
    1. Hearing loss
    2. Popping sensation with yawning/swallowing
    3. Fullness in ear
    4. Occasional dizziness
    5. Often asymptomatic

- Differential Diagnosis
    1. Acute otitis media
    2. Conductive hearing loss
    3. Meniere's disease

- Physical findings
    1. Tympanic membrane—retracted
    2. Air fluid level present, often with yellow/blue tinged fluid posterior to T.M. or bubbles of air may be seen through tympanic membrane
    3. Decreased membrane mobility with insufflation
    4. Conductive hearing loss
        a. Weber Test—lateralize to affected side
        b. Rinne Test—bone conduction greater than air conduction BC> AC

- Diagnostic Tests/Findings
    1. Audiometry—decreased hearing
    2. Tympanometry—shows middle ear effusion

- Management/Treatment
    1. If mild symptoms, may spontaneously resolve in 2 to 3 weeks
    2. Topical decongestants—phenylephrine 1 to 2 sprays to each nostril every 8 to 12 hours for 3 days only
    3. Oral decongestants may be helpful
    4. Antihistamines usually are ineffective

5. Patient education on Valsalva maneuver or chewing gum—to relieve eustachian tube blockage

6. Follow-up in 4 to 6 weeks

7. Refer if persistent hearing loss

Otitis Externa

- Definition: Inflammation of external auditory canal; commonly known as "swimmer's ear"

- Etiology/Incidence

    1. Infectious agents include:

        a. *Pseudomonas aeruginosa* (most common)

        b. *Staphylococcus aureus* or streptococcus

        c. *Proteus mirabilis*

        d. Fungi

    2. Inflammation develops from:

        a. Frequent exposure to water (most common)

        b. Mechanical trauma from bobby pins, cotton applicators, ear plugs, hearing aids

        c. Eczema, skin disorders

    3. Common in summer months, especially in hot, humid climates

    4. More common in swimmers than non-swimmers

- Signs and Symptoms

    1. Otalgia—gradual or acute onset

    2. Pruritus

    3. Purulent discharge

    4. Occasional hearing loss "plugged ear"

- Differential Diagnosis

    1. Furuncle

    2. Otitis media

    3. Mastoiditis

    4. Foreign body

    5. Eczema

    6. Cellulitis

- Physical Findings

    1. Erythema and edema of ear canal

    2. Pain on manipulation of auricle or pressure on tragus

    3. Purulent or white "cheesy" exudate may be present

    4. Preauricular adenopathy

    5. Edema may impair visualization of tympanic membrane; T.M. usually not affected

- Diagnostic Tests/Findings—culture of discharge if no response to treatment or recurrent infection

- Management/Treatment

    1. Pharmacologic

        a. Combined antibiotic, hydrocortisone and propylene glycol will effectively treat infection and reduce inflammation—cortisporin otic solution 4 to 5 gtts in ear(s) t.i.d. or q.i.d. for 7 days

        b. Antifungal and antibacterial—acetic acid otic drops

        c. Saturated cotton wick with medication facilitates entry of medication in ear canal; moisten with antibiotic as directed

        d. Severe cases often require systemic antibiotics

        e. Analgesics

    2. General measures

        a. Protect ear from additional moisture

        b. Eliminate trauma to ear canal

        c. Prevent recurrences—instill 2% acetic acid 2 to 3 drops in ear canals b.i.d. after contact with water (commercial OTC products also available)

        d. Improvement in 48 hours after initiating treatment

        e. Instruction on proper technique to clean ears

Hearing Loss

- Definition: Diminished ability to detect pure tones in decibels of 30 or greater
- Etiology/Incidence
    1. 10% of U.S. population has hearing problems
    2. Particularly common among the elderly
    3. Hearing loss may result from interference in sound conduction (conduction loss) or impaired transmission through nervous system (sensorineural) or both (mixed hearing loss)
    4. Conductive loss—decreased ability of external and middle ear to conduct sound waves to inner ear due to:
        a. Cerumen impaction
        b. Foreign body
        c. Otitis media
        d. Otosclerosis—hereditary, bony ankylosis of stapes
        e. Scarring or perforation of T.M.
        f. Congenital problems
        g. Cholesteatoma
    5. Sensorineural loss—results from changes to cochlea and/or involvement of the acoustic nerve; causes include:
        a. Acoustic neuroma
        b. Meniere's disease
        c. Presbycusis—hearing loss associated with aging
        d. Excessive noise exposure
        e. Viral syndrome—rubella, mumps
        f. Drugs—ASA, gentamicin, furosemide, erythromycin
        g. Syphilis
        h. Multiple sclerosis
- Signs and Symptoms

1. Conductive hearing loss—decreased ability to detect low tones and vowels; often history of ear disease, patient speaks softly

2. Sensorineural—impaired high tone perception, poor speech discrimination, difficulty with background noise, and high pitched female voice; patient speaks loudly

3. Presbycusis—hearing loss is bilateral; gradual in onset; loss of high frequencies first, then lower frequency sounds; tinnitus is common

- Differential Diagnosis—see Etiology
- Physical Findings

    1. Otoscopic examination of ear—usually normal

    2. Gross hearing/whisper test—diminished (acoustic nerve)

    3. Rinne test—compares air to bone conduction

        a. Normal—AC>BC

        b. Conductive loss BC>AC in affected ear(s)

        c. Sensorineural loss AC>BC

    4. Weber test

        a. Normal—sound midline

        b. Conductive loss—lateralize to affected ear

        c. Sensorineural loss—lateralize to normal ear

    5. Red flags for immediate referral:

        a. Cholesteatoma in conductive loss

        b. Acoustic neuroma in sensorineural loss

- Diagnostic Tests/Findings

    1. Pure tone audiometry by audiologist

        a. Intensity is measured in decibels (dB), frequency is measured in hertz

        b. Threshold of normal hearing O-20 dB

            (1) Mild loss—20-40 dB (soft spoken voice)

            (2) Moderate loss—40-60 dB (normal spoken voice)

            (3) Severe loss—60-80 dB (loud spoken voice)

2. Speech discrimination testing

    a. Detects clarity of hearing—impaired in sensorineural loss

    b. Results recorded as percentage correct

    c. 90 to 100% is normal

3. CT scan or MRI—to detect tumors

- Management/Treatment—dependent on etiology

1. Refer for formal audiogram

2. Refer to otolaryngologist—particularly for sensorineural loss and conductive loss unresponsive to treatment

3. Prevention

    a. Avoid loud music, machines (causes loss of high tones)

    b. Monitor ototoxic drugs carefully; if tinnitus or hearing loss discontinue use

    c. U.S. Preventive Task Force recommends routine screening after 65 years of age

4. Hearing aids—hearing amplification, beneficial to patients with correctable hearing loss

Vertigo

- Definition: Abnormal sensation of movement; disturbances of peripheral/central vestibular system which maintains spatial orientation/posture

- Etiology/Incidence

1. Causative factors include:

    a. Medications—especially aspirin and alcohol

    b. Infections—middle/inner ear, viral illness

    c. CNS disease—multiple sclerosis, syphilis

2. True vertigo is a vestibular disease

3. Diagnosis of exclusion

- Signs and Symptoms

1. "Room spinning"/weaving sensation

2. Nausea, vomiting, diaphoresis

3. Imbalance

4. Tinnitus

5. Hearing loss

6. Vague lightheadedness

- Differential Diagnosis

  1. Acoustic neuroma

  2. Meniere's disease

  3. Benign positional vertigo—in geriatric patient

  4. Cerebrovascular accident (CVA)

  5. Transient ischemic attacks (T.I.A.)

  6. Vestibular neuritis

  7. Acute labyrinthitis—associated with recent URI

  8. Medication toxicity

- Physical Findings

  1. Nystagmus with testing of extraocular movements

  3. Hearing loss

  4. Changes in blood pressure—associated with positional hypotension

  5. Carotid bruits—suggests impaired cerebral flow

  6. Cranial nerves—especially auditory changes, 5, 7, 8

  7. Romberg test—often abnormal

  8. Barany maneuver—stimulates vestibular system, reproduces vertigo

- Diagnostic Tests/Findings

  1. Audiogram if hearing impaired

  2. CT scan/MRI—to rule out tumor/neurological dysfunction

  3. VDRL and FTA—reactive in syphilis

  4. TSH, CBC with differential and glucose—to rule out infections and systemic disease

  5. Serum B_{12} to rule out pernicious anemia

- Management/Treatment

1. Immediate referral, if abnormal neurological signs

2. Bed rest

3. Antivertigo medications

   a. Meclizine—12.5 to 25 mg orally t.i.d.; causes dry mouth and sedation

   b. Dramamine 50 mg orally t.i.d.

   c. Scopolamine transdermal patch

4. Antiemetic for nausea/vomiting—promethazine 25 mg q.i.d.; or prochlorperazine 5 to 10 mg q.i.d.

5. Do not perform tests for positional vertigo on geriatric patients

6. Refer if vertigo persists

Epistaxis

- Definition: Bleeding from nostril, nasal cavity or nasopharynx

- Etiology/Incidence

  1. Anterior nosebleed most common, occurring in the vascular plexus of septum (Kisselbach plexus)

  2. Disruption of nasal mucosa due to:

     a. Trauma

     b. Infection

     c. Allergies

     d. Dry environment

     e. Medications

     f. Cocaine use

     g. Neoplasm

     h. Occasionally systemic disease (hypertension, blood dyscrasia)

  3. 10% of population will experience one significant nosebleed

- Signs and Symptoms

  1. Anterior epistaxis

     a. Unilateral bleeding from nostril

     b. Recurrent episodes last few minutes to $\frac{1}{2}$ hour

     c. Venous source of blood

  2. Posterior epistaxis—occurs more in the elderly, often difficult to correct

     a. Intermittent brisk bleeding

     b. Arterial source

     c. Blood flows into pharynx, may cause nausea and coffee ground emesis

- Differential Diagnosis: Epistaxis is a sign/symptom, not a disease; assess for significant pathology

  1. Coagulation disorders

  2. Nasal malignancy

  3. Hereditary telangiectasia

  4. Malignant hypertension

- Physical Findings

  1. Visual site—usually bleeding from one nostril; bilateral bleeding suggests trauma

  2. Skin, mucous membranes and conjunctivae with evidence of the following suggests a pathological condition:

     a. Rash

     b. Pallor

     c. Purpura

     d. Petechiae

     e. Telangiectasis

- Diagnostic Tests/Findings: Dependent on suspected etiology

  1. Hemoglobin and hematocrit are decreased if severe blood loss

  2. Low platelet count and abnormal PT/PTT suggests a bleeding disorder

- Management/Treatment

  1. Position patient sitting up and leaning forward

2. Apply continuous pinching pressure to anterior nasal septum for 10 to 15 minutes

3. If inadequate blood clotting, place a small cotton pledget of 1:1000 epinephrine or vasoconstrictor nasal drops (phenylephrine) into vestibule of nose; apply pressure for 5 to 10 minutes; this will stop most anterior venous bleeds

4. Application of ice may assist with clot formation

5. Refer to emergency room or otolaryngologist if bleeding persistent/continuous or if posterior bleed is suspected

6. General measures/prevention

    a. Warn against habitual nose picking, rubbing nose, forceful blowing

    b. Advise increased humidity, especially in winter months

    c. Use petrolatum based ointment in nostril—promotes hydration

    d. Instruct patient on how to manage simple nosebleeds

7. Recurrent episodes of epistaxis require additional investigation

Common Cold

- Definition: Minor, self-limiting viral illness of upper respiratory tract mucosa

- Etiology/Incidence

    1. Caused by rhinoviruses or corona viruses

    2. Most common reason for ''sick day''

    3. Incidence decreases with age

        a. Children average 6 to 8 colds per year

        b. Adults average 2 to 4 colds per year

    4. Transmission through hand to hand contact and airborne droplets

- Signs and Symptoms

    1. General malaise and fatigue

    2. Coryza

    3. Sore throat

4. Low grade fever

5. Nasal congestion/stuffiness

6. Watery eyes

7. Headache

8. Nonproductive cough

9. Symptoms last approximately seven days

- Differential Diagnosis

   1. Influenza

   2. *Mycoplasma pneumoniae*

   3. Otitis media

   4. Sinusitis

   5. Rhinitis

- Physical Findings

   1. Mildly elevated temperature

   2. Conjunctivae clear, possible erythema

   3. Injected nasal and pharyngeal mucosa

   4. Lungs clear

   5. Clear rhinorrhea

- Diagnostic Tests/Findings—none indicated; throat culture if streptococcal pharyngitis suspected

- Management/Treatment—palliative

   1. Rest, maintain fluid hydration

   2. Acetaminophen or ibuprofen for fever and headache

   3. Topical decongestants for nasal congestion; use 3 to 4 days only to avoid "rebound congestion"

   4. Oral decongestants for congestion

   5. Antihistamines not indicated for cold symptoms; often included in over the counter medications (OTC); sedation side effect

   6. OTC decongestants are used cautiously in diabetic, hypertensive and glaucoma patients

7. Antitussive cough medication

8. Vitamin C—may reduce days of illness

9. Frequent hand washing to prevent viral spread

10. Zinc lozenges to decrease symptoms, contraindicated in pregnancy

11. Symptoms lasting longer than 2 weeks may indicate secondary bacterial infection

Influenza

- Definition: Acute, contagious, febrile respiratory, viral infection
- Etiology/Incidence
  1. Influenza viral type A, B, C
  2. Type A influenza is most virulent, causing increased mortality
  3. Incubation 1 to 5 days
  4. Infections usually occur during epidemics in winter months
  5. Transmitted by airborne droplets
- Signs and Symptoms
  1. High fever, chills, (sudden onset)
  2. Headache
  3. Myalgia (often severe)
  4. Malaise
  5. Sore throat
  6. Nonproductive cough
  7. Nausea and vomiting
  8. Coryza
- Differential Diagnosis
  1. Upper respiratory infection (URI)
  2. Bronchitis
  3. Pertussis
  4. Pneumonia

5. Infectious mononucleosis

6. Early HIV infection

- Physical Findings

  1. Elevated temperature, rapid pulse

  2. Skin flushed

  3. Watery eyes

  4. Clear nasal discharge

  5. Occasional tender cervical lymph nodes

  6. Pharyngeal erythema

  7. Lungs—clear (occasional wheezes or rales)

- Diagnostic Tests/Findings

  1. Usually none

  2. Complete blood count (CBC) or white blood count (WBC)—mild leukopenia

  3. Chest radiography—normal

- Management/Treatment

  1. Supportive measures

     a. Increase fluid intake

     b. Humidified air

     c. Salt water gargles

     d. Analgesics and rest (for fever and myalgia)

  2. Antiviral Medications

     a. Amantadine 100 mg orally b.i.d. for 2 to 7 days

        (1) Only effective against influenza A

        (2) Shortens duration of fever, and respiratory/systemic symptoms by 50%

        (3) Needs to be administered within first 48 hours of onset of illness

        (4) Side effects—insomnia, anxiety, lightheadedness, difficulty concentrating

        (5)   Prophylaxis for high risk, unvaccinated persons—100 mg orally daily for 2 weeks

   b. Rimantadine 100 mg orally b.i.d. for 7 days; new antiviral, fewer side effects, use in patients with renal failure

3. Monitor for complications—especially in the elderly

   a. Bacterial pneumonia

   b. Otitis media

   c. Reye's syndrome

   d. Myocarditis (rare)

   e. Bronchitis

4. Prevention—Trivalent influenza vaccination 0.5cc IM deltoid

   a. Administer every fall, prior to winter months

   b. Target populations

        (1)   Over age 65

        (2)   Nursing home patients

        (3)   Patients with chronic cardiac/respiratory disorders

        (4)   Immunocompromised patients (i.e: asplenic persons, H.I.V. infection)

        (5)   Persons living in institutional settings

        (6)   Pregnant females in 2nd and 3rd trimesters

        (7)   Health care providers

   c. Contraindicated in persons allergic to eggs

   d. Administer concomitantly with pneumococcal vaccine in high risk patients

Pharyngitis

- Definition: Inflammation of pharynx, tonsils or both (sore throat)
- Etiology/Incidence

1. Viral pharyngitis (most common)

   a. Respiratory viruses—adenovirus

     b.   Rhinovirus

     c.   Herpangina—due to Coxsackie virus

     d.   Epstein-Barr (EBV), cytomegalovirus (CMV)—causes infectious mononucleosis

2.   Bacterial pharyngitis

     a.   Group A and B hemolytic streptococcus

     b.   *Neisseria gonorrhoeae*

     c.   *Corynebacterium diphtheriae*

     d.   *Haemophilus influenzae*

     e.   *Neisseria meningitidis*

3.   Other sources

     a.   *Chlamydia trachomatis*

     b.   *Mycoplasma pneumoniae*

     c.   *Candida albicans*

     d.   Trauma/irritating substance

     e.   Mouth breathing/allergies

4.   Accounts for 10% of all office visits in primary care

5.   Occurs in all age groups

- Signs and Symptoms

   1.   Sore throat

   2.   Enlarged tonsils

   3.   Dysphagia

   4.   Fever

   5.   Malaise

- Differential Diagnosis (see etiology for pathogens)

   1.   Peritonsillar abscess

   2.   Pharyngeal abscess

   3.   Epiglottitis

   4.   Stomatitis

5. Meningitis

6. Thyroiditis

- Physical Findings

    1. Elevated temperature

    2. Viral presentation (respiratory)

        a. Tonsillar enlargement with or without exudate

        b. Injected "cobblestone" appearance post-pharynx

        c. Rhinorrhea

    3. Bacterial (group A β-hemolytic streptococcus)

        a. Erythema

        b. Often exudative tonsils

        c. Enlarged tender anterior cervical lymph nodes

        d. Occasionally petechiae

        e. Scarlatina rash

    4. *Corynebacterium diphtheriae* (infrequent in immunized patients)

        a. Gray adherent membrane on tonsils and pharynx

        b. Bleeding when membrane removed

- Diagnostic Tests/Findings

    1. Viral (respiratory) pharyngitis—by clinical diagnosis *only*

    2. Throat culture—if suspect:

        a. Group A β hemolytic streptococcus (GABHS)

        b. *Neisseria gonorrhoeae* (request separately)

    3. Rapid Strep Antigen Test—positive result, detects only GABHS (5% to 10% false negatives)

    4. CBC with differential—WBC count elevated in bacterial infection

    5. Heterophil/monospot—negative

- Management/Treatment

    1. General measures

        a. Increase fluids

    b.   Gargle with warm salt water

    c.   Lozenges

    d.   Acetaminophen or ibuprofen for pain relief

2. Strep throat (GABHS)

    a.   Penicillin V 250 mg t.i.d. or q.i.d. for 10 days

    b.   Benzathine penicillin 1.2 million units IM one time only

        (1) Advantage—full treatment completed

        (2) Disadvantage—five to tenfold increase in anaphylactic reaction

    c.   Alternative for penicillin allergy—erythromycin 250 mg orally q.i.d. for 10 days

    d.   Post treatment cultures—for recurrent strep infection or rheumatic fever

    e.   Complications—if no or inadequate antibiotic treatment

        (1) Scarlet fever

        (2) Peritonsillar abscess (immediate referral)

        (3) Suppurative adenitis

        (4) Rheumatic fever

        (5) Acute glomerulonephritis

    f.   Tonsillectomy—for recurrent severe infections

3. Gonococcal pharyngitis

    a.   Ceftriaxone 125 mg IM one dose *or* cefixime 400 mg orally one dose *or* ofloxacin 400 mg orally one dose

    b.   Co-treat for chlamydia—doxycycline 100 mg orally b.i.d. *or* erythromycin 500 mg orally q.i.d. *or* azithromycin 1 g orally, single dose

4. Diphtheria (refer)

    a.   Equine antitoxin—to prevent myocarditis

    b.   Penicillin or erythromycin

Infectious Mononucleosis

- Definition: Acute viral syndrome associated with fever, pharyngitis and adenopathy—often known as "kissing" disease
- Etiology/Incidence
    1. Epstein-Barr virus (EBV)—herpes type virus causes 90% of cases
    2. Cytomegalovirus (CMV)—rare
    3. Transmission via saliva
    4. Usually occurs in adolescents and young adults (ages 10 to 35 years) in middle and upper socioeconomic populations
    5. Prolonged period of communicability—approximately 2 to 6 months after infection
- Signs and Symptoms—variable, but typically include:
    1. Fever
    2. Fatigue/malaise
    3. Nausea/anorexia
    4. Swollen lymph nodes
    5. Sore throat
- Differential Diagnosis
    1. Streptococcal pharyngitis
    2. CMV
    3. Toxoplasmosis
    4. Hepatitis A or B
    5. Lymphoma/leukemia
    6. HIV infection
- Physical Findings
    1. Marked erythema and edema of pharynx
    2. Tonsillar enlargement with exudate, occasionally palatal petechiae
    3. Enlarged lymph nodes—especially posterior cervical nodes
    4. Splenic enlargement—50% of cases

5. Hepatomegaly

6. Occasionally periorbital edema

7. Maculopapular rash

- Diagnostic Tests/Findings

  1. Complete blood count with differential

     a. WBC—leukocytosis (range of 10,000–20,000/mm^3)

     b. Increased lymphocytes (greater than 50% of leukocyte count)

     c. Atypical lymphocytes—common characteristic

     d. Thrombocytopenia (range 100,000–140,000/mm^3) 2 to 4 weeks after onset of illness

  2. Positive monospot or elevations in heterophil titer—1:224 or greater is diagnostic

  3. Liver function tests—elevations in aspartate aminotransferase (AST), alanine aminotransferase (ALT), bilirubin and LDH

  4. Throat culture—frequently secondary infection with streptococcus (GABHS)

  5. CT scan imaging—may reveal splenomegaly and/or hepatomegaly

- Management/Treatment

  1. Supportive/palliative measures

  2. Rest during acute phase of illness

  3. Avoidance of contact sports for at least one month with splenomegaly; CT scan to determine resolution of splenomegaly

  4. Avoid alcohol (ETOH) with elevated liver enzymes/hepatomegaly

  5. Corticosteriods often prescribed for significant pharyngeal edema and obstructive tonsillar enlargement

  6. Analgesics for pain relief

  7. Antiviral medications not effective

  8. Ampicillin/amoxicillin should be avoided, as patients frequently develop a maculopapular rash

  9. Existence of chronic EBV infection (chronic fatigue syndrome) is very controversial

Allergic Rhinitis

- Definition: A noninfectious symptom complex which includes perennial, or seasonal manifestations
- Etiology/Incidence
  1. Seasonal allergies—symptoms at same time each year, related to pollens
     a. Trees (April to July)
     b. Grasses (May to July)
     c. Ragweed (August to October)
  2. Perennial allergies—year round symptoms related to molds, animal dander, feathers, dust mites, cockroaches
  3. Most common allergens—pollens, molds, dust mites, animal dander
  4. 8 to 12% of U.S. population affected; onset usually before age 30
- Signs and Symptoms
  1. Nasal congestion
  2. Sneezing
  3. Clear, watery nasal discharge
  4. Itchy nose, throat, eyes
  5. Cough from postnasal drip
  6. Mouth breather/snoring
  7. Loss/alteration of smell
- Differential Diagnosis
  1. Vasomotor rhinitis
  2. Foreign body
  3. Nasal polyps/tumor
  4. Sinusitis
  5. Medications—especially overuse of topical decongestants "rebound"; oral contraceptives
  6. Deviated septum
  7. Hypothyroidism and pregnancy cause nasal congestion

- Physical Findings

  1. Pale, boggy nasal mucosa

  2. Enlarged turbinates

  3. Injected conjunctiva, tearing

  4. "Allergic shiner" under eyes

  5. No sinus tenderness

- Diagnostic Tests/Findings

  1. Nasal smear for eosinophils—elevated

  2. Serum IgE—elevated in 30 to 40% of patients

  3. Allergy testing—identify specific allergens

  4. CBC if infection suspected

- Management/Treatment

  1. Preventive measures

     a. Allergen avoidance

     b. Air conditioning/air filters

     c. Environmental control—vacuum, dust, remove carpeting, feather pillows, stuffed animals

     d. Minimize contact with animals

  2. Pharmacological

     a. Antihistamines—mainstay of treatment

        (1) OTC usually cause sedation, least expensive (diphenhyrdramine)

        (2) Nonsedating antihistamines are prescriptive drugs and expensive

           (a) Fexofenadine 60 mg orally b.i.d.

           (b) Loratadine 10 mg orally once a day on an empty stomach

        (3) Terfenadine (no longer available) and astemizole (no longer available)—potential drug interaction with erythromycin and ketoconazole; cause of cardiac dysrhythmias

    b. Decongestants (oral or topical)—vasoconstriction; decrease mucosal edema

    c. Topical corticosteriods

        (1) Beclomethasone dipropionate—2 sprays each nostril b.i.d.

        (2) Flunisolide—2 sprays each nostril b.i.d.

        (3) Steroid sprays (slow onset) up to 2 weeks before significant results appear

    d. Cromolyn sodium—one spray each nostril up to 6 times per day

    e. Immunotherapy desensitization for management failures; patients receiving desensitization must know signs/symptoms of anaphylaxis

Sinusitis

- Definition: Inflammation of one or more paranasal sinuses
- Etiology/Incidence
  1. Bacterial infections
     a. *Haemophilus influenzae*
     b. *Streptococcus pneumoniae*
     c. *Moraxella catarrhalis*
  2. Viruses
  3. Allergies
  4. Exposure to pathogen following viral URI, often a precipitating factor
  5. Deviated septum
  6. Classified as acute or chronic based upon duration of infection
  7. Maxillary sinuses most common site of infection, followed by ethmoid, sphenoid and lastly frontal involvement
- Signs and Symptoms
  1. Nasal congestion and pressure
  2. Mucopurulent nasal discharge/postnasal drip

3. Choking cough at night

4. Malaise and fever

5. Headache

6. Pain—dull to throbbing

    a. Over cheeks, worse with bending (maxillary sinus)

    b. Above and behind eye—ethmoid sinus

    c. Above eyebrows—frontal sinus

7. Periorbital edema

- Differential Diagnosis

1. Rhinitis—viral or allergic

2. Dental abscess

3. Nasal polyp/tumor

4. URI

5. Migraine/cluster headache

- Physical Findings

1. Mild to moderate elevated temperature

2. May have purulent discharge in nasal cavity

3. Percussion/palpation over frontal and maxillary sinuses—may exacerbate pain/tenderness

4. Transillumination of sinuses—may show impaired light transmission

5. Percussion of maxillary teeth—may reveal dental root infection

- Diagnostic Tests/Findings

1. None for typical presentation

2. CT scan—is preferred to conventional radiography sinus films

    a. Equal in cost to sinus films

    b. More sensitive to inflammatory changes and bone destruction

3. Sinus radiography will demonstrate opacity, air fluid levels, thick mucosa

4. Nasal culture—sinus fluid to determine actual organisms

5. CBC with differential, if patient appears toxic—elevated WBC

- Management/Treatment

    1. Antibiotics

        a. Amoxicillin—500 mg orally t.i.d. for 14 days

        b. Trimethoprim/sulfamethoxazole—1 double strength tablet b.i.d. for 14 days (penicillin alternative)

        c. Several cephalosporin options for 14 days

        d. If no response to treatment, suspect Beta lactamase producing strain—consider amoxicillin and clavulanic acid

    2. General measures

        a. Increase fluids

        b. Steam inhalation

        c. Avoid smoking

        d. Analgesics for pain relief

        e. Nasal decongestant—improves sinus drainage

    3. Topical steroids—reduce mucosal inflammation

    4. Refer to MD if no improvement after 48 hours of treatment

    5. Instruct patient to report symptoms of complications

        a. Stiff neck (meningitis)

        b. Periorbital edema (orbital cellulitis)

        c. Severe dental pain (abscess)

QUESTIONS
Select the best answer

1. The common cold is caused by:

   a. *Haemophilus influenzae*
   b. Rhinoviruses
   c. Streptococcus
   d. Herpes virus

2. Nasal congestion is a characteristic of upper respiratory infection (URI). It is best treated with:

   a. Antihistamines
   b. Nasal corticosteroids
   c. Topical decongestants
   d. Antibiotics

3. Prevention of influenza epidemics is best achieved by administration of annual "flu" vaccine. Contraindications to administering the vaccine include:

   a. Immunosuppressed patients
   b. Allergy to eggs
   c. Chronic respiratory disease
   d. Allergy to aspirin products

4. Amantadine and rimantadine are used in the treatment of influenza. Which of the following statements is true about these drugs:

   a. No significant side effects
   b. Effective against Type B influenza
   c. Decreases the duration of symptoms
   d. Best if given within 72 hours of illness onset

5. β hemolytic group A strep (GABHS) is a common pathogen in bacterial pharyngitis. It is also an infectious agent in which of the following medical conditions:

   a. Acute pyelonephritis
   b. Rheumatic fever
   c. Viral meningitis
   d. Acute mononucleosis

6. The most common physical finding associated with strep pharyngitis is:

    a. Unilateral tonsillar edema
    b. Exudative tonsils
    c. Ulcerations on buccal mucosa
    d. Injected uvula

7. Infectious mononucleosis is caused by:

    a. Coxsackie virus
    b. Herpes simplex
    c. Viral hepatitis A
    d. Epstein Barr virus

8. Earl Thomas, an 18-year-old college student, presents with fever of 101° F, sore throat, dysphagia and fatigue. Physical exam reveals periorbital edema, exudative tonsils, enlarged tender posterior cervical nodes, no hepatosplenomegaly. Your preliminary diagnosis is infectious mononucleosis. What diagnostic tests would you order to confirm your diagnosis:

    a. Throat culture
    b. Hetrophil antibody
    c. Electrolytes
    d. CMV titer

9. A 40-year-old male accountant presents with a three day history of left eye irritation. On physical examination, there is moderate conjunctival injection, watery discharge, palpable preauricular lymph nodes and visual acuity, 20/20 both eyes. The most likely diagnosis is:

    a. Acute glaucoma
    b. Bacterial conjunctivitis
    c. Blepharitis
    d. Viral conjunctivitis

10. In the history of a patient presenting with red eye, it is important to ask about:

    a. Photophobia
    b. Itchiness
    c. Cold symptoms
    d. Myopia

11. The two most important tests in assessment of a corneal abrasion are:

    a. Pupillary reaction and extraocular movements
    b. Funduscopic exam and peripheral vision
    c. Visual acuity and fluorescein stain
    d. Cover/uncover test and accommodation

12. Miss Shell presents with sinus pain, pressure and yellow nasal discharge. Your examination of this patient would include palpation and transillumination of the:

    a. Ethmoid and frontal sinuses
    b. Maxillary and sphenoid sinuses
    c. Frontal and maxillary sinuses
    d. Sphenoid and ethmoid sinuses

13. Which of the following conditions may predispose a patient to sinusitis:

    a. Tumor, gingivitis, deviated septum
    b. Nasal polyps, allergies, upper respiratory infection
    c. Temporomandibular joint syndrome, rhinitis, otitis
    d. Common cold, pharyngitis, meningitis

14. Ototoxic drugs are a potential cause of sensorineural hearing loss. Which of the following drugs may cause hearing loss:

    a. Gentamicin
    b. Penicillin
    c. Cephalexin
    d. Minocycline

15. A 60-year-old male suddenly develops headache, blurred vision and severe eye pain upon entering a dark movie theater. The most likely diagnosis is:

    a. Angle closure glaucoma
    b. Uveitis
    c. Giant cell arteritis
    d. Open angle glaucoma

16. Absent red reflex may indicate which of the following ophthalmologic conditions:

    a. Foreign body
    b. Cataracts

    c. Glaucoma

    d. Uveitis

17. Presbycusis—hearing impairment associated with aging, is characterized by:

    a. Acoustic nerve damage

    b. Cerumen impaction

    c. High frequency sensorineural loss

    d. Low frequency conductive loss

18. Macular degeneration is manifested by:

    a. Loss of peripheral vision

    b. Irregular pupils

    c. Loss of central vision

    d. Excessive tearing

19. Which condition is most likely associated with conductive hearing loss?

    a. Syphilis

    b. Meniere's disease

    c. Acute otitis media

    d. Hypothyroidism

20. A physical characteristic which differentiates otitis externa from otitis media is:

    a. Hearing loss

    b. Pain with movement of pinna

    c. Excessive cerumen

    d. Enlarged submaxillary node

21. The most common pathogen of acute otitis media in adults is:

    a. *Pseudomonas aeruginosa*

    b. *Streptococcus pneumoniae*

    c. *Mycoplasma pneumoniae*

    d. *Escherichia coli*

22. A 30-year-old housewife presents with long standing nasal stuffiness, clear watery nasal discharge and annoying sneezing. The most likely diagnosis is:

    a. Chronic sinusitis

    b. Nasal polyps

c. Common cold
d. Allergic rhinitis

23. Microscopic examination of nasal secretions of a patient with allergic rhinitis may reveal:

   a. Lymphocytes
   b. Neutrophils
   c. Eosinophils
   d. Basophils

24. Allergic rhinitis is primarily treated with:

   a. Allergy avoidance and antihistamines
   b. Systemic steroids and decongestants
   c. Topical nasal sprays and antibiotics
   d. Humidified air and cough suppressants

25. An antibiotic that is used in treating otitis media and is effective against B-lactamase producing pathogens is:

   a. Amoxicillin
   b. Erythromycin
   c. Tetracycline
   d. Trimethoprim/sulfamethoxazole

26. Topical steroids are contraindicated in patients with corneal abrasions because:

   a. They inhibit tearing
   b. They increase risk of bacterial infection
   c. They increase intraocular pressure
   d. They may lead to iritis

27. Which of the following in not a cause of epistaxis?

   a. Hypertension
   b. Diabetes mellitus
   c. Neoplasms
   d. Trauma

28. A special diagnostic test/procedure for vertigo is:

   a. Tonometry
   b. Barany maneuver

c. Pneumatic otoscopy

d. EEG

29. Mr. Jones a 32-year-old salesman presents with a complaint of frequent nose-bleeds for the last 2 months. He states they occur spontaneously 3 times a week and usually stop within ten minutes. He denies any other acute or chronic medical problems. Which of the following diagnostic tests is indicated at this time?

a. CBC

b. Hemoglobin electrophoresis

c. Prothrombin time

d. Clotting time

30. Upon further evaluation of Mr. Jones, you find he has nasal congestion, postnasal drip and scratchy throat. He uses an antihistamine at night for nasal symptoms and sleep. Your initial treatment plan for Mr. Jones should be:

a. Add a decongestant to alleviate nasal congestion

b. Increase humidity to moisten nasal mucosa

c. Have patient elevate head of bed to promote sleep

d. Discontinue antihistamine due to drying effect on nasal mucosa

31. Kyle Smith, a 21-year-old law student, presents with fatigue for 3 to 4 months, low grade fever and intermittent sore throat. You order a complete blood count. The result of the CBC is as follows: Hgb and Hct normal, elevated WBC and atypical lymphocytes. The most likely diagnosis is:

a. Hepatitis A

b. Infectious mononucleosis

c. Herpangina

d. Toxoplasmosis

32. Which of the following is *not* commonly a cause of bacterial conjunctivitis:

a. *Neisseria gonorrhoeae*

b. *Proteus mirabilis*

c. *Haemophilus influenzae*

d. *Pseudomonas aeruginosa*

33. An antibiotic which is ''the drug of choice'' in the treatment of gonococcal pharyngitis is:

a. Erythromycin

b. Ampicillin
c. Ceftriaxone
d. Amantadine

34. Hearing loss caused by cerumen impaction is considered:

    a. Conductive loss
    b. Sensorineural loss
    c. "Mixed" loss
    d. Congenital loss

35. Zeke Gilbert, a 72-year-old retired factory worker has hearing loss in his right ear due to excessive noise exposure. When performing a Weber Test, you would expect to find:

    a. Sound lateralizes equally to both ears
    b. Sound lateralizes to the left ear
    c. Sound lateralizes to the right ear
    d. Sound laterizes to neither ear

36. The most sensitive test for diagnosing sinusitis is the:

    a. CBC
    b. Nasal culture
    c. CT scan
    d. Sinus radiography

37. The most common cause/pathogen in otitis externa is:

    a. Fungi
    b. *Staphylococcal epidermidis*
    c. Alpha streptococcus
    d. *Pseudomonas aeruginosa*

38. A physical finding which differentiates conjunctivitis from glaucoma is:

    a. Injected conjunctiva
    b. Excessive tearing
    c. Clear cornea
    d. Nystagmus

39. When prescribing topical corticosteriods for patients with allergic rhinitis, it is important to discuss that:

    a. Topical steroid use may predispose to infections
    b. It may take up to two weeks before they experience significant reduction in symptoms
    c. Steroids must be taken with antihistamines to be effective
    d. After 48 hours of use, patient will experience reduction in symptoms

40. It is important to highlight the short term use of topical nasal decongestant because of this adverse effect:

    a. Rhinorrhea
    b. Confusion
    c. Somnolence
    d. Rebound congestion

30/40 75%

ANSWERS

1. b	14. a	28. b
2. c	15. a	29. a
3. b	16. b	30. d
4. c	17. c	31. b
5. b	18. c	32. d
6. b	19. c	33. c
7. d	20. b	34. a
8. b	21. b	35. b
9. d	22. d	36. c
10. a	23. c	37. d
11. c	24. a	38. c
12. c	25. d	39. b
13. b	26. b	40. d
	27. b	

BIBLIOGRAPHY

Andreoli, T. E., Bennett, J. C., Carpenter, C. J., & Plum, F. (Eds.). (1997). *Cecil essentials of medicine* (4th ed.). Philadelphia: W. B. Saunders.

Barker, L. R., Burton, J. R., & Zieve, P. D. (Eds.). (1995). *Principles of ambulatory medicine.* Baltimore: Williams & Wilkins.

Bates, B., Bickley, L. S., & Hoekelman, R. A. (Eds.). (1995). *A guide to physical examination and history taking* (6th ed.). Philadelphia: J. B. Lippincott.

Hara, J. (1996). The red eye: Diagnosis and treatment. *American Family Physician, 54*(8), 2423-2430.

Hsu, R., & Levine, S. C. (1998). Sudden hearing loss: How to identify the cause promptly. *Consultant, 38*(1), 23-32.

Institute for Clinical Systems Integration. Healthcare Guidelines Series. (1998). Viral upper respiratory tract infections in adults. *Post Graduate Medicine, 103*(1), 71-80.

Neinstein, L. S. (1996). *Adolescent health care: A practical guide* (3rd ed.). Baltimore: Williams & Wilkins.

Palay, D. A., & Krachmer., J. H. (1997). *Ophthalmology for the primary care physician.* St. Louis: Mosby.

Perkins, A. (1997). Approach to diagnosing the acute sore throat. *American Family Physician, 55*(1), 131-138.

Rosenberg, L. (1995). Glaucoma: Early detection and therapy for prevention of vision loss. *American Family Physician, 52*(8), 2289-2298.

Shannon, M. T., Wilson, B. A., & Stang, C. L. (Eds.). (1998). *Appleton & Lange's 1998 drug guide.* Stamford: Appleton & Lange.

Tierney, L., McPhee, S. J., & Papadakis, M. A. (Eds.). (1998). *Current medical diagnosis and treatment* (37th ed.). Stamford: Appleton & Lange.

Uphold, C. R., & Graham, M. V. (1998). *Clinical guidelines in family practice* (3rd ed.). Gainesville: Barmarrae Books.

Respiratory Disorders

Margaret Hadro Venzke

Pulmonary Function Tests

Proper assessment of most patients with pulmonary disease requires the use of pulmonary function testing. Understanding these tests is important in interpretation of results in relationship to the patient's diagnosis. Pulmonary function tests objectively measure the respiratory system's ability to perform gas exchange via assessment of ventilation, diffusion and mechanical properties.

- Indications for Use of Pulmonary Function Tests (PFT)
  1. Evaluation of dyspnea, cough, pulmonary dysfunction
  2. Early detection of lung dysfunction
  3. Disability assessment, including evaluation of risk factors in work settings
  4. Evaluation of response to therapy
  5. Re-evaluation of progress of restrictive or obstructive disease
  6. Pre-operative evaluation

- Types of Pulmonary Function Tests
  1. Spirometry—measure air flow rates and forced vital capacity (FVC)
     a. Forced vital capacity (FVC)—volume of air forcefully expelled from lungs after maximal inhalation
     b. Forced expiratory volume (FEV_1)—the volume of air expelled in the first second of FVC
     c. Forced expiratory flow 25-75 (FEF_{25-75})—maximal midexpiratory airflow rate
     d. Peak expiratory flow rate (PEFR)—the maximum air flow rate on forceful expulsion after maximum inspiration
     e. Maximum voluntary ventilation (MVV)—maximum volume of gas that can be breathed in one minute
  2. Lung volumes
     a. Total lung capacity (TLC)—volume of air in the lungs after maximum inspiration
     b. Functional residual capacity (FRC)—air left in lungs after a normal unforced expiration

    c. Residual volume (RV)—air remaining in lungs after maximum expiration

    d. Slow vital capacity (SVC)—volume of gas slowly exhaled after maximal inspiration

    e. Expiratory reserve volume (ERV)—the gas volume difference between the FRC and RV

- General Relationship of PFT to Pulmonary Disease

    1. Obstructive pulmonary disease is characterized by reduced air flow rates; examples include:

        a. Asthma

        b. Emphysema

        c. Chronic bronchitis

        d. Cystic fibrosis

    2. Restrictive pulmonary disease is associated with reduced lung volumes; examples include:

        a. Pulmonary infiltrate

        b. Lung resection

        c. Chest wall disorders

        d. Neuromuscular disease

Acute Bronchitis

- Definition: Acute inflammation of trachea, bronchi and bronchioles

- Etiology/Incidence

    1. Common causes

        a. Rhinovirus, coronavirus—usually short course of afebrile illness

        b. Adenovirus, influenza, *Mycoplasma pneumoniae*—more severe febrile bronchitis

        c. *Chlamydia pneumoniae*

        d. *Moraxella catarrhalis*

    2. Associated with secondary bacterial infections

      a. *Streptococcus pneumoniae*

      b. *Haemophilus influenzae*

  3. Mucous membranes become hyperemic, edematous with increased bronchial secretions

  4. Frequency and severity increase with cigarette smoking

- Signs and Symptoms

  1. Cough (hallmark symptom)

      a. Initially dry

      b. Later productive with mucopurulent sputum

  2. Fever

  3. Fatigue, malaise

  4. Chest burning or substernal pain

  5. Headache

  6. Occasional dyspnea

  7. Wheezing

  8. Generally self-limiting illness

- Differential Diagnosis

  1. Pneumonia

  2. Asthma

  3. Influenza

  4. Pertussis

  5. Upper respiratory infection

  6. Allergies

  7. Cystic fibrosis

  8. Tuberculosis

- Physical Findings

  1. Temperature less than 101° F

  2. Chest and lungs

      a. Clear to auscultation

      b.   Resonant to percussion

      c.   Wheezes

      d.   Diffuse rhonchi (often clear with coughing)

      e.   Occasional crackles

- Diagnostic Tests/Findings

   1.   Diagnosis based on clinical presentation

   2.   If diagnosis uncertain or symptoms severe

      a.   Chest radiograph—normal in acute bronchitis

      b.   Sputum cultures—not helpful in the diagnosis

      c.   CBC/WBC—normal or slightly elevated

   3.   PPD—if patient at risk for tuberculosis

- Management/Treatment

   1.   No treatment with antibiotics in otherwise healthy persons

   2.   Palliative measures

      a.   Rest

      b.   Increase fluid intake to thin secretions

      c.   Humidity/steam

      d.   Expectorants—questionable efficacy

      e.   Cough suppressants—dextromethorphan or codeine for night cough

      f.   Avoid antihistamines—dry out secretions

      g.   Decrease environmental irritants

      h.   Analgesics for pain/fever

   3.   Smoking cessation

   4.   Bronchodilator for wheezing/cough

   5.   Recovery usually in 7 to 14 days

   6.   Follow-up visit if no improvement or worsening symptoms after 72 hours

7. Secondary bacterial infections associated with high fever, productive cough with purulent sputum; treat with antimicrobial therapy

   a. Erythromycin—250 to 500 mg orally q.i.d. for 10 days for *Mycoplasma pneumoniae, Streptococcus pneumoniae* organisms

   b. Amoxicillin 250 mg orally t.i.d. for 10 days for *Streptococcus pneumoniae, Haemophilus influenzae* organisms

   c. Doxycycline 100 mg b.i.d. for 10 days for coverage of chlamydia, *Mycoplasma pneumoniae* organisms

   d. Trimethoprim/sulfamethoxazole—one double strength tablet orally b.i.d. for 10 days for coverage of *Haemophilus influenzae, Moraxella catarrhalis* organisms

8. Refer/consult with MD if no improvement after 4 to 6 weeks

Pneumonia

- Definition

  1. Acute inflammation of lung parenchyma including alveoli and interstitial tissues; usually secondary to infection

  2. Categorized as either hospital acquired (nosocomial) or community acquired regardless of causative organism

     a. Hospital acquired occurs > 48 hours after admission

     b. Community acquired encompasses all others occurring as an outpatient or within first 48 hours of hospitalization

- Etiology/Incidence

  1. Aspiration of secretions, inhalation of pathogens and/or hematogenous dissemination

  2. Common pathogens

     a. Viruses (4 to 39% of adult pneumonias, more prevalent in children)

        (1) Influenza

        (2) Parainfluenza

        (3) Adenovirus

        (4) Varicella

     b. Bacteria

(1) *Streptococcus pneumoniae* (pneumococcus)—most common

(2) *Haemophilus influenzae*—ranked 2nd to streptococcal pneumonia

(3) *Staphylococcus aureus*

(4) *Klebsiella pneumoniae*

(5) *Legionella pneumophila*—1 to 4% of community acquired pneumonia

(6) *Moraxella catarrhalis*

(7) *Chlamydia pneumoniae*

(8) *Mycoplasma pneumoniae* (most common in adolescents/young adults)

(9) *Pseudomonas aeruginosa*

(10) *Escherichia coli*

3. Hospital acquired pneumonia (nosocomial)—occurs more than 48 hours after hospital admission, more common in patients requiring intensive care and mechanical ventilation

   a. Rickettsia

   b. Protozoans

   c. Parasites

   d. Fungi

   e. *Pneumocystis carinii*—immunosupressed and HIV patients

4. Increasingly common in the elderly and patients with co-existing illness or disease

5. First ranked cause of death from infectious disease

6. Sixth leading cause of death in the U.S.

- Signs and Symptoms
   1. Fatigue, malaise
   2. Pleuritic chest pain—worsens with inspiration
   3. Fever
   4. Chills

   5. Dyspnea

   6. Cough

   7. Purulent mucus production—more common in hospital acquired

- Differential Diagnosis

   1. Types of pneumonia (see Etiology)

   2. Atelectasis

   3. Pneumothorax

   4. Lung abscess

   5. Congestive heart failure

   6. Neoplasms

   7. Chronic obstructive pulmonary disease (C.O.P.D.)

   8. Tuberculosis

- Physical Findings

   1. Elevated temperature and pulse

   2. Observe respiratory status, may have

      a. Cyanosis

      b. Nasal flaring/grunting

      c. Tachypnea

      d. Intercostal retractions

   3. Diminished localized breath sounds

   4. Evidence of consolidation

      a. Dullness to percussion

      b. Increased fremitus

      c. Egophony ''e to a'' changes

      d. Whispered pectoriloquy

      e. Rales

   5. Fine crepitant rales—do not clear with cough

- Diagnostic Tests/Findings

1. Chest radiograph may show any variety of abnormalities—findings lack specificity and are not pathognomonic

2. CBC with differential—WBC often elevated

   a. WBC differential with left shift—bacterial origin

   b. Differential useful in evaluating severity and prognosis

3. Gram stain and sputum culture—consider when atypical pathogen suspected or patient is immunocompromised

   a. Gram positive—*Streptococcus pneumoniae, Staphylococcus aureus*

   b. Gram negative—*Haemophilus influenzae,* klebsiella

4. Serum electrolytes, hepatic enzymes—important in severe cases (when considering hospitalization); hyponatremia

5. Blood cultures—severely ill, toxic patients

6. Refer for thoracentesis if pleural effusion

7. PPD to rule out tuberculosis

8. Serum cold agglutinins—for mycoplasma

- Management/Treatment

   1. General Measures

      a. Increase fluid intake

      b. Analgesics for fever and headache

      c. Avoid cough suppressants and cigarettes

      d. Humidification

   2. Empiric antimicrobial treatment of community acquired pneumonia

      a. Patients without comorbidity *and* less than 60 years old

         (1) Erythromycin 500 mg orally q.i.d. for 14 days *or*

         (2) Clarithromycin 250 mg orally b.i.d. for 7 to 14 days *or*

         (3) Azithromycin 500 mg orally day 1 then 250 mg orally daily for 4 days *or*

         (4) Tetracycline 500 mg orally q.i.d. for 14 days for macrolide allergic patients

  b. Patients with comorbidity or over 60 years old

   (1) Cefuroxime axetil 250 to 500 mg orally b.i.d. for 10 days or

   (2) Trimethoprim/sulfamethoxazole (TMP/SMX) 160 mg TMP/800 mg SMX orally b.i.d. for 14 days or

   (3) Amoxicillin-potassium clavulanate 500 mg orally t.i.d. for 10 days

   (4) Macrolides (in doses shown for patients without co-morbidity and less than 60 years old) if Legionnaire's disease suspected

  c. Patients hospitalized with community acquired pneumonia

   (1) Cefuroxime sodium 0.75 to 1.5 grams intravenously every 8 hours for 5 to 10 days or

   (2) Ceftriaxone sodium 1 to 2 grams intravenously every 12 to 24 hours for 5 to 10 days

   (3) Macrolide (in doses shown above) intravenously if Legionnaire's disease suspected

  d. Severely ill hospitalized patients require combination antibiotic therapy

3. Empiric treatment of hospital acquired pneumonia

  a. Combination antibiotic therapy required

  b. Pharmacologic selection dependent upon suspected organism

4. Discuss potential side effects of medication and stress importance of completing antibiotic treatment regimen

5. Follow-up within 24 hours by telephone

6. Schedule return visit in 3 to 4 days to evaluate progress

7. Follow-up chest radiograph in 4 to 6 weeks in patients over age 40 and all smokers

8. Prevention

  a. Pneumococcal 23 valent vaccine (pneumovax) 0.5 cc IM—indicated for patients over age 65 and those with immunosuppression or chronic disease

    b.   Influenza vaccine annually—may administer with pneumovax at the same time, at different sites

  9. Refer/consult with MD regarding:

    a.   Seriously ill, toxic patients

    b.   Persons with coexisting chronic disease

Asthma

- Definition: A reversible, episodic lung disorder characterized by increased responsiveness of the trachea and bronchi and manifested by widespread narrowing of the airways

- Etiology/Incidence

  1. Caused by a single or multiple triggers such as:

    a.   Allergies

       (1) Airborne pollens

       (2) Molds

       (3) House dust

       (4) Animal dander

       (5) Food additives/preservatives

       (6) Feather pillows

    b.   Nonallergic factors

       (1) Smoke and other pollutants

       (2) Infections

       (3) Medications—ASA, NSAID, beta-blockers

       (4) Exercise

       (5) Gastroesophageal reflux

       (6) Emotional factors

       (7) Menses, pregnancy

       (8) Thyroid disease

  2. Affects men and women equally, approximately 5% of the U.S. population

      3. Chronic disease with acute exacerbations

- Signs and Symptoms

      1. Cough—often the only symptom

      2. Wheezing—may be absent in severe exacerbation

      3. Dyspnea

      4. Chest tightness

      5. Exercise intolerance

      6. URI symptoms

      7. Conditions associated with asthma

         a. Rhinitis

         b. Sinusitis

         c. Nasal polyps

         d. Eczema/atopic dermatitis

- Differential Diagnosis

      1. Heart disease—congestive heart failure

      2. Foreign body aspiration (FOB)

      3. Chronic obstructive pulmonary disease (C.O.P.D.)

      4. Acute infection—bronchitis/pneumonia

      5. Pulmonary embolism

      6. Cough secondary to beta-blockers or ACE inhibitors

      7. Anaphylaxis due to allergen

- Physical Findings

      1. General appearance—note distress or decreased responsiveness

      2. Nasal flaring

      3. Use of accessory respiratory muscles, retraction

      4. Lungs

         a. Tachypnea

         b. Prolonged expiration

    c.   Expiratory wheezing—unilateral wheezing suggests mechanical obstruction

    d.   Generalized decreased or distant breath sounds

  5. Red flags—indicate potentially life threatening severe exacerbation requiring immediate emergency treatment

    a.   Pulsus paradoxus—an exaggerated fall in systolic blood pressure during inspiration

    b.   Diaphoresis

    c.   Inaudible breath sounds

    d.   Inability to lie flat

    e.   Cyanosis

- Diagnostic Tests/Findings

  1. Pulmonary function tests/spirometry

    a.   Peak expiratory flow rate < 80% of predicted norm for age, gender, height

    b.   Vital capacity reduced

    c.   Increase of 15% in FEV_1 or FVC after bronchodilator treatment confirms diagnosis

  2. CBC

    a.   Slight increase in WBC during acute attack

    b.   Eosinophil increase related to allergic response

  3. Chest radiograph—normal, rarely hyperinflation

  4. Arterial blood gases (ABG)

    a.   Hypoxia in severe cases

    b.   Hypocapnia

    c.   Normal pCO_2 indicates very ill patient

    d.   Hypercapnia is a medical emergency

  5. Sputum examination—positive for eosinophilia

  6. Nasal secretion—positive for eosinophilia

  7. Allergy testing

8. Broncho-provocation with methacholine, histamine, or exercise challenge induces symptoms

- Management/Treatment
    1. Indications for referral to MD or asthma specialist
        a. Newly diagnosed patients
        b. Elderly patients
        c. Lack of response to therapy
    2. Indications of acute severe exacerbations requiring emergency hospitalization
        a. Pulsus paradoxus
        b. Cardiovascular disease
        c. Nonresponse to emergency treatment
        d. Persistently low PEFR
        e. Respiratory acidosis
    3. Monitor measures of lung function with peak flow meter—establish patient's "personal best" and treat based on percent of "personal best"; "personal best" is the highest PEFR measurement after a period of maximum therapy
        a. 80 to 100%—maintain on treatment as prescribed
        b. 50 to 80%—acute exacerbation; contact clinician, adjust maintenance program
        c. Below 50%—medical alert identification; emergency treatment
    4. Goals of treatment
        a. Activity without symptoms; sleep through the night
        b. Prevention of chronic troublesome symptoms
        c. Sports and exercise participation
        d. Optimal pharmacotherapy with minimal/no adverse effects
        e. Maintain nearly normal pulmonary function
        f. Meet patient/family's expectations of, and satisfaction with asthma care

5. A stepwise approach to pharmacologic therapy is recommended to gain and maintain asthma control

6. Classes of medications

    a. Long-term control—used to achieve and maintain control of persistent asthma

        (1) Anti-inflammatory agents—inhaled corticosteroids most potent and effective

            (a) Beclomethasone

            (b) Triamcinolone

            (c) Flunisolide

            (d) Oral corticosteroids—used in severe asthma

        (2) Sympathomimetic agents—relax bronchial smooth muscle; *long acting* β_2 adrenergic agonist agents—use with anti-inflammatory therapy and for prevention of exercise induced bronchospasm (EIB)

            (a) Salmeterol—inhaled medication

            (b) Albuterol—sustained released oral medication

        (3) Antimediators—inhaled anti-inflammatory agents indicated for long-term prevention of symptoms and preventive treatment prior to exercise or allergen exposure; 4 to 6 week trial needed to determine maximal benefit

            (a) Cromolyn—nebulizer delivery may be preferred to metered dose inhaler

            (b) Nedocromil—20% of patients complain of unpleasant taste

        (4) Methylxanthines—often used as adjunct therapy to anti-inflammatory drugs for nocturnal symptoms

            (a) Theophylline—sustained release oral medication, many side effects, drug interactions

            (b) Aminophylline—IV drug, seldom used

        (5) Leukotriene modifiers—new asthma drugs, alternative to inhaled corticosteriods in mild persistent asthma for patients 12 years of age or older

        (a) Zafirlukast—take on empty stomach

        (b) Zileuton—causes elevated liver enzymes

  b. Quick-relief medications treat acute symptoms and exacerbations

    (1) Short acting β_2 adrenergic agonists—drugs of choice for relief of acute symptoms and prevention of E.I.B.

        (a) Albuterol

        (b) Bitolterol

        (c) Pibuterol

        (d) Terbutaline

    (2) Anticholinergic—Ipratropium bromide may provide additive benefit when used with inhaled β_2 adrenergic agonist; used alone when β_2 adrenergic agonists not tolerated; more effective as therapy for C.O.P.D. than asthma

    (3) Systemic corticosteroids—for moderate to severe exacerbations; prevent progression of exacerbation, speed recovery and reduce rate of relapse

        (a) Methylprednisolone

        (b) Prednisolone

        (c) Prednisone

7. Pharmacotherapy in mild intermittent asthma (step 1)

  a. Characteristics of mild intermittent asthma include one or more of the following:

    (1) Brief symptoms, no more than twice weekly

    (2) Asymptomatic between exacerbations

    (3) Nocturnal symptoms less than twice a month

    (4) PEFR 80% or greater than predicted value; variability less than 20%

  b. Medications

    (1) No daily medication

    (2) Short acting β_2 adrenergic agonist for symptom relief; if

used more than twice weekly, consider long term therapy

8. Pharmacotherapy in mild persistent asthma (step 2)

    a. Characteristics of mild persistent asthma include one or more of the following:

        (1) Symptoms > twice a week, but less than once daily

        (2) Exacerbations affect sleep and level of activity

        (3) Nocturnal symptoms more than twice a month

        (4) PEFR 80% with 20 to 30% variability

    b. Medications—one daily medication

        (1) Low dose inhaled corticosteroids (200 to 500 μg) daily divided in 2 to 4 doses; (i.e., beclomethasone 2 to 4 inhalations b.i.d.) *or*

        (2) Inhaled cromolyn or nedocromil 2 inhalations t.i.d. or q.i.d. *or*

        (3) Theophylline, sustained release tablets, 10 mg/kg per day up to 300 mg maximum; monitor theophylline level—not preferred, but may be used as alternative

        (4) Leukotriene modifier—may be considered

        (5) Short-acting inhaled β_2 adrenergic agonist agent for *quick relief;* if daily usage, need additional long term therapy

9. Pharmacotherapy in moderate persistent asthma (step 3)

    a. Characteristics of moderate persistent asthma include one or more of the following:

        (1) Daily symptoms

        (2) Daily use of short-acting β_2 adrenergic agonist

        (3) Nocturnal symptoms more than once a week

        (4) Exacerbations affect activity and sleep

        (5) Exacerbations at least twice weekly, may last for days

        (6) PEFR 60% to 80% of predicted value; variability exceeds 30%

    b.   Medications—one or two daily medications

        (1)   Medium dose inhaled corticosteroids; i.e., beclomethasone 500 to 840 mg daily in 2 to 4 divided doses *and/or*

        (2)   Medium dose inhaled corticosteroid plus long acting bronchodilator

        (3)   Quick relief—short acting β_2 adrenergic agonist; if increased or daily use, need additional long term therapy

10.   Pharmacotherapy in severe persistent asthma (step 4)

    a.   Characteristics of severe persistent asthma include one or more of the following:

        (1)   Continuous symptoms

        (2)   Frequent exacerbations

        (3)   Limited physical activity

        (4)   Frequent nocturnal symptoms

        (5)   PEFR no greater than 60% of predicted value; variability exceeds 30%

    b.   Medications—refer to asthma specialist; two or three daily medications

        (1)   High dose inhaled corticosteriods (i.e., beclomethasone greater than 840 μg in divided daily doses) *and*

        (2)   Long-acting bronchodilator (inhaled or oral β_2 adrenergic agonist or theophylline) *and*

        (3)   Oral corticosteroids—make report attempts to reduce systemic steroids and maintain control with high dose inhaled steroids

        (4)   Quick relief—short acting β_2 adrenergic agonist as needed for symptoms

11.   The stepwise approach is a general guideline to asthma therapy

    a.   Review treatment every 1 to 6 months

    b.   Rescue course of systemic corticosteroids may be needed at any time/step

    c.   Refer to asthma specialist if difficulty maintaining control of asthma

12. Environmental measures to decrease irritants

    a. Avoid outdoor allergens

    b. Eliminate indoor allergens

    c. Use of air conditioners and air filters

13. Educating the patient—key components

    a. Signs and symptoms to report

    b. Controlling asthma triggers, planning avoidance strategies

    c. Correct use of inhalers and/or spacers

    d. Use of peak flow meter

14. Written guidelines for patient concerning drug treatment, PEFR measurements, and signs and symptoms of serious exacerbation

15. Discuss adverse effects of oral steroids, including need to taper dose

16. Use of inhaled corticosteriods; rinse mouth after use to avoid oral candidiasis

17. Discuss adverse effects/drug interactions when receiving theophylline

18. Include patient's family in treatment plan

19. Avoid use of ASA and NSAIDS—may cause serious exacerbations

20. Beta-blocker medications are contraindicated

21. Stress management

22. Advise annual influenza vaccine and consider pneumococcal vaccine

Chronic Obstructive Pulmonary Disease (C.O.P.D.)

- Definition: A disease state characterized by airflow obstruction due to emphysema, chronic bronchitis, or both; may be partially reversible

    1. Emphysema—permanent abnormal distention of the terminal air spaces with destruction of alveolar walls and resultant air trapping

    2. Chronic bronchitis—excessive sputum production with chronic or recurring cough on most days for 3 months or more during 2 consecutive years

- Etiology/Incidence

    1. Occupational exposure to irritants

    2. Heredity—alpha$_1$ protease inhibitor deficiency may cause emphysema; suspect in patients under age 35 who have C.O.P.D.

    3. 10 to 15% of smokers develop C.O.P.D.

    4. Affects 14 million people in the U.S.

    5. 4th leading cause of death in the U.S.

    6. Predominantly seen over age 40

    7. Affects men more than women, but prevalence in women rising

- Signs and Symptoms

    1. Emphysema (Pink Puffer)

        a. Early stage

            (1) Mild dyspnea

            (2) Cough uncommon

            (3) Fatigue

        b. Later stage

            (1) Severe dyspnea

            (2) Dyspnea on exertion

            (3) Pursed lip breathing

            (4) Muscle wasting

            (5) Weight loss

            (6) Flushed appearance

            (7) Mild cough with clear mucoid sputum

    2. Chronic bronchitis (Blue Bloater)

        a. Mild

            (1) Productive cough of mucopurulent sputum, especially in the mornings

            (2) Intermittent dyspnea

        (3)   Copious mucus production, causing nocturnal awakening

        (4)   Frequent infections

   b.   Severe

        (1)   Cyanosis

        (2)   Edema

        (3)   Recurrent respiratory failure

- Differential Diagnosis
  1. Asthma
  2. Congestive heart failure (C.H.F.)
  3. Tuberculosis (TB)
  4. Acute bronchitis
  5. Chronic sinusitis
  6. Lung cancer

- Physical Findings
  1. Emphysema
     a. Thin
     b. Hypertrophied accessory muscles
     c. Increased anteroposterior chest diameter (barrel chest)
     d. Lungs
        (1) Hyper-resonance to percussion
        (2) Diminished breath sounds
     e. Absence of cyanosis, clubbing
  2. Chronic bronchitis
     a. Obesity
     b. Central cyanosis
     c. Normal chest diameter
     d. Lungs
        (1) Normal resonance to percussion

                (2)   Wheezes, rhonchi

       e.   Enlarged heart

- Diagnostic Tests/Findings

  1. Forced expiratory volume greater than 3 seconds in both emphysema and chronic bronchitis

  2. Decreased vital capacity and expiratory flow rates

  3. Increased respiratory volume and total lung capacity in emphysema

  4. 15 to 20% increase in expiratory flow after use of bronchodilator in C.O.P.D.

  5. Arterial blood gases

     a. Hypoxemia in chronic bronchitis

     b. Hypercapnia in emphysema

  6. Increased hematocrit indicative of polycythemia in advanced chronic bronchitis

  7. Chest radiograph

     a. Hyperinflation, occasional bullae/blebs in emphysema

     b. Increased markings and cardiac enlargement in chronic bronchitis

  8. ECG may show right ventricular hypertrophy

  9. PPD to rule out tuberculosis

- Management/Treatment

  1. Refer patients with signs and symptoms of respiratory failure to MD

  2. Discontinue smoking—consider pharmacologic interventions

  3. Avoid airway irritants and temperature extremes

  4. Maintain hydration and indoor humidity

  5. Bronchodilators

     a. Ipratropium bromide inhaler 2 to 4 inhalations every 4 to 6 hours (drug of choice)

     b. Theophylline

    c. Corticosteriods (oral) during acute exacerbations

    d. Discontinue bronchodilator if no objective improvement in PFT

6. Chest physiotherapy as needed

7. Home oxygen therapy

8. Educate regarding factors that contribute to upper respiratory infections

9. Exercise training program

10. Pursed lip breathing, diaphragmatic exercises may be helpful

11. Prevention of infection with pneumococcal and annual influenza vaccines

12. Early treatment of recurrent and chronic bacterial infections; common organisms include:

    a. *Haemophilus influenzae*

    b. *Streptococcus pneumoniae*

    c. *Moraxella catarrhalis*

13. Avoid beta-blockers, cough suppressants, and antihistamines

14. Review signs and symptoms of respiratory failure and C.H.F.

15. Teach effective cough technique

Tuberculosis (TB)

- Definition: Chronic bacterial infectious disease most commonly infecting the lungs; may occur in lymph nodes, bones, kidneys, meninges and can disseminate throughout body

- Etiology/Incidence

1. Mycobacteria of "tuberculosis complex," primarily *Mycobacterium tuberculosis,* a gram positive, acid fast bacillus

2. Usually spread by airborne droplet nuclei

3. 10 to 15 million infected in the U.S.

4. Incidence of TB is greatest in Asians, Pacific Islanders, American Indians, Alaska natives, and Hispanics

5. 90 to 95% of primary TB infections remain in a latent or dormant stage

6. High risk populations include:

    a. HIV infected individuals

    b. Close contacts of infected persons

    c. Low income populations

    d. Alcoholics and IV drug abusers

    e. Elderly

    f. Immigrants from Asia and Central/South America

    g. Persons in correctional institutions and in long term care facilities

    h. Individuals with chronic disease

- Signs and Symptoms (90% asymptomatic at the time of primary infection)

    1. Fatigue

    2. Anorexia, weight loss

    3. Fever

    4. Night sweats

    5. Productive cough with purulent sputum

    6. Hemoptysis

    7. Pleuritic chest pain

- Differential Diagnosis

    1. Pneumonia

    2. Malignancy

    3. Pleurisy

    4. Histoplasmosis

    5. Silicosis

    6. C.O.P.D.

- Physical Findings

1. Appear chronically ill

2. Weak and cachectic

3. Lungs

    a. Auscultation—apical rales, often a positive whispered pectoriloquy

    b. Palpation—increased tactile fremitus over consolidated areas

    c. Percussion—dull

- Diagnostic Tests/Findings

1. Chest radiograph—pulmonary infiltrates with hilar adenopathy

2. PPD

    a. Positive with active disease or prior exposure

    b. BCG may produce positive PPD for one year; then interpretation is standard

    c. AIDS patients and immunosupressed patients have diminished reactivity

3. PPD Interpretation (record induration, not erythema)

    a. A reaction of 5 mm is considered positive in patients with:

        (1) Recent close contact with infected person

        (2) Evidence of inactive disease

        (3) HIV infection

    b. A reaction of 10 mm is considered positive in patients with:

        (1) Diabetes mellitus, cancer or end stage renal disease

        (2) Immigrants from Asia, Africa, Latin America

        (3) Medically underserved, low income populations

        (4) High risk minorities

        (5) Residents of nursing homes and prisons

        (6) Health care workers

    c. A reaction of 15 mm is considered positive for all populations

    d. False-negative result

(a) PPD administered after live virus vaccine (e.g., postponed for 4 to 6 weeks following measles vaccination)

(b) Immunosuppressed

(c) Elderly

e. False-positive result

(1) Recent BCG vaccine

(2) Nontuberculosis mycobacterium

f. "Positive converter"—previous negative PPD, turns positive within a two year period, person is asymptomatic for active disease and has negative chest radiograph

4. Sputum culture

a. Essential to confirm diagnosis of TB—three specimens advised

b. Takes 3 to 6 weeks for results to be obtained

5. Gastric aspirate culture

a. Alternative to bronchoscopy

b. Use for culture only—not stained smear

- Management/Treatment

1. Prevention

a. Bacillus Calmette-Guérin (BCG) vaccine intended for prophylaxis of noninfected persons; not routinely used in the U.S.

b. Positive PPD converter—prescribe isoniazid 300 mg orally every day for 6 to 12 months

2. Pharmacotherapy—consult/refer to MD or specialist prior to initiating therapy

a. Medications (for sensitive organisms)

(1) Isoniazid daily 5 mg/kg up to 300 mg per day for 2 months, together with

(2) Rifampin daily 10 mg/kg up to 600 mg per day for 2 months

(3) Pyrazinamide 15 to 30 mg/kg up to 2 grams per day for 2 months

      (4)   After 2 months of triple therapy above, follow with 4 months of daily or twice weekly isoniazid and rifampin

  b. Medication (for resistant bacilli) in addition to above, until sensitivities to drugs are known

      (1)   If isoniazid resistance suspected, ethambutol added first 2 months 15 to 20 mg/kg for 2 months or

      (2)   Pyrazinamide 15 to 30 mg/kg for 2 months or

      (3)   Streptomycin 15 mg/kg IM

3. Order baseline liver function tests prior to initiating antituberculosis medications

4. Perform baseline color vision (red-green) test prior to ethambutol therapy

5. Follow-up on contacts of persons with active disease

6. Reportable disease—report to state and local health departments

7. BCG vaccine may be recommended for skin test negative individuals who have repeated exposure

8. After therapy completion, follow up in one year; monitor for recurrence

9. Stress importance of compliance; Direct Observed Therapy (DOT)—one method of ensuring adherence

10. Review symptoms of drug side effects and toxicity

  a. Isoniazid

      (1)   Peripheral neuropathy (prevent with daily pyridoxine)

      (2)   Hepatitis

      (3)   Hypersensitivity

  b. Rifampin

      (1)   Orange discoloration of secretions and urine

      (2)   Permanent orange stain to contact lenses

      (3)   Nausea

      (4)   Vomiting

  c. Pyrazinamide

            (1)   Hepatotoxicity

            (2)   Hyperuricemia

       d. Ethambutol

            (1)   Fever

            (2)   Rash

            (3)   Optic neuritis

       e. Streptomycin—ototoxicity

11. Stress importance of nutritious diet and education regarding selection of food

Lung Cancer

- Definition: Primary malignant neoplasm of the lung; cell types involved include squamous cell, adenocarcinoma, large cell carcinoma and small cell carcinoma

- Etiology/Incidence

  1. Cigarette smoking accounts for 95% of lung cancer in men and 85% of those in women

  2. Cigarette smoke in combination with other environmental pollutants (e.g., asbestos) influences increased incidence

  3. Most common in 50 to 70 year olds

  4. Occurs in males more frequently than females

  5. Leading cause of cancer death in men and women in the U.S.

- Signs and Symptoms: Depend on the area of tumor location and involvement of nodes or other organs; only 10 to 25% of patients are asymptomatic at time of diagnosis; symptoms occur with advanced disease

  1. "Smoker's cough"—most common early symptom

  2. Anorexia/weight loss

  3. Dyspnea—related to obstruction of major bronchus

  4. Hemoptysis—20% of all patients with hemoptysis have lung cancer

  5. Wheezing

  6. Fever

7. Chest pain—related to extension beyond parenchyma

8. Fatigue

9. Hoarseness

10. Bone pain

11. Neurological deficits

- Differential Diagnosis

  1. Pneumonia

  2. Lung abscess

  3. Bronchitis

  4. Tuberculosis

- Physical Findings

  1. Examination may not reveal significant changes

  2. Tumor obstructing bronchus—may cause atelectasis

  3. Visible or palpable supraclavicular lymph nodes

  4. Hepatomegaly

- Diagnostic Tests/Findings

  1. Chest radiograph

     a. Negative in 15% of patients with lung cancer

     b. Not diagnostic in itself, but indicates need for additional work up

     c. Manifestations—hilar or enlarging mass, infiltrate, atelectasis, cavitation or pleural effusion

  2. Laboratory

     a. CBC

     b. Liver function tests

     c. Serum electrolytes and calcium

  3. Definitive diagnosis requires cytologic or histologic evidence

  4. Sputum for cytology—positive in 40 to 60% of patients

  5. Bronchoscopy with biopsy

    6. MRI/CT scan

  • Management/Treatment

    1. Surgery—25% of patients with lung cancer are candidates for surgery

    2. Chemotherapy

    3. Radiation therapy—generally palliative

    4. Refer to MD when lung cancer suspected

    5. Encourage patient to stop smoking

    6. Decrease exposure to pollutants

    7. Realistic assessment for patient and family of prognosis, pros and cons of therapy—essential to patient's decision for treatment

    8. Discuss side effects of chemotherapy/radiation

    9. Encourage nutritious diet

    10. Effective pain control

    11. Hospice care

Questions
Select the best answer

1. Which of the following drugs is contraindicated in the treatment of severe asthma?

    a. Propranolol
    b. Theophylline
    c. Amoxicillin
    d. Albuterol

2. The most common organism causing community-acquired pneumonia is:

    a. *Eschericia coli*
    b. *Staphylococcus aureus*
    c. *Streptococcus pneumoniae*
    d. *Klebsiella pneumoniae*

3. Which of the following is not a part of the differential diagnosis of chronic cough?

    a. Tuberculosis
    b. Gastroesophageal reflux disease
    c. Allergies
    d. Pneumonia

4. The most common side effect of isoniazid is:

    a. Idiopathic splenomegaly
    b. Seizures
    c. Gynecomastia
    d. Peripheral neuropathy

5. Alpha$_1$ antitrypsin deficiency is associated with which of the following conditions?

    a. Chronic bronchitis
    b. Asthma
    c. Emphysema
    d. Cystic fibrosis

6. A 25-year-old nurse presents to employee health for her annual physical examination. Her previous PPD, one year ago, is negative. A PPD is repeated and results 3 days later show 14 mm of induration. The nurse is asymptomatic and

her chest radiograph is normal. The most appropriate management at this time would be:

   a. Repeat chest radiograph yearly
   b. Prescribe isoniazid for 6 to 12 months
   c. Prescribe rifampin for 6 to 12 months
   d. Repeat PPD in two months

7. Which of the following statements is true in the treatment of moderate persistent asthma?

   a. Inhaled corticosteroids are the cornerstone of therapy
   b. Beta-blockers should be used vigorously
   c. Cromolyn is used during acute attacks
   d. Theophylline should not be used with steroid therapy

8. Which of the following signs/symptoms are not associated with chronic bronchitis?

   a. Productive cough
   b. Obesity
   c. Dyspnea
   d. Pursed lip breathing

9. The most important measurement of pulmonary function in asthma is:

   a. The total lung capacity
   b. The forced vital capacity
   c. The residual volume
   d. The peak expiratory flow rate

10. The most common cause of pneumonia in adolescents and young adults is:

   a. Pneumococcal
   b. Mycoplasma
   c. Varicella
   d. Chlamydia

11. Outpatient treatment of pneumonia for a 50-year-old healthy male would be:

   a. Amoxicillin
   b. Trimethoprim/sulfamethoxazole
   c. Erythromycin
   d. Cephalexin

12. Physical findings in bacterial pneumonia would include:

    a. Hyper-resonance to percussion
    b. Rales that clear with cough
    c. Decreased fremitus
    d. Positive egophony

13. Max Murphy, a 30-year-old postal worker, presents with malaise, fatigue and dry cough. Physical exam findings include low grade fever 100° F, right tympanic membranes with bullae, lungs clear, no lymphadenopathy. The most likely diagnosis for this patient is:

    a. Influenza
    b. Legionnaire's Disease
    c. Acute bronchitis
    d. Asthma

14. Pneumococcal vaccine is considered a preventive measure to bacterial pneumonia. It is indicated for which populations?

    a. Patients with acute bronchitis
    b. Patients with C.O.P.D.
    c. Adolescents and young adults
    d. Persons over age 45

15. An indicator of a severe asthma attack requiring emergency treatment includes:

    a. Prolonged expiration
    b. Bilateral rales
    c. Chest tightness
    d. Inaudible breath sounds

16. When ordering a CBC in a person with acute exacerbations of asthma, you would expect to see:

    a. Moderate elevation in WBCs and atypical lymphocytes
    b. Decrease in WBCs and lymphocytosis
    c. Increased hematocrit and increased platelets
    d. Mild elevation in WBCs and eosinophilia

17. Albuterol is an example of:

    a. Antihistamine
    b. β_2 adrenergic agonist

    c. Corticosteroid

    d. Antitussive

18. Which of the following is not a risk factor for lung cancer?

    a. Radon exposure

    b. Passive cigarette smoking

    c. Allergen irritant

    d. Asbestos exposure

19. The leading cause of cancer deaths in the U.S. is:

    a. Gastric cancer

    b. Malignant melanoma

    c. Breast cancer

    d. Lung cancer

20. The drug of choice in treatment of chronic bronchitis is:

    a. Theophylline

    b. Erythromycin

    c. Cromolyn sodium

    d. Ipratropium bromide

21. Pulsus paradoxus is:

    a. Increase in diastolic blood pressure on expiration

    b. Decrease in systolic blood pressure on inspiration

    c. Increase in systolic blood pressure on expiration

    d. Decrease in diastolic blood pressure on inspiration

22. Mary is a 44-year-old housewife with mild intermittent asthma since she was age 7. She requests you renew her β_2 adrenergic agonist inhaler and states she has heard how she should test her lung function with a peak flow meter at home. What is the most important rationale for home measurement of peak expiratory flow rate?

    a. It improves total lung capacity

    b. It is the most objective measure of respiratory status

    c. It measures the effectiveness of β_2 adrenergic therapy

    d. It improves the inspiratory/expiratory ratio

23. Which of the following groups are *not* at high risk for tuberculosis?

    a. HIV infected individuals
    b. Asian immigrants
    c. Homeless individuals
    d. College students

24. The serum cold agglutinins test is used to diagnose:

    a. *Haemophilus influenzae* pneumonia
    b. Legionella pneumonia
    c. Rickettsia infection
    d. Mycoplasma pneumonia

25. The problem with diagnosing early stage lung cancer is that:

    a. The CBC lab result is normal
    b. It mimics the symptoms of asthma
    c. Patients are often asymptomatic until late in the disease
    d. Pulmonary function tests are normal

26. Signs and symptoms of C.O.P.D. correlate with which one of the following:

    a. Emphysema with decreased total lung capacity (TLC)
    b. Asthma and right sided heart failure
    c. Chronic bronchitis and airway obstruction
    d. Hemoptysis and hypoxemia

27. Larry Bates, a 32-year-old accountant with moderate persistent asthma, presents with dyspnea and wheezing for 2 days. His current medications include beclomethasone 2 inhalations b.i.d. and theophylline 300 mg at hs. His PEFR is approximately 60% of his personal best. Based on this information, what treatment would you prescribe for Larry?

    a. Add cromolyn sodium inhaler to regimen
    b. Give albuterol inhaler 2 inhalations q.i.d. for acute symptoms
    c. Add salmeterol inhaler for daytime symptoms
    d. Give antihistamine to decrease symptoms

28. Additional history reveals that Larry's girlfriend has just acquired a kitten. He noticed his asthma got worse after playing with the kitten. The best intervention for Larry to do at this time is:

    a. Wash hands before and after playing with the kitten
    b. Consider allergy shots
    c. Avoid contact with the kitten

    d. Take an antihistamine/decongestant approximately 30 minutes prior to exposure to the kitten

29. Young Chow, an 18-year-old Chinese exchange student, presents to student health for immunization update. He states he had BCG vaccine as a young child and therefore will never get tuberculosis. You administer a PPD and the result is positive. Your next best intervention would be to:

    a. Assume the positive result is due to BCG vaccine, no further evaluation needed
    b. Assume the positive result is related to TB exposure or infection, order a chest radiograph
    c. Begin isoniazid therapy immediately
    d. Repeat PPD test in one month to verify results

30. The most common side effect of the anti-tuberculin drug rifampin is:

    a. Hepatotoxicity
    b. Optic neuritis
    c. Fever
    d. Orange discoloration of secretions

Answers

1. a	11. c	21. b
2. c	12. d	22. b
3. d	13. c	23. d
4. d	14. b	24. d
5. c	15. d	25. c
6. b	16. d	26. c
7. a	17. b	27. b
8. d	18. c	28. c
9. d	19. d	29. b
10. b	20. d	30. d

Bibliography

Abrams, W. B., Beers, M. H., & Berkow, R. (Eds.). (1995). *The Merck manual of geriatrics.* Whitehouse Station, NJ: Merck & Co.

Clinician reviews supplement. (1996) Therapeutic spotlight: Acute exacerbations of chronic bronchitis. (Special issue, Dec. 1, 1996). Clinicians Publishing Group.

Dambro, M. R. (Ed.). (1998). *Griffith's 5 minute clinical consult.* Baltimore: Williams & Wilkins.

Fenstermacher, K., & Hudson, B. (1997). *Practice guidelines for family nurse practitioners.* Philadelphia: W. B. Saunders.

Goroll, A. H., May, L. A., & Mulley, A. G., Jr. (Eds.). (1995). *Primary care medicine* (3rd ed.). Philadelphia: J. B. Lippincott.

Ham, R. J., & Sloane, P. D. (Eds.). (1997). *Primary care geriatrics: A case based approach* (3rd ed.). St. Louis: Mosby.

Highlights of the expert panel report #2. *Guidelines for the diagnosis and management of asthma.* (1997). National Institutes of Health/National Heart, Lung and Blood Institute. Publication #97-4051A.

Leiner, S. (1997). Acute bronchitis in adults: Commonly diagnosed but poorly defined. *The Nurse Practitioner, 22*(1), 104-119.

Moffitt, M. P., & Wisinger, D. B. (1996). Tuberculosis: Recommendations for screening, prevention and treatment. *Postgraduate Medicine, 100*(4), 201-218.

Philp, E. B. (1997). Chronic cough. *American Family Physician, 56*(5), 1395-1402.

Report of U. S. Preventive Services Task Force (1996). *Guide to clinical preventive services* (2nd ed.). Baltimore: Williams & Wilkins.

Richman, E. (1997). Asthma diagnosis and management. *Clinician Reviews, 7*(8), 76-112.

Tierney, L., McPhee, S. J., & Papadakis, M. A. (Eds.). (1998). *Current medical diagnosis and treatment* (37th ed.). Stamford: Appleton & Lange.

Cardiovascular Disorders

Sally K. Miller

Hypertension (HTN)

- Definition: Persistent elevation of systolic blood pressure (SBP) > 140 mm Hg or diastolic blood pressure (DBP) > 90 mm Hg based upon an average of two or more blood pressure readings at each of two or more visits after an initial screening visit, or persons taking antihypertensive medication; important to perform blood pressure measurements under nonstressful circumstances, i.e., well rested, empty bladder, no immediate psychosocial stressors; hypertension should not be diagnosed based upon one blood pressure measurement unless that measurement is greater than 180/110 or is accompanied by end organ damage (National Heart, Lung, and Blood Institute, 1997)

    1. Blood Pressure Classification Guidelines

Classification	SBP		DBP
Optimal	< 120	and	< 80
Normal	< 130	and	< 85
High-normal	130-139	or	85-89
Hypertension			
Stage 1	140-159	or	90-99
Stage 2	160-179	or	100-109
Stage 3	≥ 180	or	≥ 110

- Etiology/Incidence: 95% due to unknown etiology; currently several proposed theories, including hyperactivity of the sympathetic nervous system (SNS); hypertension of unknown etiology is known as primary, essential, or idiopathic hypertension; remaining 5% of cases are attributable to secondary causes

    1. Theories of Etiology of HTN
        SNS hyperactivity
        Renin-angiotensin system
        Defect in natriuresis
        Elevated intracellular Na+

        Etiology of Secondary HTN
        Renal disease
        Renal vascular disease
        Hyperaldosteronism
        Cushing's syndrome
        Pheochromocytoma
        Coarctation of the aorta
        Pregnancy

    2. Incidence
        a. 10% to 15% of Caucasian adults
        b. 20% to 30% of African-American adults
        c. Heredity

      d.   Cigarette smoking

      e.   Increased salt intake

      f.   Obesity

      g.   Affects over 50 million Americans

- Signs and Symptoms

    1. Often no symptoms—known as "silent killer"

    2. Symptoms of underlying cause may present in secondary hypertension

        a. Flushing

        b. Palpitations

        c. Pallor

        d. Tremor

        e. Profuse perspiration

    3. Suboccipital pulsating headache occurring early in morning and improving throughout the day in severe hypertension

    4. Chronic hypertension may result in ventricular hypertrophy and the associated symptoms of heart failure

    5. Oliguria, nocturia, or hematuria may present

    6. Epistaxis in severe hypertension

    7. Severe hypertension may present with signs and symptoms of hypertensive encephalopathy

        a. Nausea and vomiting

        b. Somnolence and confusion

        c. Visual disturbances

- Differential Diagnosis: Secondary causes of hypertension must be ruled out

    1. Multiple renal diseases may cause hypertension, i.e.

        a. Medical renal disease

        b. Diabetic nephropathy

        c. Acute tubular necrosis

2. Endocrine disorders

   a. Cushing's syndrome

   b. Hyperaldosteronism

   c. Pheochromocytoma

   d. Diabetes mellitus (DM)

   e. Acromegaly

   f. Hyperthyroidism

3. Structural disorders

   a. Coarctation of the aorta

   b. Carotid artery stenosis

   c. Renal artery stenosis

4. Pregnancy

- Physical Findings

1. Most significant is elevated pressure noted in definition

2. S_4 gallop due to decreased left ventricular compliance is common

3. Displaced point of maximal impulse (PMI) when left ventricular hypertrophy present

4. Diffuse anterior chest wall heave when right ventricular hypertrophy present

5. Peripheral pulses may be abnormal in some secondary cases

   a. Coarctation of the aorta

   b. Stenosis of major arteries

6. Diastolic murmur of aortic stenosis may be heard

7. Dependent edema in chronic, uncontrolled cases

8. Renal artery bruit in cases of renal artery stenosis

9. May see neurologic evidence of previous cerebral infarcts

10. Flame hemorrhages and/or fluffy exudate on ophthalmoscopic examination

- Diagnostic Tests/Findings

    1. In uncomplicated essential hypertension, laboratory findings usually normal

    2. May see hematuria and/or proteinuria when secondary to renal disorder

    3. Rapid sequence intravenous pyelogram (IVP) to rule out renal vascular disease

    4. Chest radiograph

        a. Rule out coarctation of the aorta

        b. Cardiac hypertrophy in chronic, uncontrolled cases

    5. Plasma lipids may be elevated

    6. Hormone levels to evaluate underlying endocrine cause

        a. Elevated serum aldosterone levels—primary hyperaldosteronism

        b. Elevated adrenocorticotropic hormone or serum cortisol—Cushing's syndrome

        c. Low thyroid stimulating hormone and elevated T_3—hyperthyroidism

        d. Elevated serum and urine catecholamines—pheochromocytoma

- Management/Treatment

    1. Nonpharmacologic treatment should be instituted in all patients diagnosed with hypertension according to the definition presented

        a. Weight reduction

        b. Low sodium diet (2 g)

        c. Cessation of smoking

        d. Avoidance/reduction of alcohol intake

        e. Stress management

        g. Relaxation/exercise

        h. Lipid control

    2. Pharmacologic therapy should be instituted in all patients with stage

2 or greater hypertension. The decision to begin pharmacologic therapy in patients with stage 1 hypertension is controversial, but should be considered in all clients with any of the risk factors noted or the presence of end organ damage.

a. Diuretics are the most widely used antihypertensive medication

   (1) Hydrochlorothiazide 12.5 to 50 mg once daily

   (2) Furosemide 20 to 320 mg in daily or divided daily doses—not ordinarily used in the treatment of hypertension except in the presence of renal dysfunction

   (3) Use cautiously in patients with osetoporosis, gout, and diabetes

b. Beta-blockers, calcium channel blockers, alpha-adrenergic blockers, and angiotensin converting enzyme (ACE) inhibitors are also first line choices; physiologic responses to medication groups vary in response to demographic factors; accompanying illness is also factor in medication selection

   (1) Beta-blockers produce good response in older Caucasians and African-Americans

      (a) Atenolol 25 to 200 mg daily

      (b) Labetalol 200 to 1200 mg daily in two divided doses

      (c) Metoprolol 50 to 200 mg daily in one or two divided doses

      (d) Contraindicated in patients with CHF, type 1 DM, and bronchial asthma

      (e) Use cautiously in patients with conduction disorders and hypertriglyceridemia

   (2) Calcium channel blockers widely effective

      (a) Diltiazem 90 to 360 mg daily in two divided doses

      (b) Verapamil 180 to 480 mg daily in two divided doses

      (c) Contraindicated in the presence of disorders of

conduction; use cautiously when baseline heart rate less than 50 beats per minute (bpm)

(d) Contraindicated in the presence of sick sinus syndrome, and 2nd or 3rd degree atrioventricular block

(e) Generally contraindicated in patients with C.H.F.—may be used in specialized cases of mild diastolic failure

(3) ACE inhibitors have little effect as monotherapy in African-Americans—are effective in Caucasians

(a) Captopril 50 to 300 mg daily in two or three divided doses

(b) Lisinopril 5 to 40 mg once daily

(c) Agent of choice in patients with type 1 DM or renal dysfunction

(d) Contraindicated in bilateral renal artery stenosis

(e) 15% of patients develop cough as side effect

c. Alpha$_2$ agonists are second line option

d. Angiotensin II receptor antagonists for patients who cannot tolerate side effects of angiotensin converting enzyme inhibitors

e. Combination therapy often utilized

3. Counseling regarding medication side effects, compliance, follow-up and lifestyle modifications

4. Consult physician when instituting pharmacologic therapy and when patient does not respond to first-line pharmacotherapy

Coronary Artery Disease (C.A.D.)

- Definition: Clinical syndrome also known as angina pectoris that occurs from atherosclerotic changes to the coronary vasculature; the result is decreased blood flow through vessels either due to partial obstruction (sclerosis) or vasospasm (may happen in a nonsclerotic vessel); when tissue ischemia and pain occurs as a result of decreased blood flow, angina occurs

- Etiology/Incidence

1. Hypertension (2 times greater risk than general population)

2. Tobacco use (2 to 3 times greater risk than general population)

3. Total serum cholesterol > 260 mg/dL (2 times greater risk than general population)

4. Diabetes mellitus (2 times greater risk than non-diabetic population)

5. Family history with a first degree relative (2 to 5 times greater risk than general population)

6. Sedentary lifestyle

7. Use of oral contraceptives

8. Gender prevalence depends upon age

    a. Overall more prevalent in men by a 4:1 ratio

    b. Under age 40, ratio is 8:1

    c. Over age 70, ratio is 1:1

9. Obesity

10. Personality type is less certain risk factor

- Types of Angina

    1. Exertional—occurs with activity, generally subsides with rest

    2. Variant threshold occurs at various times, including rest

    3. Prinzmetal's angina occurs only at rest

        a. Chest pain occurs without the usual precipitating factors

        b. Often affects women under age of 50

        c. Characteristically occurs in early morning, awakening patient from sleep

        d. Tends to involve right coronary artery

- Signs and Symptoms

    1. Characteristic chest discomfort

        a. Sensation of tightness, squeezing, burning, pressure

        b. 80% to 90% of cases discomfort is felt behind or slightly to the left of the mid-sternum

        c. Radiates most often to left shoulder and upper arm, traveling down inner aspect of arm to elbow, forearm, wrist, and fourth or fifth finger

   d. May be felt in lower jaw, back of neck, or upper left side of back

   e. Typically lasts 15 to 20 minutes, may resolve more quickly but usually lasts at least several minutes; pain lasting > 30 minutes is unstable angina

2. Anxiety

3. Dyspnea

- Differential Diagnosis

   1. Gastroesophageal reflux (heartburn)

   2. Anxiety

   3. Depression

   4. Costrochondral pain

   5. Pneumothorax

   6. Congestive heart failure

   7. Pneumonia

   8. Pericarditis

   9. Asthma

   10. Aortic dissection

   11. Myocardial infarction

- Physical Findings

   1. Systolic and diastolic blood pressures usually elevated during attack

   2. May hear apical systolic murmur due to transient mitral regurgitation

   3. Transient S_3 and/or S_4 not uncommon

   4. May detect signs of disease that contribute to or accompany C.A.D.

      a. Diabetes mellitus

      b. Hypertension

      c. Aortic stenosis

      d.   Hypertrophic cardiomyopathy

      e.   Mitral valve prolapse

5.   Pulse and respirations may be elevated

6.   May see tobacco stained teeth or fingers

7.   May see signs of peripheral artery disease

      a.   Diminished distal pulses

      b.   Pale skin

      c.   Poor hair growth

8.   Levin's sign (clenched fist over sternum) highly suggestive of angina

9.   May not have any remarkable physical findings

- Diagnostic Tests/Findings

1.   Serum lipid levels—LDL cholesterol must be lowered to < 100 mg/dL

2.   The electrocardiogram (ECG)

      a.   Normal in 25% patients with angina

      b.   Characteristic finding is down sloping of S-T segment or T wave peak or inversion during attack; reverses after attack

      c.   May show signs of old myocardial infarction or hypertrophy

3.   Exercise electrocardiography (stress testing)

      a.   Ischemic changes or angina during exercise test—clinically diagnostic

      b.   Markedly positive test is any one of the following

         (1)   S-T segment depression after start of exercise

         (2)   > 2 mm of new S-T segment depression in multiple leads

         (3)   New S-T segment elevation

         (4)   Decreased systolic blood pressure with exercise

         (5)   Development of heart failure with exercise

         (6)   Inability to exercise for > 2 minutes

       (7)   Prolonged interval after exercise for return to normal ECG

  4. Nuclear medicine studies to evaluate presence, location and extent of coronary disease

     a. Exercise thallium imaging

       (1)   Especially useful in patients with pre-existing ECG abnormalities and patients taking digoxin

       (2)   Areas of diminished uptake indicate hypoperfusion

       (3)   Should be conducted at experienced center

     b. Radionuclide ventriculography

       (1)   Images left ventricle and measures ejection fraction

       (2)   Resting abnormalities represent infarction

       (3)   Abnormalities with exercise indicate stress induced ischemia

     c. Coronary angiography

       (1)   Definitive test for diagnosis of C.A.D.

       (2)   Indicated in high risk patients

          (a)   With refractory unstable angina

          (b)   With spontaneous or exercise induced ischemia after myocardial infarction

- Management/Treatment (see Table 1)

  1. Treatment of acute attack

     a. Sublingual or buccal spray nitroglycerin

     b. Dose may be repeated three times at five minute intervals

     c. Pain unrelieved after three doses is unstable and should be evaluated in emergency room

  2. Prevention of further attacks

     a. Reduction of risk factors when possible

       (1)   Weight reduction

       (2)   Smoking cessation

       (3)   Exercise program

  b. Lowering LDL cholesterol to < 100 mg/dL is of paramount importance

       (1)   If LDL cholesterol is between 100 to 160 mg/dL—diet modification program may be implemented

       (2)   If LDL cholesterol is > 160 mg/dL or remains > 130 mg/dL after three months of diet modification—pharmacologic therapy should be instituted

          (a)   Nicotinic acid

          (b)   Bile acid binding resins

          (c)   Hydroxymethylglutaryl co-enzyme A (HMG CoA) reductase inhibitors

          (d)   All patients whose risk for CAD warrants pharmacologic therapy should also take aspirin daily

  c. Beta-blockers prevent angina by reducing myocardial oxygen requirements

       (1)   Metoprolol 50 to 200 mg daily in two divided doses

       (2)   Atenolol 25 to 200 mg once daily

       (3)   Major contraindications are bronchospastic disease, bradydysrhythmias, and heart failure

  d. Calcium channel blockers prevent angina by reducing myocardial oxygen demand and inducing coronary vasodilation

       (1)   Nifedipine 30 to 120 mg daily

       (2)   Verapamil 180 to 480 mg in one or two doses daily

       (3)   Diltiazem 360 mg in two daily doses

  e. Long acting nitrates prevent angina by inducing coronary vasodilation

       (1)   Isosorbide dinitrate 10 to 40 mg three times daily

       (2)   Sustained release nitroglycerin 6.25 to 25 mg daily in two to four divided doses

  f. Coronary revascularization is indicated in the following:

Table 1

TREATMENT ALGORITHM FOR STABLE ANGINA

History of heart failure or ejection fraction < 35%?

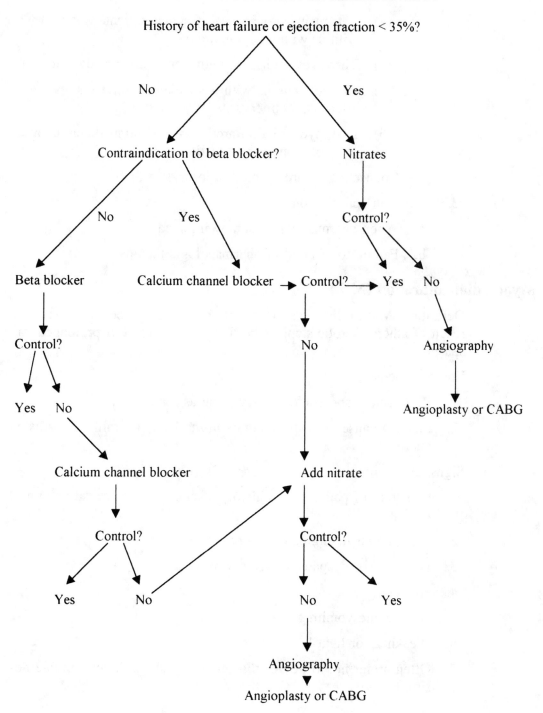

(1) Unacceptable symptoms despite medical therapy to its tolerable limits

(2) Left main coronary artery stenosis greater than 50% with or without symptoms

(3) Three vessel disease with left ventricular dysfunction

(4) Unstable angina with ischemia on exercise stress test after symptom control

(5) Post myocardial infarction with continued angina or ischemia on noninvasive testing

    g. Counseling regarding medication side effects

3. Physician consultation

    a. When pharmacologic therapy initiated

    b. Failure to respond to pharmacologic therapy

Myocardial Infarction (M.I.)

- Definition: Myocardial necrosis due to inadequate blood flow, usually a result of atherosclerotic stenosis but may be the result of prolonged vasospasm

- Etiology/Incidence

    1. Risk factors and epidemiology same as for C.A.D.

    2. Leading cause of death in adults in the U.S.; 1.5 million deaths annually

- Signs and Symptoms

    1. One-third of patients give history of alteration in typical pattern of angina

    2. Pain similar to angina but more severe

    3. Diaphoresis, dyspnea, cough and wheeze

    4. Anxiety

    5. Nausea and vomiting

    6. Weakness or light-headedness

    7. Often prefer not to lie quietly—continuously seek comfortable position

8. Women may present with atypical symptoms, i.e., burning sensation in chest, indigestion, weakness

- Differential Diagnosis

    1. Angina

    2. Gastroesophageal reflux

    3. Pulmonary embolus

    4. Costochondral pain

    5. Pericarditis

    6. Dissecting aortic aneurysm

    7. Anxiety

- Physical Findings

    1. Heart rate may range from bradycardia to tachycardia

    2. Dysrhythmias common

    3. Low grade fever may appear after 12 hours and persist for several days

    4. S_4 and murmur of mitral regurgitation common

    5. S_3 less common—when present indicates severe left ventricular dysfunction

    6. Blood pressure may be elevated or abnormally low

    7. May see findings consistent with heart failure; jugular vein distention, rales

    8. Cyanosis and cold temperature indicate low cardiac output

- Diagnostic Tests/Findings

    1. ECG is essential—most patients have ECG changes

        a. Convex S-T segment elevation with peaked upright or inverted T waves indicative of acute M.I.

        b. S-T segment depression may indicate non-Q-wave M.I.

        c. Development of Q waves generally considered diagnostic of M.I.

    2. Leukocytosis 10,000 to 20,000/μL on second day

3. Cardiac isoenzymes progressively increase as necrosis evolves

    a. Creatine kinase-muscle brain (CK-MB) increases within 4 to 6 hours of pain onset, peaks in 10 to 20 hours, returns to baseline in 36 to 48 hours

    b. Lactic dehydrogenase (LDH) elevations detectable 12 hours after pain onset, peak in 24 to 48 hours, and remain elevated for 10 to 14 days—LDH_1: LDH_2 ratio > 1.0 consistent with M.I.

    c. Troponin T and Troponin I demonstrate high specificity and sensitivity and remain elevated for 5 to 7 days post M.I.

4. Echocardiography for assessment of cardiac wall motion and valvular/structural defects post M.I.

5. Technetium 99 pyrophosphate scintigraphy used in diagnosis of M.I. for patients hospitalized late in the course

6. Radionuclide ventriculography allows assessment of regional wall motion and ejection fraction

7. Coronary angiography is definitive test to visualize the coronary vasculature

- Management/Treatment: Immediate hospitalization

1. Immediate goals are to provide oxygen, relieve pain, and treat dysrhythmia

    a. Oxygen by nasal cannula, face mask, or endotracheal tube

    b. Morphine sulfate 2 to 4 mg at 5 to 10 minute intervals p.r.n.

    c. Nitroglycerin sublingual or intravenously

    d. Heparin 5,000 unit bolus followed by intravenous infusion

    e. Chewable aspririn 160 mg

    f. Treat dysrhythmia as indicated

2. Thrombolytics to reperfuse coronary arteries within 4 to 6 hours of pain onset

    a. Evaluate for contraindications i.e., bleeding disorders, recent surgery

    b. Tissue plasminogen activator (tPA)

    c. Streptokinase

3. Percutaneous transluminal coronary artery angioplasty (PTCA)

4. Other medications have varying levels of effectiveness in the acute setting

   a. Beta blockers

   b. Calcium channel blockers

   c. ACE inhibitors

5. Patient education regarding cardiac rehabilitation and risk factor reduction

6. Physician consultation when acute M.I. suspected

Congestive Heart Failure (C.H.F.)

- Definition: Clinical syndrome that results when cardiac output is insufficient to meet metabolic demands of body; any condition that affects heart rate or contractile function can precipitate C.H.F.

- Etiology/Incidence

   1. Acute myocardial infarction; dysrhythmia

   2. Chronic hypertension

   3. Valvular stenosis or regurgitation

   4. Cardiomyopathy

   5. Medication toxicity

   6. 2,000,000 estimated cases in the U.S.—400,000 new cases diagnosed annually

- Types of C.H.F.

   1. Acute

      a. Abrupt onset usually follows acute M.I. or valve rupture

      b. Also known as "left sided failure"

      c. Symptoms are produced by acute diffusion of water into the pulmonary air spaces

   2. Chronic

      a. Develops as a result of inadequate compensatory mechanisms that have been employed over time to improve cardiac output

      b.   Also known as "right sided failure"

      c.   Symptoms are produced by increased hydrostatic pressure in the venous system and subsequent diffusion of water into the interstitium

   3.   Systolic—contractile dysfunction results in decreased cardiac output

   4.   Diastolic—inability to relax and fill with blood results in decreased cardiac output

- Signs and Symptoms

   1.   Acute C.H.F.

      a.   Dyspnea at rest

      b.   Frothy cough worse in the recumbent position

      c.   Feeling of anxiety and/or impending doom

   2.   Chronic C.H.F.

      a.   Dyspena on exertion; easily fatigued

      b.   Chronic non-productive cough

      c.   Abdominal fullness

      d.   Weight gain

      e.   Paroxysmal nocturnal dyspnea

      f.   Oliguria, nocturia

      g.   Peripheral cyanosis

- Differential Diagnosis

   1.   Acute M.I.

   2.   Pulmonary embolus

   3.   Pneumonia

   4.   Asthma

   5.   Chronic venous insufficiency

- Physical Findings

   1.   Acute

      a.   Coarse rales over all lung fields

      b.   Wheezing over all lung fields

      c. S_3 gallop very common

      d.   Appears generally healthy except for the acute event

      e.   Systolic murmur of mitral regurgitation

      f.   Usually no edema or systemic signs of fluid overload

2.   Chronic

      a.   Lungs may be clear or may exhibit rales at the bases

      b.   Dependent edema

      c.   Appears chronically ill

      d.   Jugular venous distention

      e.   Hepatosplenomegaly

      f.   Point of maximal impulse displaced to the left

      g.   Diffuse anterior chest wall heave

      h. S_3 and/or S_4

      i.   Any variety of stenotic or regurgitant murmurs

- Diagnostic Tests/Findings

1.   Acute

      a.   Hypoxemia and hypocapnia on arterial blood gas

      b.   Serum multichemical analysis (SMA) 7 (sodium, potassium, chloride, carbon dioxide, blood urea nitrogen, creatinine, and glucose) usually normal

      c.   Urinalysis usually normal

      d.   Chest radiograph shows pulmonary edema, Kerley's lines, effusions

      e.   Echocardiogram will show contractile, relaxation, and valve function

2.   Chronic

      a.   SMA 7 may show electrolyte abnormalities

      b.   Mild hypoxemia on arterial blood gas—pCO_2 usually normal

      c.   Chest radiograph shows redistribution of flow, enlarged heart

        d.   Echocardiogram will show contractile, relaxation, and valve function

- Management/Treatment

   1. Of primary importance is identification and treatment of underlying cause

   2. Nonpharmacologic

        a.   Sodium/fluid restriction

        b.   Rest/activity balance

        c.   Weight reduction in the obese

   3. Pharmacologic

        a.   Angiotensin converting enzyme (ACE) inhibitors

            (1)   Captopril 6.25 to 50 mg three to four times daily

            (2)   Enalapril 2.5 to 40 mg daily in two divided doses

            (3)   Lisinopril 2.5 to 10 mg daily

        b.   Diuretics

            (1)   Hydrochlorothiazide 12.5 to 25 mg daily

            (2)   Furosemide 20 to 160 mg daily in one or two daily doses

        c.   Inotropic

            (1)   Beneficial in mild to moderate systolic failure

            (2)   Digoxin 0.125 to 0.25 mg daily

        d.   Calcium channel blockers

            (1)   Beneficial in mild to moderate diastolic failure

            (2)   Nicardipine 20 to 40 mg b.i.d.

        e.   Vasodilators—useful as adjunct therapy in heart failure refractory to initial therapies

   4. Patient counseling

        a.   Lifestyle modification

        b.   Medication toxicities and side effects

   5. Physician consultation

a. When pharmacologic therapy initiated

b. When patient unresponsive to initial medications

Arteriosclerotic Occlusive Disease

- Definition: Narrowing and eventual obstruction of the arterial lumen usually caused by atherosclerosis; occlusion tends to be segmental; result is decreased blood supply to limbs

- Etiology/Incidence: Same as those for coronary artery disease

- Signs and Symptoms

  1. Intermittent claudication usually presenting symptom

  2. Distance patient can walk is indicative of degree of circulatory impairment

  3. Cold and/or numbness of the extremity

  4. Pain or ache at night/rest suggestive of severe disease

- Differential Diagnosis

  1. Sciatica

  2. Myopathies

  3. Acute arterial emboli

- Physical Findings

  1. Reduced or absent pulses distal to obstruction

  2. Dependent rubor

  3. Skin pallor or cyanosis

  4. Poor hair/nail growth

  5. Dry ulceration/gangrene in severe disease

- Diagnostic Tests/Findings

  1. Radiography of affected extremity may show calcification

  2. Doppler ultrasound will demonstrate reduced pressures distal to occlusion

  3. Arteriography will show location and extent of block

- Management/Treatment
  1. Control risk factors as possible
  2. Walk daily to develop collateral circulation—walking to point of pain followed by a three minute rest should be done eight times daily
  3. Aspirin 80 to 325 mg has theoretical value and should be given to all patients with severe disease
  4. Surgical revascularization

Thrombophlebitis

- Definition: Partial or complete occlusion of a vein by a thrombus with secondary inflammation of venous wall—may be superficial or deep
- Etiology/Incidence
  1. Trauma, particularly if venous stasis present
  2. Venous stasis
  3. Prolonged bedrest
  4. Hypercoagulation states
  5. Use of oral contraceptives (particularly in smokers)
  6. Post-operative period
  7. More prevalent in females
- Signs and Symptoms
  1. Sudden onset of pain (superficial)
  2. Pain, tenderness, ache, or tightness especially with activity (deep)
- Differential Diagnosis
  1. Muscle strain or contusion
  2. Cellulitis
  3. Arterial disease
  4. Lymphatic obstruction
- Physical Findings
  1. Localized heat and erythema (superficial)
  2. Edema distal to occlusion (deep)

3. Distention of superficial venous collateral vessels

4. Low grade temperature

5. Cool skin

6. Palpable cords

- Diagnostic Tests/Findings

    1. Doppler ultrasound and impedance plethysmography to evaluate venous flow

    2. Contrast venography is definitive study to identify location and extent

- Management/Treatment

    1. Elevation of extremity and warm compress (superficial)

    2. Bedrest with extremity elevated (deep)

    3. Anticoagulation therapy for deep thrombosis

        a. Heparin infusion for 7 to 10 days

        b. Coumadin therapy for 12 weeks

        c. Consult physician when anticoagulation initiated

Chronic Venous Insufficiency

- Definition: Impaired venous return with resultant chronic lower extremity edema

- Etiology/Incidence

    1. Destruction of valves in deep venous channels of lower legs secondary to deep thrombophlebitis

    2. Neoplastic obstruction of pelvic veins

    3. Leg trauma

    4. Sustained elevation of venous pressure

    5. More common in women than men

- Signs and Symptoms

    1. Aching of lower extremities relieved by elevation

    2. Edema at end of day or after prolonged standing

    3. Night cramps

- Differential Diagnosis

    1. Lymphedema

    2. Congestive heart failure

    3. Renal disease

    4. Liver disease

- Physical Findings

    1. Edema of lower extremities

    2. Trophic changes with brownish discoloration

    3. Cool to touch

    4. Thin, shiny, atrophic skin

    5. Wet ulcerations on the medial or anterior aspect of the leg

- Diagnostic Tests/Findings

    1. BUN/creatinine to rule out renal disease

    2. Liver function tests to rule out liver disease

    3. Chest radiograph to rule out congestive heart failure

    4. Doppler ultrasound to rule out thrombosis

- Management/Treatment

    1. Bedrest with legs elevated to diminish chronic edema

    2. Use of elastic stockings

    3. Weight reduction in the obese

    4. Hydrocortisone cream for stasis dermatitis

Questions
Select the best answer

1. When is it appropriate to diagnose and treat hypertension based upon one blood pressure?

    a. When there is a strong family history
    b. When the diastolic pressure is > 100 mm Hg
    c. When there is end organ damage
    d. When there is suboccipital headache

2. Which of the following is not a cause of secondary hypertension?

    a. Sympathetic nervous system hypersensitivity
    b. Renal vascular disease
    c. Pheochromocytoma
    d. Coarctation of the aorta

3. What is the percentage of Caucasian adults afflicted with hypertension?

    a. < 10%
    b. 10-15%
    c. 20-30%
    d. > 50%

4. The patient with chronic hypertension presents with lower extremity edema, abdominal pain and fatigue. Physical exam findings reveal a diffuse chest wall heave and displaced point of maximal impulse. This makes you suspicious that the patient has:

    a. Biventricular hypertrophy
    b. Renal vascular stenosis
    c. Hypertensive encephalopathy
    d. Malignant hypertension

5. Which of the following endocrine disorders is not a cause of secondary hypertension?

    a. Cushing's syndrome
    b. Diabetes mellitus
    c. Hyperthyroidism
    d. Addison's disease

6. Pharmacologic therapy should be started in any patient who is diagnosed with

hypertension and has end organ damage. The most widely used antihypertensive medications are:

   a. Beta blockers
   b. Calcium channel blockers
   c. Diuretics
   d. Angiotensin converting enzyme inhibitors

7. Which of the following medications is more effective in Caucasians than other races in the treatment of hypertension?

   a. Lisinopril 5 mg p.o. q.d.
   b. Furosemide 20 mg p.o. q.d.
   c. Metoprolol 50 mg p.o. b.i.d.
   d. Diltiazem 90 mg p.o. b.i.d.

8. Which of the following risk factors puts a client at greatest risk for coronary artery disease?

   a. Stage 3 hypertension
   b. Serum cholesterol of 300 mg/dL
   c. A parent with history of myocardial infarction
   d. Type I diabetes mellitus

9. Prinzmetal's angina typically occurs:

   a. During periods of emotional stress
   b. Early in the morning
   c. In men under age 50
   d. In extremes of temperature

10. Your patient complains of chest pain just to the left of the mid-sternal area that occurred while mowing the lawn. As you pursue the history of present illness in an effort to rule out angina, which of the following characteristics of the pain experience makes angina less likely?

   a. The pain was also felt in the back of the neck
   b. The pain felt like a burning sensation
   c. The pain lasted 15 minutes
   d. The pain was a stabbing, knife like sensation

11. Aortic stenosis can be a contributing cause of coronary artery disease. Which of the following heart sounds is suggestive of aortic stenosis?

a. A systolic murmur loudest at the second intercostal space, right sternal border

b. A diastolic murmur loudest at the second intercostal space, left sternal border

c. An extra heart sound heard early in diastole

d. An extra heart sound heard early in systole

12. Exercise electrocardiography (ECG) is clinically diagnostic for coronary artery disease. Which of the following is not a positive finding on exercise ECG?

   a. > 2 mm of new S-T segment depression in multiple leads
   b. Decreased systolic blood pressure with exercise
   c. S-T segment depression after start of exercise
   d. Inability to exercise for > 5 minutes

13. You diagnosed coronary artery disease in Mrs. J. three months ago. At that time her LDL cholesterol was 160 mg/dL, and so your teaching interventions included ways to lower fat in her diet. Today her LDL cholesterol is 125 mg/dL. The most appropriate intervention is to:

   a. Begin lovastatin 10 mg q.d. and re-evaluate in one month
   b. Continue diet modification and re-evaluate in three months
   c. Begin enteric coated aspirin 325 mg q.d. and re-evaluate in one month
   d. Begin cholestyramine 12 gm b.i.d. and re-evaluate in three months

14. Which of the following pharmacological agents prevents angina by reducing myocardial oxygen demand and inducing coronary vasodilation?

   a. Diltiazem
   b. Isosorbide dinitrate
   c. Atenolol
   d. Aspirin

15. Mr. L. is a 64-year-old patient with difficult to control angina. His initial therapy was atenolol 25 mg q.d., and increased until his dose was 200 mg daily. When angina persisted diltiazem 180 mg b.i.d. was added to the regimen, but even the combination of medications is not controlling symptoms. At this point the next appropriate step would be to:

   a. Recommend cardiac angiography
   b. Begin nifedipine 30 mg q.d.
   c. Begin isosorbide dinitrate 10 mg. t.i.d.
   d. Recommend radionucleide ventriculography

16. Patients having a myocardial infarction (M.I.) may report that the chest pain they are experiencing is different from their usual anginal pain. Which of the following is also suspicious for M.I. rather than angina?

    a. Pain lasting > 15 minutes
    b. Nausea and vomiting
    c. Elevated systolic blood pressure
    d. Presence of S_3 or S_4 heart sounds

17. Which of the following diagnostic findings is most suggestive of myocardial infarction?

    a. 15,000/μL leukocytes
    b. Development of Q waves
    c. LDH 500 U/L
    d. S-T segment depression

18. Acute congestive heart failure produces symptoms as a function of the diffusion of water into the pulmonary air spaces. Acute failure is most commonly caused by:

    a. Chronic hypertension
    b. Valvular stenosis
    c. Medication toxicity
    d. Myocardial infarction

19. When increased hydrostatic pressure in the venous system causes water to diffuse into the interstitium, resultant physical findings would most likely include:

    a. Weight gain
    b. S_3 gallop
    c. Coarse rales in all lung fields
    d. Dyspnea at rest

20. Kerley's lines on chest radiography are suggestive of:

    a. Inadequate compensatory mechanisms when cardiac output fails
    b. Hydrostatic pressure increase in the peripheral vascular system
    c. Diffusion of water into pulmonary air spaces
    d. Prinzmetal's angina

21. Congestive heart failure is a syndrome that results when the cardiac output is insufficient to meet the metabolic demands of the body. This can be either an acute or chronic state. Causes of chronic failure include:

a. Hypertension
b. Mitral valve rupture
c. Myocardial infarction
d. Cardiac ischemia

22. Typical laboratory findings in acute C.H.F. include:

a. Red blood cells in urinalysis
b. Blood urea nitrogen (BUN) 70mg/dL; serum creatinine 2.0 mg/dL
c. PaO_2 64 mm Hg by arterial blood gas
d. Redistribution of flow by chest radiography

23. Calcium channel blockers may be useful therapy in congestive heart failure when:

a. Failure is due to the inability of the ventricle to relax
b. Failure is severe and refractory to digoxin
c. Failure is due to cardiomyopathy
d. Failure is severe and refractory to vasodilators

24. Dependent rubor is a physical finding associated with:

a. Chronic venous insufficiency
b. Arteriosclerotic occlusive disease
c. Deep vein thrombosis
d. Superficial thrombophlebitis

25. Which of the following physical findings is not associated with thrombophlebitis?

a. Low grade temperature
b. Cool skin
c. Heat and erythema
d. Reduced or absent peripheral pulses

26. Edema of the lower extremities is a physical finding associated with a variety of medical conditions. A diagnosis of chronic venous insufficiency is made when other causes are ruled out. When chronic venous insufficiency is diagnosed, the appropriate treatment includes:

a. Heparin infusion for 7-10 days
b. Use of elastic stockings
c. Aspirin 325 mg daily
d. Surgical revascularization

27. Which of the following blood pressures would be classified as stage 2?

 a. 170/100 mm Hg
 b. 180/95 mm Hg
 c. 200/110 mm Hg
 d. 146/98 mm Hg

Answers

1. c	10. d	19. a
2. a	11. a	20. c
3. b	12. d	21. a
4. a	13. b	22. c
5. d	14. a	23. a
6. c	15. c	24. b
7. a	16. b	25. d
8. c	17. b	26. b
9. b	18. d	27. a

Bibliography

Donaldson, M. C., & Olin, J. W. (1996). Peripheral arterial disease: 5 steps to a better outcome. *Patient Care, 30*(1), 224-6, 226, 231.

Eftychiou, V. (1996). Clinical diagnosis and management of the patient with deep vein thrombophlebitis and acute pulmonary embolism. *Nurse Practitioner: American Journal of Primary Health Care, 21*(3), 50, 52, 58.

Khan, M. G. (1996). *Heart disease diagnosis and therapy: A practical approach.* Baltimore, MD: Williams & Wilkins.

Mancia, G., & van Zweiten, P. A. (1996). How safe are calcium channel antagonists in hypertension and coronary heart disease? *Journal of Hypertension, 14*(1), 13-7.

Massie, B. M., & Amiden, T. A. (1998). Heart. In L.M. Tierney, Jr., S. J. McPhee, & M. A. Papadakis (Eds.). *Current medical diagnosis and treatment* (37th ed., pp. 333-428). Stamford, CT: Appleton & Lange.

McGovern, P. G., Pankow, J. S., Shahar, E., Doliszny, K. M., Folsom, A. R., Blackburn, H., & Luepker, R. V. (1996). Recent trends in acute coronary heart disease and mortality, morbidity, medical care and risk factors. *New England Journal of Medicine, 334*(14), 884-901.

Miller, S. K. (1997). Clinical assessment and pharmacologic management of congestive heart failure in the acute and chronic phases. *Advance for Nurse Practitioners, 5*(6), 16-26.

National Heart, Lung, and Blood Institute. (1997). The sixth report of the Joint National Committee on Detection, Evaluation and Treatment of High Blood Pressure, (DHHS) (NIH Publication No. 98-4080). Bethesda, MD: National Institutes of Health.

Peters, S. (1997). On the trail of a killer: New developments in heart disease. *Advance for Nurse Practitioners, 5*(5), 45-49.

Sadowski, A. V., & Redeker, N. S. (1996). The hypertensive elder: A review for the primary care provider. *Nurse Practitioner: American Journal of Primary Health Care, 21*(5), 99-100, 105-12.

Hematological and Oncological Disorders

Sister Maria Salerno

Common Anemias

Anemia describes a symptom of abnormally low red blood cell count, quality of hemoglobin, and/or volume of packed cells. The World Health Organization defines it in terms of peripheral blood hemoglobin < 13.0 grams(g) [hematocrit < 42%] for men and < 12.0 grams [hematocrit < 36%] for women. Anemias are classified on the basis of red cell morphology (microcytic, normocytic, or macrocytic) and amount of pigment they contain (hypochromic, normochromic), or the etiology.

Microcytic Anemias (MCV < $80\mu^3$)

Iron Deficiency Anemia

- Definition: A microcytic, hypochromic anemia with a mean corpuscular volume (MCV) < $80\mu^3$ caused by insufficient iron for hemoglobin synthesis; may be normocytic, normochromic in early stage

- Etiology/Incidence

   1. Inadequate iron intake (< 1 to 2 mg/day), e.g., infants on milk only diets, persons on vegetarian diets, alcoholics, pregnant women or adolescents whose demand is increased

   2. Impaired absorption of iron, e.g., after gastrectomy, in Celiac disease

   3. Slow, persistent blood loss, e.g., menorrhagia, gastritis, aspirin ingestion, polyps, GI neoplasms, peptic ulcer disease, esophageal varices, hemorrhoids; in adult males and postmenopausal females acute or chronic hemorrhage is most common cause

   4. One of the most common anemias throughout the world; particularly prevalent in women of childbearing age; estimated 20% of adult women, 50% of pregnant women, and 3% of adult males in the U.S. have iron deficiency

- Signs and Symptoms

   1. Depend on:

      a. Rate at which anemia develops

      b. Age of the individual

      c. Individual's compensatory mechanisms

    d. Activity level

    e. Underlying disease state

    f. Severity of the anemia

  2. General signs and symptoms

    a. Easily fatigued

    b. Dyspnea on exertion

    c. Dizziness

    d. Listlessness

    e. Pallor (conjunctiva, nail beds, mucous membranes)

    f. Faintness

    g. Weakness

    h. Headaches

    i. Tachycardia

    j. Wide pulse pressure

    k. Heart murmurs

    l. Myocardial hypertrophy

    m. Angina

    n. Anorexia

    o. Pica

- Differential Diagnosis

  1. Thalassemia

  2. Sideroblastic anemia

  3. Anemia of chronic disease

  4. Lead poisoning

- Physical Findings

  1. General appearance—pale, lethargic; no overt signs if anemia is mild

  2. Vital signs—pulse and respirations may be increased in moderate to severe anemia; in severe cases postural hypotension may be evident

3. Integumentary—pallor and dryness of skin and mucous membranes; brittle, flattened, ridged, concave, or spoon shaped nails (koilonychia); brittle, fine hair

4. HEENT—smooth, shiny, beefy-red appearance of the tongue with atrophy of the papillae; angular stomatitis or cheilitis; pale conjunctiva and gums

5. Cardiovascular—tachycardia, mild cardiac enlargement; functional systolic murmurs in severe anemias

6. Abdominal—may be some hepatic enlargement

7. Neurological—usually within normal limits; in severe anemia confusion may be evident

- Diagnostic Tests/Findings

    1. See Table 1 and 2 for laboratory tests used in diagnosis of common anemias

    2. Routine CBC (with peripheral smear)

        a. Hemoglobin— < 14 g/dL in males; < 12 g/dL in females

        b. Hct— < 42% in males; < 36% in females

        c. Low MCV (microcytic) and MCHC (hypochromic)

        d. Low erythrocyte count (RBC)

        e. Increased red cell distribution width (RDW)

    3. Iron status determinants—serum ferritin is considered the most sensitive and most specific for iron deficiency; bone marrow studies are done if the diagnosis is unclear and/or there is a lack of response to a three week therapeutic trial

        a. High total iron binding capacity (TIBC)—usually normal or low in anemia of chronic disease (ACD)

        b. Low serum ferritin < 12 μg/L—infection, chronic disease, and liver disease may raise ferritin levels and mask coexisting iron deficiency; in these cases a serum ferritin level < 30 μg/L is consistent with iron deficiency

        c. Serum iron—low < 50 μg/dL; may be normal in early stages (oral contraceptives may cause false elevation)

Table 1

Common Laboratory Tests Used in Diagnosing Anemia

Hematocrit (Hct)	Relative amount of plasma to total red blood cell mass; measure of RBC concentration. Normal 40-54% males; 38-47% females
Hemoglobin (Hgb)	Basic screening test for anemia. Main component of erythrocytes. Vehicle for transport of O_2 & CO_2 Normal 13.5-18 g/100 mL males; 12.0-15 g/100 mL females
Red Blood Cell Count (RBC)	Measure of number of Hgb carrying red blood cells (RBC, erythrocytes); needed to calculate other RBC indices
Mean Corpuscular Volume (MCV)	Mathematical measure of average RBC size; expressed in micro cubic millimeters; value classifies cells as microcytic, normocytic, macrocytic; normal $80\text{-}100\mu^3$
Mean Corpuscular Hgb (MCH)	Mathematical measure of hemoglobin concentration of average RBC; expressed in picograms; calculated by dividing Hgb in grams by number of RBC; allows for classification of RBC as hypochromic, normochromic; normal 27-31 pg/cell
Mean Corpuscular Hgb Concentration (MCHC)	Mathematical measure of concentration of Hgb in grams per 100 mL of RBC; normal 32-36 g/dL or 32%-36%; little help in identifying hypochromia or microcytosis
Red Cell Distribution width (RDW)	Mathematical coefficient of width variation in red cell size—RDW increase indicates greater variation in cell size
Serum Iron (SI)	Concentration of iron bound to transferrin; inverse correlation with TIBC; normal 50-150 μg/dL in adults; insensitive to early iron deficiency
Total Iron Binding Capacity (TIBC)	Measures amount of iron that transferrin can still bind; inverse correlation with serum iron; normal 250-450 μg/dL in adults
Bilirubin (indirect)	Fractionation of total bilirubin; reflects breakdown of hemoglobin; elevated levels indicate hemolysis
% Transferrin Saturation (% SAT)	100 X SI/TIBC; low sensitivity for iron deficiency Normal 20-50%
Serum Ferritin	Correlates roughly with total iron stores; no diurnal variation; not affected by exogenous ingestion or injection, or specimen contamination; most sensitive and specific for iron deficiency Normal males 16-300 μg/L; females 4-161 μg/L (Nicoll, 1998)
Coombs Indirect	Detects free antibodies in patient's serum and certain RBC antigens
Peripheral Blood Smear	Smear of whole blood stained with Wright's stain; variations in cell morphology and staining characteristics important to diagnosis of hematologic conditions
Bone Marrow	Marrow aspirated for microscopic examination; indicated when anemia not obviously due to iron deficiency; iliac crest preferred to sternum site

NOTE: Laboratory values differ in different labs. Check normals in laboratory where tests are conducted

Table 2

**Select Morphological and Etiologic Categories
of Anemia and Related Laboratory Findings**

	Macrocytic (MCV> 100)		Microcytic (MCV <80)		Normocytic (MCV 80-100)
	B_{12} Deficiency	*Folate Deficiency*	*Iron Deficiency*	*Thalassemia*	*Anemia of Chronic Disease*
Reticulocyte Ct	low	low	low	normal/sl. high	normal/low
MCH	normal	normal	low	low	normal
Fe	high	high	normal/low	normal/sl. high	low-high
TIBC	normal	normal	high	normal	normal/low
Bilirubin	sl. high	sl. high	normal	high	normal
Ferritin	high	high	low	normal	normal/high
B_{12}	low	normal	normal	normal	normal
Folate	normal	low	normal	normal/low	normal/low

      d.   Low serum transferrin saturation — < 20%

      e.   Bone marrow studies

         (1) Show depletion of iron (on staining), normocytic hyperplasia

         (2) Usually not part of initial work up

  4. Bilirubin—normal

• Management/Treatment

  1. Diagnostic

      a.   Once diagnosis is established underlying cause must be identified and if possible, corrected; bleeding must be suspected in the absence of clearly identifiable nutritional intake deficiency or increased body need

      b.   Search for infection, trauma, neoplasm, GI disorders

      c.   Stool guaiac, bilirubin, and additional studies may be needed to establish etiology

      d.   Obtain physician consult on any patient with:

         (1) Hct < 25%/dL

         (2) Positive stool guaiac or history of bleeding

       (3)   Family history of anemia

       (4)   Suspected underlying inflammatory, infectious, or malignant disease

       (5)   Failure to respond to iron supplementation

2. Therapeutic

   a.   Oral iron replacement

       (1)   Oral is safer and much less expensive than IM or IV

       (2)   Begin six month trial of ferrous sulfate tablets, 300 to 325 mg (depending on brand) three times a day after meals

       (3)   Determine effectiveness of iron replacement therapy during the first two weeks of therapy (increased reticulocyte count)

       (4)   Refer those on oral iron replacement therapy to a physician if 2 g/100 mL increase in Hgb is not seen in 3 to 4 weeks; in uncomplicated iron deficiency, a 1 g per week increase is expected

       (5)   Levels return to normal within two months, 3 to 6 months more needed to replace stores

       (6)   Response failure usually due to noncompliance

   b.   Parenteral iron is indicated if patient can not tolerate or absorb oral iron or if iron loss exceeds oral replacement; IM or IV iron dextran is used (very rarely used)

       (1)   More expensive

       (2)   Associated with significant side effects

          (a)   Anaphylaxis

          (b)   Phlebitis

          (c)   Regional adenopathy

          (d)   Serum-sickness type reaction

          (e)   Staining of IM injection sites

       (3)   Dose based on the patient's weight

3. Education

    a.   Cause of iron deficiency and treatment plan

    b.   Purpose, dosage, side effects, toxic effects of iron replacement

        (1)   Side effects of nausea, GI irritation, constipation, diarrhea, and black stools

        (2)   Food and fluid taken concurrently may interfere with absorption but may be warranted to alleviate gastric distress

        (3)   Taking with orange juice or other source of vitamin C (ascorbic acid) will enhance absorption

        (4)   Milk and antacids will interfere with absorption

        (5)   Monitor and discuss with patients concurrent use of over the counter medications—some products such as urine and stool deodorizers often used by elderly with incontinence problems can lead to iron overdose and heart failure

        (6)   Therapy should continue for six or more months to replenish tissue stores

    c.   Medication should be kept out of reach of children as iron overdose can be fatal to them

    d.   Nutrition—foods high in iron include organ and lean meats, egg yolk, shellfish, apricots, peaches, prunes, grapes, raisins, green leafy vegetables, iron fortified breads and cereals

    e.   Activity—frequent rest periods as needed

Thalassemia

- Definition: Thalassemia is a group of genetic inherited syndromes of abnormal hemoglobin synthesis

- Etiology/Incidence

    1.   Inherited, autosomal recessive disorder that results in impaired synthesis of either the alpha or beta chain of adult hemoglobin; four genes control alpha chain production, two control beta chain production

    2.   Second most common cause of microcytic anemia

    a. Alpha Thalassemia more common in Blacks, Chinese, Vietnamese, Cambodians, and Laotians

    b. Beta Thalassemia more common in those of Mediterranean descent (Italians, Greeks, some Arabs and Sephardic Jews)

  3. In U.S. more common than iron deficiency in African-Americans, Asian-Americans, and Italian-Americans

- Signs and Symptoms: The severity of the anemia can range from mild to severe depending on the number of hemoglobin controlling genes involved; forms seen in adults include:

  1. Alpha trait (carrier state) (1 of 4 alpha chain-forming genes affected)—usually asymptomatic

  2. Alpha-Thalassemia Minor (2 of 4 alpha chain-forming genes affected) and Beta-Thalassemia minor (heterozygous form)—both are usually asymptomatic and have mild presentations with mild to moderate microcytic, hypochromic anemia, enlarged liver and spleen, bronze coloring of the skin, and bone marrow hyperplasia

  3. Beta Thalassemia Major (homozygous form affecting both beta chain-forming genes) also called Cooley's anemia—severe anemia with significant cardiovascular burden; high output congestive failure is common; fractures related to bone marrow expansion; retarded growth and maturation; in addition to general signs and symptoms presented in section on Iron Deficiency Anemia

  4. Hemoglobin H disease (3 of 4 alpha hemoglobin chain-forming genes affected)—occurs predominantly in Chinese; moderate to severe microcytic anemia with splenomegaly

- Differential Diagnosis

  1. Iron deficiency anemia

  2. Sideroblastic anemia

  3. Anemia of chronic disease

  4. Lead poisoning—not common in adults unless occupation related

- Physical Findings: Will generally be within normal limits unless the more severe forms of thalassemia are encountered

  1. General appearance—pallor or bronze appearance; mild listlessness

  2. Abdominal—enlarged liver, enlarged spleen

3. Cardiovascular—tachycardia, widened pulse pressure, systolic murmur if anemia is moderate or severe

4. Respiratory—may have increased respiratory rate

5. Musculoskeletal—some bone deformity of the face (chipmunk deformity) related to expansion of bones caused by hyperplastic marrow

6. Neurologic—within normal limits

- Diagnostic Tests/Findings

  1. Hgb—decreased

  2. MCV—low

  3. Serum iron—normal or increased

  4. TIBC—normal

  5. Ferritin—normal or increased

  6. RDW—normal

  7. Reticulocyte count—may be normal or increased

  8. Hemoglobin electrophoresis—demonstrates decreased alpha or beta hemoglobin chains

  9. Peripheral smear will show microcytosis, variable hypochromia, target cells (thin, fragile RBC), basophilic stippling

  10. Skull and skeletal radiographs—widened marrow spaces in skull and long bones; osteoporosis

- Management/Treatment

  1. No specific treatment for mild to moderate forms

  2. Iron supplementation generally contraindicated in all thalassemias since iron overload can result—patients with alpha trait and co-existing iron deficiency should be referred to physician for iron supplementation

  3. Sometimes chronic folate supplementation is used

  4. Severe forms should be referred to a hematologist for treatment which often includes transfusions and chelation therapy to avoid fatal iron overload (hemochromatosis)

  5. Refer for genetic counseling

6. Stress overall good nutrition without additional iron supplementation

7. Discuss signs and symptoms of iron overload

   a. Weakness/lassitude

   b. Loss of body hair

   c. Weight loss

   d. Palmar erythema

   e. Gynecomastia

   f. Loss of libido

   g. Abdominal pain

   h. Thinning, darkening skin

   i. Pain and or stiffness in joints

   j. Blurred vision or other symptoms related to onset of diabetes

   k. Shortness of breath

   l. Swelling in ankles

8. Document findings to avoid

   a. Unnecessary repeated work-ups

   b. Inappropriate iron supplementation

Macrocytic Anemias (MCV > $100\mu^3$)

Pernicious Anemia

- Definition: A megaloblastic, macrocytic, normochromic anemia caused
  by a deficiency of intrinsic factor produced by the stomach which results
  in malabsorption of vitamin B_{12} necessary for DNA synthesis and maturation of RBC

- Etiology/Incidence

  1. Possibly due to an autoimmune reaction involving the gastric pari-
     etal cell that results in nonproduction of intrinsic factor and atrophy
     of gastric mucosa

  2. Can also occur secondary to other factors which lead to decreased
     production of intrinsic factor or decreased absorption of B_{12}

        a. Loss of parietal cells post-gastrectomy

        b. Overgrowth of intestinal organisms

        c. Ileal resection or abnormalities

        d. Fish tape worm

        e. Congenital enzyme deficiencies

    3. Common in Caucasians of Northern European descent

    4. Both sexes equally affected

    5. Usually presents around age 60

    6. Increased incidence in those with other immunologic disease

- Signs and Symptoms

    1. Weakness

    2. Sore tongue or glossitis

    3. Peripheral paresthesia—numbness, burning, tingling

    4. Palpitations

    5. Dizziness

    6. Swelling of legs

    7. Anorexia

    8. Diarrhea

    9. Mucositis

    10. Dementia and spinal cord degeneration in advanced stages

- Differential Diagnosis

    1. Folate deficiency

    2. Anemia of liver disease

    3. Myelodysplastic syndromes

- Physical Findings

    1. Vital signs—temperature may be slightly elevated, wide pulse pressure, pulse and respirations may be elevated if anemia is severe

    2. General appearance—premature aging; premature graying of hair

3. HEENT—smooth beefy red tongue; sclera and skin may be slightly icteric

4. Cardiovascular—systolic flow murmur, tachycardia, and cardiomegaly if anemia is severe

5. Abdomen—hepatomegaly and splenomegaly may be evident

6. Neurological—deep tendon reflexes increased or decreased; diminished position sense; poor or absent vibratory sense in lower extremities; ataxia; poor finger-nose coordination; positive Romberg and Babinski; mental status changes ranging from mild forgetfulness and irritability to psychotic behavior

- Diagnostic Tests/Findings

1. Hgb and Hct—decreased

2. RBC—decreased

3. Reticulocytes—normal or low

4. MCV—increased > 100 μ^3

5. MCHC—normal

6. Serum B_{12}—decreased < 100 pg/mL

7. Increased LDH

8. Serum folate and/or RBC level—normal or decreased

9. Serum bilirubin—increased

10. Urinalysis—increased urobilinogen

- Management/Treatment

1. Diagnostic—consult with physician regarding those:

    a. With other immunologic diseases

    b. With a history of B_{12} replacement

    c. Suspected of having pernicious anemia for further testing, e.g., those with neurological symptoms but without macrocytosis or overt anemia; might include:

        (1) GI radiographic studies

        (2) Gastric analysis—absence of free hydrochloric acid after histamine or pentagastrin injection

       (3) Bone marrow aspiration—hyperplastic, megaloblastic marrow

       (4) Schilling test (tests absorption of radiolabeled vitamin B_{12} both with and without administration of intrinsic factor on basis of 24 hour urine excretion) to distinguish between primary and secondary causes

  2. Therapeutic

    a. B_{12} (cyanocobalamin) 100 μg IM daily for 1 week; decrease frequency and administer a total of 2,000 μg during the first 6 weeks of therapy; maintenance treatment requires lifelong administration of 100 μg IM monthly

    b. In select cases, oral cobalamin in high doses (1,000 μg per day) can replace parenteral for maintenance, but must be taken daily and consistently

    c. If anemia is severe may need K^+ supplementation to avoid hypokalemia

    d. Follow up elderly and those with cardiovascular symptoms 48 hours after initiating therapy; rapid increase in RBC production can lead to hypervolemia in these persons

    e. Consider concomitant iron supplementation during first month of therapy; rapid blood cell regeneration increases iron requirement and may lead to iron deficiency

  3. Education

    a. Teach client about etiology and nature of the disease

    b. Discuss need for lifelong B_{12} replacement by injection

    c. Provide client with information on side effects of B_{12} injections

       (1) Pain and burning at injection site

       (2) Peripheral vascular thrombosis

       (3) Transient diarrhea

    d. CNS symptoms/signs are reversible if present < 6 months prior to treatment

    e. Teach client or family member to administer injections or refer to home care agency to provide injections

    f.   Teach comfort and safety measures to clients with neurological involvement (can be arrested but not reversed with treatment)

  4.   Follow-up—check initial hematologic response in 4 to 6 weeks; then every 6 months for Hct and stool for occult blood; endoscopy every 5 years; incidence of gastric cancer increased in persons with pernicious anemia

Folic Acid Deficiency Anemia

- Definition: Macrocytic, normochromic, megaloblastic anemia caused by a deficiency of folic acid needed for DNA synthesis, RBC maturation, and maintenance of gastric mucosa

- Etiology/Incidence

  1. Inadequate intake may be relative to malabsorption syndrome or increased demand as in pregnancy and infancy; body stores depleted more rapidly than B_{12}

  2. Drugs that may cause decreased folic acid levels include oral contraceptives, phenytoin, antimalarials, estrogen, chloramphenicol, phenobarbital; trimethoprim/sulfamethoxazole, and sulfasalazine

  3. Found in all races and in all age groups

  4. More common than pernicious anemia, especially in alcoholics and other chronically malnourished persons, e.g., anorexics, many elderly, and those who do not eat fresh fruits and vegetables (especially green leafy) or overcook them

- Signs and Symptoms

  1. Similar to those of B_{12} deficiency but more severe; neurological signs are absent

  2. General signs and symptoms

     a. Easily fatigued

     b. Dyspnea on exertion

     c. Dizziness

     d. Listlessness

     e. Pallor (conjunctiva, nail beds, mucous membranes)

     f. Faintness

     g. Weakness

     h. Headaches

     i. Tachycardia

     j. Wide pulse pressure

     k. Heart murmurs

     l. Myocardial hypertrophy

     m. Angina

     n. Anorexia

     o. Pica

- Differential Diagnosis

  1. Pernicious anemia

  2. Anemia of liver disease

  3. Myelodysplastic syndromes

- Physical Findings: Similar to those found in most anemias

  1. General appearance—pale, lethargic or no overt signs if anemia is mild

  2. Vital signs—pulse and respirations may be increased in moderate to severe anemia; in severe cases postural hypotension may be evident

  3. Integumentary—pallor and dryness of skin and mucous membranes; brittle nails; brittle, fine hair

  4. HEENT—glossitis, angular stomatitis or cheilitis; pale conjunctiva and gums

  5. Cardiovascular—tachycardia; mild cardiac enlargement; functional systolic murmurs in severe anemias

  6. Abdominal—may be some hepatic enlargement

  7. Neurological—usually within normal limits

- Diagnostic Tests/Findings

  1. Hct—decreased

  2. Reticulocyte count—normal or decreased

  3. MCV—elevated

4. MCHC—normal

5. RBC folate level— < 150 ng/mL and/or RBC level decreased

6. Serum folate— < 3 ng/mL; less reliable than RBC folate

7. Schilling test—normal

8. Serum B_{12}—normal

- Management/Treatment

  1. Diagnostic—consult with physician regarding clients with suspected folate deficiency for differential diagnosis of concurrent B_{12} deficiency and treatment

  2. Therapeutic—folate 1 mg orally or parenterally per day

     a. Duration of treatment dependent on etiology and its elimination

     b. If related to malabsorption (e.g., Sprue) up to 5 mg/day

     c. Large doses of folic acid will correct hematologic abnormalities of B_{12} deficiency but not arrest neurological abnormalities.

  3. Education—especially important for women of childbearing age as deficiency during first trimester is associated with neural tube defects in the fetus

     a. Nature and cause of anemia

     b. Need for and purpose of therapeutic replacement

     c. Teach dietary sources of folic acid which include asparagus, bananas, fish, green leafy vegetables, peanut butter, oatmeal, red beans, beef liver, wheat bran

        (1) Encourage daily intake from these foods

        (2) Instructions in preparation as overcooking can destroy folic acid

        (3) Provide client with list of foods high in folic acid

     d. Need for frequent rest periods until anemia is corrected

     e. Importance of good oral hygiene

  4. Follow-up

     a. Check initial hematologic response with Hct and reticulocyte count in 4 to 6 weeks

        (1)   Reticulocyte count should begin to increase within 2 to 3 days after therapy is begun and should peak in 5 to 7 days

        (2)   Hct begins to rise after the second week

        (3)   Total correction expected within 2 months

    b.   Individuals with a good response can be followed every 6 to 12 months if they must continue therapy

Normocytic Anemias (MCV 80–100 μ^3)

- Hypoproliferative—reticulocyte count normal or decreased < 3% secondary to decreased bone marrow production

- Hyperproliferative—reticulocyte count increased > 3% secondary to increased hemolysis or bleeding

Anemia of Chronic Disease (ACD)

- Definition: A chronic, normochromic, normocytic, hypoproliferative anemia associated with chronic inflammatory disease, e.g., systemic lupus, rheumatoid arthritis; infection, e.g., bacterial endocarditis, tuberculosis, AIDS, Crohn's disease, and some malignancies; *often progresses to a hypochromic anemia*

- Etiology/Incidence

  1. Etiology not fully understood but involves decreased erythrocyte life span, ineffective erythropoiesis, and disturbances of the iron cycle

  2. Most common cause of hypoproliferative, normocytic anemia

  3. Exact incidence unknown, however association with so many other disorders probably ranks it second to iron deficiency in incidence

- Sign and Symptoms

  1. General symptoms common to all anemias such as fatigue, weakness, exertional dyspnea, lightheadedness, and anorexia

  2. Usually fewer and milder than most other anemias

  3. Other signs and symptoms are usually related to the specific underlying disease and may be more overt than those of anemia

- Differential Diagnosis

1. Aplastic anemia

2. Pure red blood cell aplasia

3. Infiltration marrow diseases

4. Exclude reversible causes

- Physical Findings

  1. General appearance—may appear thin, pale, toxic

  2. Vital signs—increased pulse and respirations

  3. Skin—may be pale, jaundiced, moist

  4. HEENT—sclera may be icteric, tongue may be coated

  5. Cardiovascular—cardiomegaly, tachycardia, systolic murmurs

  6. Abdomen—splenomegaly, hepatomegaly

- Diagnostic Tests/Findings

  1. Hct—low

  2. Hgb—low (if < 9g/dL consider other causes)

  3. MCV—normal or slightly low

  4. Serum iron—low

  5. TIBC—normal or low

  6. Serum ferritin—normal or increased

  7. Percentage of iron saturation (FE/TIBC)—30% or more rules out iron deficiency

- Management/Treatment

  1. Treatment of associated disease

  2. Adequate nutritional intake; use of B_{12}, folic acid, and liver extract have not been effective in treatment of this type anemia

  3. Adequate rest

  4. Consult with physician regarding clients with suspected anemia of chronic disease for further testing (bone marrow biopsy), and treatment of underlying disorder

5. Education—patient education will most likely be centered on etiology and treatment of the underlying chronic disease and its relationship to anemia

6. Follow-up—will depend on identified etiology

Sickle Cell Anemia

- Definition: A chronic hemolytic anemia characterized by sickle-shaped RBC

- Etiology/Incidence

  1. Autosomal recessive genetic disorder; individual is homozygous for hemoglobin (Hb SS)

  2. Abnormal hemoglobin (Hb S) develops in place of hemoglobin A (Hb A)

  3. Some individuals may have *sickle cell trait* (heterozygous with about $\frac{1}{4}$ of their hemoglobin in abnormal S form and remainder as normal A

  4. Mutation that causes Hb S to develop involves one amino acid; one valine amino acid is substituted for a glutamic acid

  5. Prevalent in black persons of African or African-American ancestry; also found at a lower frequency in persons of Mediterranean ancestry

- Signs and Symptoms

  1. Sickle Cell Trait

     a. Essentially asymptomatic except in extreme conditions

     b. Symptoms from vaso-occlusion occur only in cases of severe hypoxia

  2. Sickle Cell Anemia

     a. Manifestations due to anemia, vaso-occlusive events, and to secondary end-organ damage:

        (1) Osteomyelitis

        (2) Retinopathy

        (3) Renal disease—hematuria

        (4) Cardiomegaly

       (5)   Nonpalable spleen in adults

  b. Increased susceptibility to infection

  c. Vaso-occlusive crises

       (1)   Due to an increased rate of sickling

       (2)   Precipitating factors include conditions that cause hypoxia or deoxygenation of the RBC, e.g., viral or bacterial infections, high altitudes, emotional or physical stress, surgery, blood loss, dehydration; occasionally crisis occurs spontaneously

       (3)   Episodes characterized by sudden onset of excruciating pain in back, chest, or extremities

       (4)   Occasionally low-grade fever may occur 1 to 2 days following attack

       (5)   Pain may last from hours to days

       (6)   Severe abdominal pain with vomiting may be present

- Differential Diagnosis

  1. Acute pulmonary infarction without sickle β thalassemia
  2. Acute hepatitis
  3. Choledocholithiasis
  4. Cholecystitis

- Physical Findings

  1. During vaso-occlusive crises, there may be no external findings such as heat, swelling or tenderness over the affected bones; if bone infarction occurs close to a joint an effusion can develop

  2. Chronic findings

     a. Skin ulcers/jaundice

     b. Mild scleral icterus; retinal hemorrhage or detachment, neovascularization

     c. Cardiomegaly, systolic murmur

     d. Hepatomegaly

     e. Degenerative arthritis

- Diagnostic Tests/Findings
    1. Peripheral smear
        a. Sickle Cell Trait—normal
        b. Sickle Cell Anemia—partially or completely sickled cells
    2. Sickle Cell preparation/Sickledex
        a. Sickle Cell Trait—sickle cells
        b. Sickle Cell Anemia—sickle cells
        c. Used for initial screening
        d. Can not differentiate between anemia/trait
    3. Hemoglobin electrophoresis
        a. Sickle Cell Trait—Hb S and Hb A
        b. Sickle Cell Anemia—Hb S
        c. Used for confirmation and discrimination between anemia/trait
- Management/Treatment
    1. Physician referral for suspected cases and consultation for management
    2. Therapeutic—primarily supportive
        a. Chronic folic acid supplementation
        b. Use of cytotoxic agents to reduce frequency of painful episodes
        c. Antibiotic prophylaxis
    3. In acute painful episodes
        a. Analgesia
        b. Large volume IV fluids
        c. Oxygen to treat hypoxia
        d. Antibiotics to treat associated bacterial infections
        e. Blood transfusions reserved for aplastic or hemolytic crises, and during third trimester of pregnancy
    4. Patient education

a. Basis of disease and reasons for supportive care

b. Methods to avoid crises

c. Pain control

d. Availability of support groups

5. Referral for genetic counseling of identified heterozygotes (sickle cell trait) and prenatal diagnostic services for pregnancies at risk for sickle cell anemia

Leukemia

- Definition: Acquired, neoplastic, myeloproliferative disorder of hematopoietic stem cells
- Etiology/Incidence
  1. In most cases no known cause can be found
  2. Possible causes include:
     a. Exposure to ionizing radiation and certain chemicals, e.g., benzene, prior exposure to alkylating agents
     b. Genetic and congenital factors
  3. Incidence of all leukemias is approximately 13 per 100,000/per year
  4. More frequent in males than females
- General features of the four common forms of leukemia are shown in Table 3
- Differential Diagnosis
  1. Viral induced cytopenia, lymphadenopathy
  2. Immune or drug-induced cytopenia
  3. Aplastic anemia
- Diagnostic Tests/Findings (see Table 3)
  1. CBC/differential—subnormal RBC, neutrophils and occasionally subnormal platelets
  2. Sedimentation rate—elevated
  3. Reticulocyte count— < 0.5
  4. Bone marrow studies—confirmatory for final diagnosis

Table 3

Comparison of Most Common Types of Leukemia

Type	Age of Onset	Signs & Symptoms Physical Findings	Diagnostic Tests/Findings	Prognosis
Acute Lymphocytic	Childhood More gradual rise in frequency in later life; 20% of acute adult	Fever; pallor; bleeding; anorexia; fatigue; generalized lymphadenopathy and infection, joint pain etc.	Cytopenia, pancytopenia WBC—H, L, or N RBC, Hgb, Hct-L Platelets-L Bone marrow-lymphoblasts	Good response to treatment 80% of adults have complete remission
Acute Myelogenous	Increase with age; 50% under age of 50	Fatigue; weakness; headache; mouth sores; bleeding; fever; sternal tenderness; occasional lymphadenopathy	RBC, Hgb, Hct-L Platelet ct—very low WBC—H to L Myeloblasts—many	Remission rates range from 50 to 85%; patients >50 years are less likely to achieve complete remission
Chronic Lymphocytic	Middle and old age	May be asymptomatic; may have fatigue anorexia, weight loss, dyspnea on exertion; splenomegaly; lymphadenopathy; hepatomegaly	Hallmark is sustained absolute lymphocytosis 40,000-150,000/μL; Bone marrow—increased lymphocytes	Median survival—approximately 10 yrs
Chronic Myelogenous	Occurs most often at median age of 42	May be asymptomatic; or insidious onset of nonspecific symptoms, e.g., fatigue, weakness, anorexia, weight loss, fever, night sweats, splenomegaly; blurred vision; resp. distress; priapism, sternal tenderness	RBC, Hgb, Hct-L Platelet count—H early, L later; WBC-H; leukocytosis with immature granulocytes WBC— about 150,000-200,000/μL in symptomatic pt; Bone marrow—Ph[1] chromosome presence is significant	No advantage to early therapy if asymptomatic; 60% of young adults with allogenic bone marrow transplants complete cure; median survival in non-transplanted patients is 3 to 4 years.

L = low; N = high

5. Chest radiograph—identification of mediastinal mass

6. Ultrasound or CT—organomegaly

- Management/Treatment

  1. Physician referral for suspected cases

     a. Goal of treatment is remission

     b. Chemotherapy

     c. Bone marrow transplantation

  2. Assistance in meeting psychosocial needs

3. Assistance for patient and families in adjusting to chronic effects of illness, e.g., dependence, withdrawal, changes in role responsibilities, alterations in body image

4. Patient education

   a. Importance of compliance with chemotherapy regimens; side effects and management

   b. Disease process and rationale for treatment

   c. Adaptation to any physical limitations

Non-Hodgkin's Lymphoma

- Definition: Heterogenous group of lymphocytic malignancies with absence of giant Reed-Sternberg cells characteristic of Hodgkin's Disease

- Etiology/Incidence

  1. Etiology unclear; animal studies have suggested a viral etiology

  2. Other factors associated with increased incidence include:

     a. Ionizing radiation

     b. Hereditary predisposition

     c. Congenital or acquired immunodeficiency

     d. Exposure to pesticides

  3. Approximately 45,000 new cases occur each year in the U.S., and appear to be increasing (Freedman & Nadler, 1997)

  4. Most common neoplasm between ages of 20 and 40; with increased incidence of AIDS, number of cases has sharply increased

- Signs and Symptoms

  1. More than $\frac{2}{3}$ of patients present with persistent painless peripheral lymphadenopathy

  2. Some patients may present with persistent cough and chest discomfort (mediastinal involvement)

  3. If abdominal contents involved, chronic pain, abdominal fullness, early satiety or viscus obstruction may be presenting symptoms

  4. Diffuse disease may present with skin lesions, testicular masses

  5. Fever, night sweats, weight loss.

- Differential Diagnosis
    1. Infectious mononucleosis
    2. Cytomegalovirus infection
    3. Human immunodeficiency virus involvement
    4. Toxoplasmosis
    5. Other malignant tumors
    6. Cat-scratch disease
    7. Tuberculosis
    8. Syphilis
    9. Sarcoidosis
- Physical Findings
    1. Painless peripheral lymphadenopathy may be initial finding
    2. May present with abdominal mass, massive splenomegaly
    3. Early systemic findings usually absent
- Diagnostic Tests/Findings
    1. Requires skilled interpretation of adequate tumor tissue to determine tumor architecture and cell type
    2. B cell and T cell typing—complements pathologic interpretation
    3. Bone marrow biopsy—pathologic confirmation of disease process
    4. Staging procedures conducted once diagnosis established—no perfect classification system exists; various types include the Rappaport classification, Luke and Collins classification, the International Panel Working Formulation (NCI), Ann Arbor staging system
    5. Chest radiograph may show mediastinal mass
- Management/Treatment (Based on grade and extent of disease)
    1. Radiotherapy
    2. Chemotherapy
    3. Bone marrow transplantation

4. Newer modalities include MAbs alone and combined with radionuclides or toxins to produce cytotoxic effects; cytokines, e.g., interferons, tumor necrosis factor and interleukin 2 are currently under study

5. General considerations

    a. Prognosis not usually as good as with Hodgkin's disease

    b. Both family and patient require supportive therapy during diagnosis and treatment stages

    c. Education and necessity of drug compliance important factor

    d. Increased susceptibility to infection

Hodgkin's Disease

- Definition: Malignant disorder with lymphoreticular proliferation
- Etiology/Incidence

  1. Cause is unknown

  2. Approximately 8,000 new cases are diagnosed each year in the U.S.

  3. Average age is 32 years; peaks at 15 to 35 years and again after age 50

  4. More common in males

- Signs and Symptoms

  1. Most patients present with a painless, enlarging mass, most often in the neck or occasionally in axilla or inguinal region; often the only manifestation at time of diagnosis

  2. Older patients may present with:

      a. Fatigue

      b. Weight loss

      c. Persistent fever and/or night sweats

  3. Pruritus—may be mild and localized, but may be progressive; rarely occurs in the absence of fever

  4. An unexplained symptom is immediate pain in diseased areas after consuming alcoholic beverages

- Differential Diagnosis

1. Infectious mononucleosis
2. Toxoplasmosis
3. Cytomegalic inclusion disease
4. Non-Hodgkin's lymphoma
5. Leukemia
6. Bronchogenic carcinoma
7. Sarcoidosis
8. Cat-scratch disease

- Physical Findings

    1. Initial findings are usually enlargement of cervical, axillary, or inguinal lymph nodes (movable, nontender)
    2. Other findings may include hepatomegaly and splenomegaly; usually not present unless the disease is advanced

- Diagnostic Tests/Findings

    1. Presence of characteristic Reed-Sternberg giant cell on biopsy of lymph node tissue or other sites (needle aspiration not sufficient)
    2. WBC—polymorphonuclear leukocytosis may be present
    3. CBC—hypochromic, microcytic anemia in advanced disease
    4. Low serum iron, low iron binding capacity
    5. Chest radiologic examinations—to determine mediastinal involvement

- Management/Treatment

    1. Physician referral for suspected cases

        a. Radiotherapy

        b. Chemotherapy

        c. Autologous bone marrow transplant for chemotherapy failures

    2. For treatment to be precise, Hodgkin's disease needs to be staged which involves determining the extent and involvement of the disease

    3. Psychosocial considerations for patient and family

4. Since prognosis is usually good, patients need to be helped to deal with the disease realistically even though it is a malignant disorder

5. Once patient is in remission, ongoing maintenance treatment is usually not needed; patients need to be instructed in the importance of returning for follow-up visits

6. Patient education

    a. Gonadal side effects of treatment

    b. Consideration of sperm banking for males

    c. Risk of secondary malignancy

Questions
Select the best answer

A 50 year old male of Italian descent comes in for a routine work related health assessment. He has no complaints. His history and physical examination are unremarkable. A routine CBC indicates Hgb 11.2 g/100 mL, MCV 72μ^3, WBC 5.7 × 10^3, Hct 35%, MCH 25

1. Based on this information how would his anemia be classified?

    a. Normocytic, normochromic
    b. Microcytic, hypochromic
    c. Macrocytic, hypochromic
    d. Microcytic, normochromic

2. Which aspect of this patient's history would provide the least useful information for diagnostic decision making?

    a. Diet (including alcohol use)
    b. Social history
    c. Family history
    d. Medical history

You find that this patient has a diet with regular daily intake of lean red meats, vegetables, and fruits and he denies alcohol use except once or twice a year. He does use Maalox almost daily for indigestion. He says that weak blood runs in his family, although he has never had this problem. He has no surgical history and has never been treated for any medical problems except high cholesterol which was treated with diet and exercise

3. This information helps rule out which of the following as cause for his anemia?

    a. Folate deficiency
    b. Inadequate dietary intake
    c. GI bleeding
    d. Malabsorption of vitamins and minerals

4. This patient's lack of abnormal physical signs and symptoms:

    a. Probably indicates a lab error in the blood work
    b. Is not unusual given the degree of his anemia
    c. Is not unusual in a patient of this age
    d. May be masked by use of Maalox

5. Your next step would be to:

    a. Order B_{12} and folate serum levels
    b. Order serum iron and TIBC
    c. Obtain a urine culture
    d. Order a Schilling test

6. What other test would be essential at this point?

    a. Stool guaiac
    b. GI series
    c. Bilirubin
    d. Liver function tests

7. Which is the most likely etiology of the type of anemia exhibited in this patient?

    a. B_{12} or folate deficiency
    b. Chronic disease
    c. Dehydration
    d. GI bleeding

8. If you obtain a negative stool guaiac in a male patient with a microcytic, hypochromic anemia who has a low serum iron and a high TIBC, you would:

    a. Begin ferrous sulfate 300 mg orally t.i.d.
    b. Order a Schilling test
    c. Repeat the stool guaiac
    d. Refer to a hematologist

Mrs. M. is a 30-year-old graduate student from Morocco with a family and personal history of "weak blood" who presents with a complaint of abdominal pain, increasing fatigue, and weight loss. She has never needed treatment for her blood problem but has been supplementing her usually well balanced diet with high potency vitamin and mineral supplements because of the increased stress of graduate studies in a foreign country. A routine CBC indicates a mild microcytic, hypochromic anemia.

9. It is likely that this patient's "weak blood" is:

    a. Thalassemia Minor
    b. Thalassemia Major
    c. Related to an unidentified chronic disease
    d. Related to an iron deficiency from gastrointestinal bleeding

10. You need to consider which of the following as a strong etiology for her current symptoms?

    a. Iron deficiency
    b. Folate deficiency
    c. Peptic ulcer
    d. Iron overload

11. If further blood studies indicate a decreased TIBC and increased serum iron your next step should be which of the following?

    a. Tell Mrs. M. to discontinue her vitamin/mineral supplements; obtain hematologic consult
    b. Refer her for genetic counseling
    c. Refer for hemoglobin electrophoresis
    d. Begin chelation therapy and refer for a GI consult

Ms. Z is a 26 year old, black female who comes in complaining of fatigue, shortness of breath, and lightheadedness. Her history reveals no significant medical problems but several years of fad dieting without vitamin supplementation. Physical findings are unremarkable except for pallor of the mucous membranes, tachycardia, and a systolic flow murmur

12. Your next step would be to:

    a. Start B_{12} injections
    b. Order a CBC, reticulocyte count
    c. Order a TIBC and serum iron
    d. Start on multivitamins with iron

13. Further testing of Ms. Z. reveals a low reticulocyte count and macrocytic cells. Your next step should be to:

    a. Start B_{12} injections
    b. Order serum iron and TIBC
    c. Order RBC-folate and B_{12} levels
    d. Order a Schilling test

14. Which of the following would help in your differential diagnosis?

    a. Patient's history of ice pica
    b. Patient's use of oral contraceptives
    c. A confirmed diagnosis of sickle cell trait
    d. Family history of iron deficiency

15. The anemias most often associated with pregnancy are:

    a. Folic acid and iron deficiency
    b. Folic acid deficiency and Thalassemia
    c. Iron deficiency and Thalassemia
    d. Thalassemia and B_{12} deficiency

16. Neural tube defects in the fetus have been primarily associated with which type deficiency in the mother?

    a. Iron
    b. Folic Acid
    c. Vitamin B_{12}
    d. Vitamin E

17. Most common causes of megaloblastic, macrocytic anemia are:

    a. Folate and or B_{12} deficiency
    b. Chronic disease
    c. Iron deficiency and infection
    d. Hemolysis of blood cells

18. Patients with iron deficiency anemia should be instructed that:

    a. Return of normal blood values will occur within a week of oral iron supplementation
    b. Iron supplements will need to be taken for the rest of their life
    c. Taking iron preparations with milk will enhance absorption
    d. Iron preparation may be taken with meals

19. Elderly persons with pernicious anemia should:

    a. Be instructed to increase their dietary intake of foods high in B_{12}
    b. Be told they will not need to return for follow-up for at least a month after initiation of treatment
    c. Be told that oral B_{12} is safer and less expensive than parenteral replacement
    d. Be told that diarrhea can be a transient side effect of B_{12} injections

20. Which of the following would be included in a diet rich in iron?

    a. Peaches, eggs, beef
    b. Cereals, kale, cheese
    c. Red beans, enriched breads, squash

    d. Legumes, green beans, eggs

21. A woman taking folic acid supplements for Folic Acid Deficiency will need to know that:

    a. It will take several months before she will feel better
    b. Folic acid should not be taken with meals and may cause diarrhea
    c. Iron supplements are contraindicated while one is on folic acid
    d. Oral contraceptives, pregnancy and lactation increase dietary requirements for folic acid

22. In alcoholics with anemia:

    a. Pernicious anemia is more common than folic acid deficiency
    b. Iron deficiency, folic acid deficiency may coexist
    c. The alcohol interferes with iron absorption
    d. Oral vitamin replacement is contraindicated

23. Hypoproliferative normocytic anemia:

    a. Is marked by a normal or decreased reticulocyte count
    b. Is usually secondary to hemolysis or bleeding
    c. Is relatively rare and usually only associated with malignancies
    d. Is only associated with chronic infections

24. In normocytic anemia of chronic disease:

    a. Treatment is purely symptomatic
    b. Long term supplementation of folic acid and B_{12} is needed
    c. Treatment is focused on the associated disease
    d. Serum iron and TIBC are the most specific and sensitive diagnostic tests

25. Which of the following is true of anemia of chronic disease?

    a. A Hgb of < 9 g/dL confirms the diagnosis
    b. Symptoms associated with the anemia may be masked by the symptoms of the underlying disease
    c. Is manifested by more severe signs than most of the other common anemias
    d. Is never associated with reversible causes

26. Sickle Cell Anemia is caused by:

    a. Replacement of hemoglobin A with hemoglobin CS

   b. Transposition of glutamic acid on hemoglobin A molecule
   c. Abnormal hemoglobin S in place of hemoglobin A
   d. Sickle cell trait

27. The test used to differentiate sickle cell anemia/sickle cell trait is:

   a. Sickle cell preparation
   b. Peripheral smear
   c. Sickledex
   d. Hemoglobin electrophoresis

28. Chronic myelogonous leukemia usually presents with the following:

   a. Increased platelets and leukocytosis
   b. Presence of Reed-Sternberg cells in bone marrow aspirate
   c. Ph^1 chromosome in bone marrow
   d. With typical fatigue, weakness, anorexia and frequent nosebleeds

29. A 32-year-old male presents in the office with concerns about a lump in the area of his collar bone. He states that someone told him that it might be a sign of some kind of cancer. Your best response at this time would be to:

   a. Examine him and tell him to come back in two weeks to be re-evaluated
   b. Inquire whether he has any cats which might cause Cat Scratch fever
   c. Work him up for a possibility of infectious mononucleosis
   d. Examine him with referral to physician for possible Hodgkin's disease work-up

30. Diagnosis of Hodgkin's disease is based upon:

   a. Hepatomegaly with fatigue, weight loss, pruritus, and night sweats
   b. Presence of Ph^1 chromosome in lymphoid tissue
   c. Extensive lymphadenopathy with elevated WBC count
   d. Presence of Reed-Sternberg cells in lymph node tissue

Answers

1. b		16. b	
2. b		17. a	
3. b		18. d	
4. b		19. d	
5. b		20. a	
6. a		21. d	
7. d		22. b	
8. c		23. a	
9. a		24. c	
10. d		25. b	
11. a		26. c	
12. b		27. d	
13. c		28. c	
14. b		29. d	
15. a		30. d	

80%

24/30

Bibliography

Campbell, E. W., & Smith, M. R. (1996). Hematology for primary care physicians. *Disease Monthly*, *42*(3), 131–34.

Clinical guidelines. (1997). Adult screening for anemia and hemoglobinopathies. *The Nurse Practitioner*, *20*(12), 48, 50–51.

Davenport, J. (1996). Macrocytic anemia. *American Family Physician*, *53*, 155–162.

Freedman, A. S., & Nadler, L. M. (1997). Malignancies of lymphoid cells. In A. S. Fauci, E. Braunwald, K. J. Isselbacher, J. D. Wilson, J. B. Martin, D. L. Kasper, S. L. Hauser & D. L. Longo (Eds.). *Harrison's principles of internal medicine* (14th ed., pp. 695–712). NY: McGraw-Hill.

Green, R. (1996). Macrocytic anemias. In J. W. Hurst, M. Markman, & A. E. Lichtin (Eds.). *Medicine for the practicing physician* (4th ed., pp. 821–828). Stamford, CT: Appleton & Lange.

Griffith, C. J. (1996). Evaluation and management of anemia. *ADVANCE for Nurse Practitioners*, *4*(5), 29–35.

Hawley, K. (1996). Pernicious Anemia. *American Journal of Nursing*, *96*(11), 52.

Linker, C. A. (1998). Blood. In L. M. Tierney, S. J. McPhee, & M. A. Papadakis (Eds.). *Current medical diagnosis and treatment* (37th ed., pp. 479–533). Stamford, CT: Appleton & Lange.

Newton, W. (1995). Laboratory diagnosis of iron deficiency anemia. *Journal of Family Practice*, *41*, 404–405.

Nicoll, C. D. (1998). Appendix: Therapeutic drug monitoring & laboratory reference ranges. In L. M. Tierney, S. J. McPhee, & M. A. Papadakis (Eds.). *Current medical diagnosis and treatment* (37th ed., pp. 1529–1537). Stamford, CT: Appleton & Lange.

Richer, A. (1997). A practical guide for differentiating between iron deficiency anemia and anemia of chronic disease in children and adults. *The Nurse Practitioner*, *22*(4), 82, 85–98.

Schilling, R. F., & Williams, W. J. (1995). Vitamin B_{12} deficiency: Underdiagnosed, overtreated? *Hospital Practice*, *30*(7), 47–52, 54.

Gastrointestinal Disorders

Sister Maria Salerno

Peptic Ulcer Disease (PUD)

- Definition: Ulceration of the GI mucosa in areas bathed by acid pepsin; stomach, duodenum, and esophagus are common sites

- Etiology/Incidence

    1. Infection with *Helicobacter pylori* leading to imbalance between mucosal protective factors and corrosive effects of acid and pepsin is considered primary cause

    2. Steroidal and nonsteroidal anti-inflammatory drug (NSAID) therapy, particularly aspirin, or other processes or factors leading to

        a. Hypersecretion of gastric mucosa

        b. Increased parietal cell mass

        c. Increased secretion of gastrin and hydrochloric acid

        d. Increased gastric emptying time

    3. Precipitating or aggravating factors include:

        a. Steroidal and nonsteroidal anti-inflammatory drug therapy, particularly aspirin

        b. Physiologic stress—severe trauma, burns, shock

        c. Psychological stress

        d. Alcohol and nicotine use; caffeine, coffee

        e. Presence of alcoholic liver cirrhosis, chronic pancreatitis, chronic lung disease, hyperparathyroidism, rheumatoid arthritis

    4. Lifetime prevalence about 10% for adult population

        a. Duodenal

            (1) 80% are duodenal

            (2) Higher incidence in males

            (3) Without antibiotic treatment 80% recur in year following initial healing

            (4) Incidence decreasing in U.S.

            (5) Familial disposition—more frequent in persons with type O blood

            (6) Peak incidence between 30 and 55 years of age

    b. Gastric

        (1) Occur with about the same incidence in males and fe-males

        (2) About 5% are malignant

        (3) Peak incidence—age 55 to 65 years of age; rare < 40 years of age

- Signs and Symptoms

    1. Intermittent epigastric pain—gnawing, burning, boring, nagging

    2. Pain begins 1 to 3 hours after eating, frequently awakens person at night

    3. Pain relieved by food or antacids

    4. Food sometimes aggravates pain of gastric ulcer

    5. Weight loss frequent in persons with gastric ulcer

    6. Dyspepsia (bloating, nausea, anorexia, excessive flatulence)

- Differential Diagnosis

    1. History of typical pain-food-relief pattern is most important criterion for diagnosis of duodenal ulcer

    2. History not helpful in distinguishing gastric from duodenal

    3. Rule out other causes of epigastric pain

        a. Pancreatitis

        b. Biliary tract disease

        c. Neoplasms

        d. Liver disease

        e. Gastritis

        f. Pneumonia

        g. Functional problems

        h. Cardiovascular disease, e.g., angina

- Physical Findings

    1. Usually none

    2. Epigastric tenderness in advanced disease

- Diagnostic Tests/Findings

    1. Barium radiograph of the upper GI tract will detect 90% of peptic ulcers—indications include:

        a. Diagnosis of atypical cases

        b. Typical presentations with failure to respond to treatment in 3 to 4 weeks; cases of recurrence

        c. Differentiating gastric from duodenal

        d. Differentiating malignant from nonmalignant gastric ulcers

        e. Documentation of healing

    2. Endoscopy

        a. Expensive but more sensitive and specific than barium radiographs; becoming test of choice in many settings

        b. Indicated if clinical symptoms persist despite negative barium studies

        c. Rule out malignancy in gastric ulcers

        d. For those with diagnosed or suspected blood loss, perforation, vomiting, early satiety, or weight loss

    3. Stool for occult blood—positive if bleeding is present

    4. CBC

        a. Hgb and Hct may be decreased

        b. With chronic slow bleeding—hypochromic, microcytic anemia is likely

        c. If bleeding is acute—normocytic, normochromic anemia

    5. Tests for helicobacter

        a. Urea breath test

            (1) 95% to 98% sensitivity and specificity; results comparable to endoscopic biopsy

            (2) Ingested drugs can cause false negatives; perform four weeks after last antibacterial treatment

        b. Serological tests

            (1) IgA, IgG antibodies, ELISA

(2) Inexpensive; sensitivity and specificity about 95%

(3) Not useful for follow up testing because of slow decline after treatment

(4) High serum lipid levels can interfere with results

   c. Histological evaluation

     (1) Requires endoscopic biopsy

     (2) Invasive and expensive

   d. Culture of biopsy

     (1) Grows slowly and requires selective medium and environment

     (2) Primary use in research

- Management/Treatment

  1. Goals

   a. Relief of symptoms

   b. Healing

   c. Prevention of recurrence

   d. Eradication of bacteria

  2. Nonpharmacological

   a. Stop smoking

   b. Avoid ASA and nonsteroidal anti-inflammatory drugs

   c. Reduce stress

   d. Reduce use of alcohol and caffeine (conflicting data, but still recommended until healing is documented)

  3. Pharmacological

   a. Antimicrobials to eradicate *H. pylori*

     (1) Options include:

       (a) Standard triple therapy—metronidazole 250 to 500 mg q.i.d. plus amoxicillin or tetracycline 500 mg q.i.d, with bismuth subsalicylate 4 cc or 2 tablets q.i.d. and omeprazole for 7 to 14 days

        (b) MOC—metronidazole 500 mg b.i.d., omeprazole 20 mg b.i.d., with clarithromycin 250 to 500 mg b.i.d.

        (c) RBC—ranitidine and bismuth citrate 400 mg b.i.d. for 28 days with clarithromycin for first 14 days

        (d) Dual therapy—omeprazole 40 mg once a day for 4 weeks with clarithromycin 500 mg for 2 weeks

    (2) Bismuth compounds act as topical antimicrobial, complementing antibiotics

    (3) Compliance with combination therapies a problem

    (4) Acquired resistance of microbe to metronidazole, and to lesser extent, clarithromycin often occurs with either if given alone

    (5) Standard therapy currently least expensive

    (6) Side effects of antimicrobial treatment

        (a) Candida

        (b) Rash

        (c) Pseudomembranous colitis

        (d) Photosensitivity

    (7) No one "right" regimen

b. Proton pump inhibitors _Prilosec_

    (1) Omeprazole 20 mg per day for 4 to 8 weeks

        (a) Not approved for maintenance therapy

        (b) Short term use with duodenal ulcers, esophagitis

    (2) Lansoprazole _Prevacid_

        (a) Long-term management of hypersecretory conditions

        (b) Short term use with duodenal ulcers, esophagitis

        (c) Inactivated by acid: enteric coated, take with food

    (3) Like H_2 antagonists interfere with cytochrome P450 with similar drug interactions/precautions

(4) Create less acidic environment suppressing but not eradicating *H. pylori*

(5) Particularly useful in prevention/treatment of NSAID induced ulceration

c. H$_2$ receptor antagonists ~Tagamet

    (1) Cimetidine—300 mg orally t.i.d. with meals and at bedtime for 4 to 6 weeks (more recent studies indicate similar healing with 400 mg b.i.d. or 800 mg at bedtime)

        (a) May be given IV in inpatient settings

        (b) Side effects

            (i) Frequently associated with acute confusional states in elderly or very ill patients.

            (ii) Muscular pain; mild, transient diarrhea; impotence; gynecomastia; leukopenia; mildly elevated creatinine and transaminase levels are rare and tend to be seen only with long-term use

        (c) Interferes with metabolism and increases blood levels of benzodiazapines, lidocaine, metronidazole, phenytoin, theophylline, and warfarin

        (d) Should not be taken within an hour of taking antacids

    (2) Ranitidine—150 mg orally b.i.d. or 300 mg orally at bedtime for active PUD; 150 mg orally at bedtime for maintenance

        (a) Also available for IV use

        (b) Side effects—rise in transaminase levels (ALT, formerly SGPT); dizziness; headache; tachycardia; malaise; constipation; diarrhea; rash; and rarely confusion

        (c) No significant drug interactions

        (d) May cause false-positive protein on urinary dipstick analysis

Zantac

pepcid

(3) Famotidine—20 mg orally twice a day or 40 mg at bedtime

    (a) As efficacious as ranitidine

    (b) Least risk of drug interaction

(4) Nizatadine—150 mg orally twice a day or 300 mg at bedtime for up to 8 weeks

acid

    (a) No safer than cimetidine

    (b) More expensive than cimetidine

d. Antacids

(1) Should give dose equivalent to 80 to 100 mEq acid neutralizing capacity; for most, 30 to 40 mL given 1 and 3 hours after each meal; see Table 1 for comparison of various antacid preparations

Table 1

Antacids

Content Comments	Brand Name	Dose required for 80–100 mEq of acid neutralizing effect per dose	mEq of sodium per dose
Low Buffering Capacity			
CaCO$_3$ Rebound hyperacidity	Tums Alka II Chooz	8–10 tablets	0.5–0.6
Al(OH)$_3$ Constipating; high sodium	Amphogel	60–75 mL	1.2–1.5
Al(OH)$_3$ & Mg(OH)$_3$ Only for esophageal reflux	Gaviscon	94–118 mL	10.6–13.2
Moderate Buffering Capacity			
Al(OH)$_3$ & Mg(OH)$_3$ Low Sodium	Gelusil Mylanta Maalox Plus Riopan	35–44 mL 32–40 mL 30–38 mL 30–38 mL	0.23–0.29 0.20–0.25 0.36–0.45 0.08–0.1
High Buffering Capacity			
Al(OH)$_3$ & Mg(OH)$_3$ Liquid more effective than tablets.	Geluxil II Maalox TC Mylanta II	17–21 mL 14–18 mL 16–20 mL	0.2–0.25 0.1–0.13 0.15–0.2

Note: Sodium Bicarbonate, Alka Seltzer have a very short duration of action; acid rebound, systemic alkalosis are problems

    (2) Primarily aluminum, calcium, or magnesium containing agents; sodium bicarbonate very short acting and systemic absorption can cause alkalosis (not recommended)

    (3) Length of effect dependent on gastric emptying time; 30 minutes on an empty stomach, longer when taken with meals

    (4) Side effects

        (a) Diarrhea with magnesium hydroxide based agents

        (b) Constipation with aluminum hydroxide containing agents

        (c) Hypophosphatemia in aluminum containing agents due to aluminum phosphate binding and decreased GI absorption

        (d) Osteopenia with long-term use of agents containing aluminum

        (e) Rebound acid secretion and hypercalcemia with calcium containing agents

    (5) Drug interactions

        (a) Interfere with taste; absorption of iron, digoxin, and some antibiotics, e.g., tetracyclines

        (b) Interfere with effectiveness of oral contraceptives

e. Anticholinergics

    (1) Rarely used in contemporary treatment and only with advice of physician

    (2) Primarily for relief of refractory pain

    (3) High dosage with severe side effects required to achieve antisecretory effect

f. Sucralfate (mucosal protectant)—1 g orally q.i.d. on an empty stomach

    (1) No significant side effects

    (2) Drug Interaction

        (a) Decreases absorption of digoxin, tetracycline, phenytoin, cimetidine, theophylline and other drugs

(b) Antacids interfere with effectiveness and should not be given within 1 hour of sucralfate administration

g. Treatment with antacids, H_2 receptor antagonists, or sucralfate results in 90 to 95% cure rate in 8 to 12 weeks

4. General considerations

a. Consult with physician regarding:

(1) Additional diagnostic studies for persons with suspected underlying disease or failure to respond to treatment in 2 to 4 weeks

(2) Persons with concurrent weight loss

(3) Persons with indications of peritonitis (rigidity, rebound tenderness, fever)

b. Refer to physician persons with confirmed or suspected complications

(1) Bleeding occurs in about 10% to 15% of persons with PUD

(a) Immediate medical emergency with possible surgical intervention required

(b) Signs and symptoms—heartburn, belching, epigastric discomfort, vomiting of bright red or coffee ground liquid

(c) Sudden relief of epigastric pain may be related to bleeding as blood acts as an acid buffer

(d) Diarrhea may also be evident; blood is a cathartic

(2) Perforation occurs in about 5% to 10% of persons with duodenal and 2% to 5% of those with gastric ulcers

(a) Surgery is the indicated treatment

(b) Signs and symptoms include acute pain, fever, leukocytosis, hypotension, peritoneal irritation

(c) Peritoneal irritation is evidenced by abdominal rigidity, guarding, rebound tenderness, decreased or absent bowel sounds

(3) Gastric outlet (pyloric) obstruction is seen in less than 5% of all patients diagnosed with PUD and is most often associated with duodenal ulceration

    (a) Surgical intervention may be indicated

    (b) Signs and symptoms include worsening pain; vomiting of undigested food; dehydration; hypokalemia; and metabolic alkalosis

c. Patient education

    (1) Disease and therapeutic management

    (2) Purpose, dosage, side effects of medications

    (3) Diet

        (a) No evidence to support need for bland diet or small frequent meals

        (b) Encourage avoidance of known gastric acid stimulants, e.g., coffee, cola, and other caffeine containing beverages

        (c) Avoidance of any foods or beverages which aggravate symptoms

        (d) Avoid eating within three hours of bedtime to avoid nocturnal stimulation of acid secretion

    (4) Stress reduction

    (5) Need to report to health care provider lack of response to medications, rectal bleeding, weight loss, increased weakness or dizziness, increasing pain

d. Follow up

    (1) In 2 to 4 weeks to review:

        (a) Symptom response to medications

        (b) GI bleeding

        (c) Side or toxic effects of medications

    (2) For those with gastric ulcers document healing with upper GI barium radiograph or endoscopy—in 6 weeks for small ulcers; 12 weeks for large; imperative in gastric ulcers; unnecessary in uncomplicated duodenal

Table 2

Foods And Other Substances That Decrease Lower Esophageal Sphincter Tone

Anticholinergics
Benzodiazepines
Calcium channel blockers
Diazepam
Meperidine
Narcotics
Progesterone
Alcohol
Caffeine
Nicotine
Chocolate
Fatty foods
Peppermint
Yellow onions

Gastroesophageal Reflux Disease

- Definition: Reflux of stomach and duodenal contents into the esophagus leading to a spectrum of clinical manifestations predominated by inflammation of the esophagus; classified with gastric and duodenal ulcers as a peptic ulcer disease

- Etiology/Incidence

  1. Most often related to inappropriate relaxation of the lower esophageal sphincter (LES) which allows reflux of gastric acid and pepsin into the distal esophagus

     a. Idiopathic

     b. Foods and other agents (see Table 2)

  2. Inflammation can also be caused by ingestion of caustic agents such as lye, or infectious agents such as candida, herpes simplex, or cytomegalovirus which directly attacks esophageal mucosa

  3. Infectious agents most often noted in immunosupressed individuals, e.g., persons with AIDS, diabetes, and persons receiving chemotherapy

  4. Incidence not known, however, a daily prevalence rate of heartburn, the major symptom of esophagitis, has been estimated to be 7% in a normal adult population

- Signs and Symptoms

  1. Retrosternal aching or burning heartburn (pyrosis) occurring 30 to

60 minutes after eating; associated with large meals, and aggravated by lying down or bending over

2. Chest heaviness, pressure radiating to neck or jaw, or shoulders

3. Regurgitation of fluid or food particles

4. Nocturnal aspiration

5. Recurrent pneumonia or bronchospasm

6. Pain or difficulty swallowing

- Differential Diagnosis

   1. Myocardial infarction/angina

   2. Esophageal spasm

   3. Cholelithiasis

   4. Neoplasms

   5. Chemical or infectious esophagitis

   6. Conditions leading to gastric dysmotility, e.g., scleroderma, diabetes

- Physical Findings—generally insignificant

- Diagnostic Tests/Findings

   1. Usually only needed in atypical or severe cases

   2. Barium radiograph of upper GI tract

      a. To rule out strictures or other acid-peptic disease indicated in patients with:

         (1) Dysphagia

         (2) Painful swallowing

         (3) Significant weight loss

         (4) Occult blood loss

      b. Usually normal, but may show inflammation, ulcer, or stricture

   3. Endoscopy becoming more routine than barium radiography in most settings—is indicated in same instances as barium radiography; may show visible mucosal damage which can be confirmed by biopsy; in cases of caustic ingestion or suspected infectious etiology endoscopy is usually first diagnostic test

4. Bernstein acid perfusion—rarely needed with classic history; requires alternating infusion of 0.1 N hydrochloric acid and normal saline into the esophagus; positive reproduction of symptoms with the hydrochloric acid infusion and not the saline is usual in esophageal reflux

5. Esophageal motility and 24 hour esophageal pH tests are more specialized and reserved for atypical cases; consult with or refer patient to gastroenterologist

- Management/Treatment

    1. Phase I—implement general measures

        a. Weight reduction if obese

        b. Elevation of head of bed

        c. Avoid large meals and carbonated beverages particularly three hours prior to going to bed; no indication that fruit juices aggravate the problem

        d. Limit fats and carbohydrates

        e. Avoid straining at stool

        f. Avoid agents that decrease LES tone—nicotine, alcohol, chocolate, caffeine, theophylline, calcium channel blockers, anticholinergics

        g. Antacids—(see Table 1)

            (1) Mainstay of therapy

            (2) 80 to 100 mEq of neutralizing activity (30 cc for most agents) after meals and at bedtime

            (3) Liquid preferred to tablet forms

    2. Phase II—if general measures are ineffective add H_2 antagonist cimetidine or ranitidine in same dosages as in peptic ulcer disease

    3. Phase III—if Phase II measures are ineffective consult with physician regarding further testing and use of more aggressive therapies which might include:

        a. Higher dose of H_2 blockers or omeprazole

        b. H_2 blocker and a prokinetic to increase LES tone, esophageal motility, and gastric emptying

     (1)   Metoclopramide—10 to 15 mg before meals and at bedtime

        (a)   High frequency of side effects

        (b)   Include fatigue, anxiety, confusion, and extrapyramidal reactions

     (2)   Cisapride—10 mg before meals and at bedtime

        (a)   Works synergistically with H_2 receptor antagonists to promote healing

        (b)   Fatal cardiovascular events may occur when taken with drugs that inhibit the cytochrome P450 3A4 enzymes and/or when co-morbidities that predispose to dysrhythmias

     (3)   Bethanechol 25 mg 30 minutes before meals

        (a)   To date has shown limited effectiveness

        (b)   Contraindicated in asthma, ischemic heart disease, or urinary retention

4.   Phase IV—surgical intervention reserved for patients with stricture, bleeding, pulmonary aspiration, or severe refractory symptoms

5.   General considerations

   a.   Consult with physician regarding persons

     (1)   With atypical presentation

     (2)   Refractory to simple treatment

     (3)   With dysphagia and or weight loss in addition to heartburn

   b.   Education

     (1)   Mechanism of esophageal reflux and goals of management

     (2)   Aggravating factors

     (3)   Correction of misconceptions regarding causes (hiatal hernia seldom a cause) and treatment

     (4)   Proper use, dosage, side effects of pharmacologic agents

Cholecystitis

- Definition: Acute or chronic inflammation of the gallbladder
- Etiology/Incidence
  1. About 90% related to presence of pigmented or cholesterol calculi which can vary in diameter from 1 mm to 4 cm; when a stone becomes impacted in the cystic duct, inflammation develops behind the obstruction; if not relieved, pressure builds up in the gallbladder and leads to distension, ischemic changes, gangrene, and perforation with subsequent abscess formation and less frequently generalized peritonitis
  2. Occurs subsequent to bile stasis, bacterial infection, or ischemia
  3. Most common form of gallbladder disease; affects more than 15 million Americans
  4. Being 50 to 70 years old, female over 40 years old and obese are all risk factors
  5. Pregnancy, sedentary lifestyle, low fiber diet, use of oral contraceptives or antilipemics also associated with the development of cholecystitis
- Signs and Symptoms
  1. Episodic occurrences of postprandial fullness, heartburn, nausea, flatulence, regurgitation of bitter fluid, vomiting often precipitated by a large or fatty meal
  2. Anorexia (inability to finish an average size meal)
  3. Recurrent episodes of biliary colic—sudden appearance of severe pain in the epigastrium or right hypochondrium which subsides relatively slowly (12 to 18 hours)
     a. Tenderness of the same area may persist for days
     b. Accompanied by vomiting in 75% of the cases
  4. Constant aching pain or pressure in the right upper quadrant or epigastrium that radiates to the back or right shoulder
- Differential Diagnosis
  1. Perforated peptic ulcer
  2. Acute pancreatitis

3. Appendicitis

4. Salpingitis

5. Diverticulitis

6. Perforated hepatic carcinoma

7. Liver abscess

8. Hepatitis

9. Pneumonia with right sided pleurisy

10. Myocardial infarction

- Physical Findings

  1. General appearance—unremarkable between attacks; ill during attack

  2. Vital signs—mild temperature elevation, tachycardia, and increased respiratory rate during acute attack

  3. Integument—mild jaundice occurs in about 20% of cases

  4. Abdomen—guarding, rebound tenderness in right hypochondrium; palpable, tender sausage shaped mass in RUQ during acute attack in 20% to 30% of cases

  5. Positive Murphy's sign—inspiratory arrest secondary to extreme tenderness when subhepatic area is palpated during deep inspiration

- Diagnostic Tests/Findings

  1. CBC—mild leukocytosis with increased bands (shift to the left)

  2. ECG—normal, important in ruling out myocardial infarction as cause of symptoms

  3. Chest radiograph—normal, important in ruling out pneumonia as cause of symptoms

  4. Flat plate radiograph of abdomen—gallstones

  5. Ultrasound (study of choice with 95% sensitivity 98% specificity for stones)—gallstones, thickened gallbladder wall stones

  6. Technetium T_c99_m PIPIDA (HIDA) scan—cystic duct occlusion and nonvisualized gallbladder

  7. Alkaline phosphatase—elevated

8. Serum amylase—elevated, > 1,000 suspect concomittant pancreatitis

9. Serum aspartate aminotransferase (AST, formerly termed SGOT) and serum alanine aminotransferase (ALT, formerly SGPT) may be transiently elevated

10. Bilirubin—mildly increased

11. Old age, lymphoma, malnutrition, and immunosuppression may alter laboratory tests

12. CT scan has no advantage over ultrasound in diagnosis of acute attack

13. Oral cholecystography not used for acute attack

- Management/Treatment

   1. Elective cholecystectomy recommended for:

      a. Symptomatic patients with radiologic or ultrasound evidence of gallbladder disease

      b. Those at high risk for complications such as those with:

         (1) A calcified gall bladder

         (2) Gallstones > 2 cm in diameter

         (3) Diabetes

   2. Conservative treatment for those who are asymptomatic

      a. If on clofibrate (an antilipemic) or oral contraceptives stop or decrease dosage

      b. Avoid foods that seem to precipitate symptoms, otherwise no need to alter diet or restrict fats

      c. Anticholinergics not helpful

      d. Treat dyspeptic symptoms with antacids (25% to 50% of patients will respond)

      e. Some patients may be put on a trial of chenodiol 750 mg orally per day

         (1) Best results are obtained in patients with small floating cholesterol stones

         (2) Contraindicated in patients with inflammatory bowel disease or peptic ulcer disease

      (3)   Approximately 50% recurrence rate within five years after treatment

      (4)   Side effects—hepatotoxicity, diarrhea, and increased LDL cholesterol

      (5)   Expensive

3.   Lithotripsy or destruction of stones with extracorporeal shock waves has limited application at present

4.   General considerations

   a.   Refer all persons with suspected cholecystitis to physician for further evaluation, possible hospitalization, and possible surgery

   b.   Patient education

      (1)   Disease course, expected outcomes, and treatment

      (2)   Changes in symptoms which necessitate contact of health professional, e.g., change in pain pattern or pain accompanied by fever, chills

      (3)   Teach purpose, dosage, side effects of medications

      (4)   Nutrition

         (a)   If fatty foods seem to precipitate symptoms a low-fat diet may be helpful

         (b)   Some research has shown that increased fiber in the diet reduces incidence of gallstone formation

         (c)   If obese, a reducing diet is indicated; avoid rapid weight loss and fad diets which may actually increase risk of gallstone formation and precipitate acute symptoms

      (5)   Encourage regular physical exercise; sedentary life style is associated with stone formation as well as obesity

   c.   Follow-up annually and for acute attacks

   d.   Complications include empyema, gangrene, and perforation

Appendicitis

- Definition: Inflammation of the vermiform appendix

- Etiology/Incidence

  1. Obstruction of the appendix with hardened feces (fecalith), stricture, inflammation, foreign body, or neoplasm

  2. Occurs in all age groups, but more common in males between 10 and 30 years of age

  3. Higher mortality rate due to complications in children, adolescents, and person over 55 years of age

  4. One of the leading causes for abdominal surgery

- Signs and Symptoms

  1. Acute onset of periumbilical or epigastric pain which ranges from mildly diffuse to severe

  2. Anorexia, nausea, and vomiting (usually subsequent to pain onset)

  3. Shifting of pain to right lower quadrant (McBurney's point) after several hours; aggravated by walking or coughing

  4. Occasional radiation of pain into the ipsilateral testicle or labia

  5. Spasm of abdominal muscles

  6. Constipation usual; diarrhea rare

  7. Elderly clients may present with mild symptoms of unexplained weakness, anorexia, tachycardia, and abdominal distention with little pain

  8. After 24 hours may progress to perforation with sudden cessation of pain and subsequent peritonitis manifested by

     a. Abdominal rigidity

     b. Generalized abdominal tenderness

     c. High fever

     d. Vomiting

     e. Dehydration

     f. Decreased bowel sounds

     g. Shock

- Differential Diagnosis

  1. Gastroenteritis

2. Pneumonia

3. Ruptured ovarian cyst

4. Tubal pregnancy

5. Acute cholecystitis

6. Neoplastic perforation of the colon

7. Renal calculi

8. Pyelonephritis of the right kidney

- Physical Findings

    1. General appearance—may or may not appear ill

    2. Vital signs—fever 100 to 102° F

    3. Slight tachycardia related to pain and fever

    4. Abdominal—point and rebound tenderness in RLQ; decreased or absent bowel sounds

    5. Positive psoas and obturator signs

    6. Rectal/pelvic exams—tenderness in the right perirectal area

    7. Musculoskeletal—abdominal pain (RLQ) with hip extension and with straight leg raise

- Diagnostic Tests/Findings

    1. CBC with differential—leukocytosis with increased band cells (shift to the left); in the elderly shift may be present without leukocytosis

    2. Radiograph of the abdomen may show fecalith

- Management/Treatment: All persons with suspected or diagnosed appendicitis should be immediately referred to a physician for hospitalization and surgery. Appendicitis that has progressed to perforation or peritonitis will be associated with longer morbidity and higher mortality

Diverticulitis

- Definition: Inflammation of one or more diverticula in the bowel wall with microperforation and abscess formation in the pericolic fat

- Etiology/Incidence

    1. Inflammatory process similar to etiologic agents in appendicitis

2. Occurs in about 33% of persons with diverticula (estimated to be 5% to 20% of the adult population)

   a. Incidence increases over age 40

   b. More frequent in females than males

   c. Higher incidence in persons with low fiber dietary habits

   d. Diverticula found most often in the sigmoid colon but may occur anywhere in the GI tract

3. Free perforation with signs of peritonitis is rare

- Signs and Symptoms

  1. Acute left lower quadrant pain—steady and severe lasting for several days or crampy and intermittent

  2. Constipation more usual than diarrhea

  3. Pain increased with defecation

  4. Flatulence

  5. Nausea

  6. Low grade fever

- Differential Diagnosis

  1. Appendicitis

  2. Carcinoma of the colon

  3. Crohn's disease

  4. Ischemic colitis

  5. Gynecologic disorders, e.g.,

     a. Ectopic pregnancy

     b. Ovarian abscess

- Physical Findings

  1. Vital signs—mild fever, tachycardia

  2. Abdomen—guarding, rebound tenderness, rigidity especially over LLQ; if abscess has formed, a tender palpable mass may be noted

  3. Rectal examination—tender painful mass may be present

- Diagnostic Tests/Findings

1. CBC—slight leukocytosis

2. Sed rate—elevated

3. Stool guaiac—positive in about 25% of cases

4. Urine—normal unless colovesicular fistula present then bacteriuria, leukorrhea, hematuria

5. Barium enema will confirm presence of diverticulosis and help rule out other etiologies, however not indicated during acute phase

6. Proctoscopic examination—negative

7. Sigmoidoscopy—inflamed mucosa

8. Stool for ova/parasites—negative

- Management/Treatment: For most patients with mild disease outpatient treatment will be indicated and includes:

    1. Clear liquids for 1 to 2 days followed by a bland diet once symptoms have subsided

    2. Antibiotic therapy with one of the following:

        a. Ampicillin 500 mg orally every 6 hours

        b. Tetracycline 500 mg orally every 6 hours

        c. Amoxicillin/clavulanate potassium 500 mg every six hours

        d. A combination of ampicillin and an aminoglycoside is common

    3. Bedrest to promote colon rest recommended until symptoms subside

    4. General considerations

        a. Consult with physician regarding

            (1) Those who fail to improve in 72 hours

            (2) Those with a temperature > 102° F

            (3) Need for additional testing

        b. Patients with severe disease require hospitalization, antibiotics, bowel rest, and IV hydration

        c. Patient education

            (1) Etiology/incidence and usual clinical course of the disease and rationale for recommended treatment

(2) Instruction on recommended dietary guidelines

(a) After acute phase, high fiber diet to include foods such as bran, whole grains, cereals, raw, cooked or died fruit, raw vegetables, cooked high residue vegetables

(b) High fiber diet may cause bloating and flatulence during the first two weeks of use; this resolves with continued high fiber intake

(3) Avoid laxatives, enemas, antidiarrheal agents and uncooked high residue foods

(4) Report fever, bleeding, increasing pain to health care provider immediately

(5) Bulk forming agents such as psyllium hydrophilic muciloid and use of stool softeners such as docusate sodium may help prevent frequent recurrence

d. Follow-up—return visit or phone follow-up in 24 to 48 hours to verify relief with initiating therapy; and then again after completion of antibiotic therapy

Viral Hepatitis

- Definition: Inflammation of the liver

- Etiology/Incidence

1. Type A (infectious)

a. Infection with hepatitis A virus (HAV), a small RNA enterovirus

(1) Spread primarily by fecal-oral route; also parenterally

(2) Found in infected water, food, shellfish

(3) Intimate contact and poor sanitation and personal hygiene seem to be contributing factors

(4) Incubation period 2 to 6 weeks

(5) Infectivity—2 to 3 weeks in late incubation and early clinical phase

b. Common in crowded situations such as low income housing, school, military, and prison dormitories; can occur in any age group; common in immigrants from under developed countries, school age children, and young adults

    (1)   Self limiting in > 99% of cases

    (2)   No carrier state or chronic infection

    (3)   Severity increases with age

    (4)   In U.S. seroprevalence of Anti-HAV in adults indicates 40% to 50% have had the disease

2. Type B (Serum)

    a. Infection with hepatitis B virus (HBV), a DNA virus with core and surface components

        (1) HB_sAg (Hepatitis B surface antigen) found in serum, saliva, semen, stool, and urine

        (2)   Core contains HB_cAg (Hepatitis B core antigen) and when present, HB_eAg (secretory form of HB_cAg present only in HB_sAg positive sera); HB_eAg associated with high virus titer and high infectivity

        (3)   Incubation period 6 weeks to 6 months

        (4)   Transmission by blood, blood products, and other body fluids, such as saliva and semen

        (5)   Mother-infant transmission if mother infected during 3rd trimester

        (6)   Approximately 10% of infected individuals become chronic carriers

    b. Common in drug addicts, homosexual males, those with multiple sexual partners and densely populated urban neighborhoods; higher risk individuals include persons exposed to needle punctures and blood products such as IV drug abusers; those on hemodialysis; those requiring blood transfusions, or IV chemotherapy; and health care personnel such as nurses, laboratory workers, surgeons, and hemodialysis personnel

        (1)   Considered to be a sexually transmitted disease

        (2)   Accounts for about 40% of acute hepatitis cases/annually

3. HDV (hepatitis delta virus) incomplete RNA virus

     a.   Requires antecedent or simultaneous HBV infection

     b.   Common in IV drug users and recipients of multiple transfusions

     c.   Concomitant infection usually results in more severe manifestations than HBV alone

     d.   Immunity to HBV protects against HDV

4.   Type C (parenteral non-A, non-B)

     a.   Infection with Hepatitis C Virus (HCV), an RNA virus.

         (1)   Incubation variable—5 to 10 weeks

         (2)   Chronic liver disease develops in 10% to 40%

         (3)   Related to development of hepatocellular carcinoma in 10%

     b.   Leading cause of post transfusion hepatitis

     c.   High risk population—IV drug users, hospital personnel, male homosexuals, and those receiving multiple transfusions

5.   Type E (enteral or epidemic non-A, non-B)

     a.   Infection with Hepatitis E Virus (HEV), a single stranded RNA virus

         (1)   Viral particles found in stool of infected persons

         (2)   Does not progress to chronic liver disease

         (3)   Incubation—2 to 9 weeks

         (4)   Usually mild disease in adults > 15 yrs

         (5)   Mortality as high as 10% to 20% in pregnant woman

     b.   Rare in the U.S.

6.   Type G (HGV)

     a.   Infection with a flavivirus

         (1)   Transmitted percutaneously

         (2)   Most infections asymptomatic

         (3)   May result in chronic viremia but chronic disease rare

     b.   Risk groups include transfusion recipients, IV drug users

      c.   Frequent co-infection with HCV

- Signs and Symptoms: Clinical manifestations for all types are similar and can vary from a minor flu-like illness to fatal liver failure.

   1.   HAV may present with nonspecific or "flu" syndrome

   2.   HBV clinical course more variable than HAV and associated with extrahepatic manifestations, e.g., urticaria, other rashes, arthritis

   3.   HCV acute illness variable, flu-like and subsides spontaneously

   4.   Prodromal phase or preicteric phase (lasts approximately two weeks)

      a.   Fatigue, malaise

      b.   Anorexia

      c.   Nausea/vomiting

      d.   Headache

      e.   Hyperalgia

      f.   Cough, coryza, pharyngitis

      g.   Changes in taste with aversion to alcohol and smoking

      h.   Right upper abdominal pain

      i.   Weight loss of 2 to 4 kg

   5.   Active or icteric phase (lasts 2 to 6 weeks)

      a.   Jaundice—sclera and skin (never manifested in some patients)

      b.   Dark urine

      c.   Clay-colored stools; often precedes jaundice

      d.   Enlarged tender liver

      e.   Pruritus, urticarial rash more often associated with HBV

   6.   Post-icteric or recovery phase

      a.   Resolving jaundice, increasing sense of well-being, and decrease in symptomatology

      b.   Chronic active hepatitis in those with HBV may begin at this point and is manifested by persistence of symptoms

- Differential Diagnosis

1. Infectious mononucleosis

2. Choledocholithiasis

3. Hepatotoxic drugs, e.g., chloramphenicol, acetaminophen, methyldopa

4. Carcinoma of the head of the pancreas

5. Alcoholic cirrhosis

6. History and serological tests assist in differentiating type

- Physical Findings

  1. General appearance—mildly ill to generally debilitated

  2. Vital signs—mild fever

  3. Integumentary—slight jaundice; rash

  4. HEENT—yellow sclera, lymphadenopathy

  5. Abdomen—enlarged, tender liver; splenomegaly (in about 10% of cases); normal bowel sounds

- Diagnostic Tests/Findings

  1. CBC with differential—WBC low to normal

  2. Urinalysis—proteinuria; bilirubinuria

  3. Abnormal liver function tests

     a. Elevated AST (formerly SGOT), ALT (formerly SGPT) typically 500 to 2000 IU/L

     a. Rise 7 to 10 days before jaundice

     b. Begin to fall shortly after onset of jaundice; should return to normal after 6 months

     c. Degree of increase does not necessarily parallel disease severity

     d. LDH, serum bilirubin, alkaline phosphatase, prothrombin time normal or slightly increased

  4. Serology tests—refer to Table 3

- Management/Treatment

  1. Consult with physician regarding patient management

2. Approach is primarily supportive in uncomplicated cases

    a. Activity/rest

        (1) Rest recommended during active phase

        (2) Resumption of full activities during the recovery period does not appear to prolong illness, cause relapse or development of chronic disease

        (3) Avoidance of activity that might cause trauma to liver or spleen

    b. Adequate fluid and dietary intake

        (1) 3,000 to 4,000 mL fluid per day; high carbohydrate fluids such as fruit juices, carbonated beverages are encouraged but not always well tolerated

        (2) Foods high in protein, carbohydrates, and calories

        (3) Low fat diet not shown to be beneficial

        (4) Most important to eat whatever is tolerated

Table 3

Serology Tests for Viral Hepatitis

IgM antibody to HAV — appears during acute or early convalescent phase and disappears in about 8 weeks; implies recent infection with HAV
IgG antibody to HAV implies previous infection with HAV; confers immunity
HB$_S$Ag (Hepatitis B surface antigen) — positive throughout the active phase of illness; first test to obtain if acute HBV infection is suspected; will remain positive in asymptomatic carriers and in chronic hepatitis
Anti-HB$_S$ (Antibody specific to HB$_S$Ag [Hepatitis B surface antigen])—positive indication of non-infectious state and recovery, and immunity; appears after HB$_S$Ag disappears
Anti-HB$_C$ (Antibody to HB$_C$Ag [Hepatitis B core antigen])—present at onset of acute illness; remains present for years, and is found in asymptomatic carriers; in many patients there is a period (window) between the disappearance of HB$_S$Ag and the appearance of Anti-HB$_S$ Antibody, usually during late stages of acute phase or early convalescence; during this period, Anti-HB$_C$ will be the only serological marker of the infection
Anti-HDV (Antibody to Hepatitis D) — marker of co/or superinfection by hepatitis D in persons with Hepatitis B; appears late and is short lived
HB$_e$Ag (Protein derived from HBV core) — indicates circulating HBV and highly infectious sera
Anti-HB$_e$ (Antibody to HB$_e$Ag) — appears weeks-months after HB$_e$Ag and HBV are no longer detecable in blood; presence indicates substantially less infectious sera
Anti-HCV (Antibody to HCV) — appears 6 months after initial infection, remains elevated indefinitely, considered infectious and capable of transmission
HCV-RNA (Hepatitis C RNA) can detect circulating virus in 1–2 weeks after infection; becoming the gold standard for HCV detection.

    c. Antiemetics may be prescribed 30 minutes before meals to control nausea and vomiting; rectal administration may be better tolerated than oral

    d. Patients with elevated PT may be given vitamin K

    e. Symptomatic relief of pruritus with colloidal baths, soaps, and lotions

    f. Avoid alcohol and other drugs detoxified or metabolized by the liver

    g. Avoid birth control pills and C-17 alpha alkyl-substituted androgenic steroids during acute phase; may increase bilirubin levels

3. For HCV—interferon alfa-2B (Intron A) 3 million units SC or IM three times a week for six months

    a. Exact mechanism of action unknown

    b. Produces clinical remission in 40% to 60%

    c. 70% to 80% of those with remission have recurrence of active disease in 6 to 12 months post-treatment

    d. Most positive response with:

        (1) Low serum titer HCV RNA

        (2) Younger age

        (3) Female

        (4) Absence of cirrhosis

    e. No data to date showing better survival rates or inhibition of progress to chronic active hepatitis

4. General considerations

    a. Refer for possible hospitalization and further testing

        (1) Complicated cases

        (2) Severely ill patients

        (3) Persons with signs of fulminating hepatitis or encephalitis

        (4) Dehydrated persons

        (5) Those with a PT > 15 seconds

(6) Those suspected of having another underlying disease process

b. Newly diagnosed cases reported to health department

c. Patient education

   (1) Disease course and expected outcomes

   (2) Verify any drug use including over the counter medications and vitamin supplements with the healthcare provider until completely recovered

   (3) Maintain proper hygiene; proper hand-washing, disposal of all body wastes

      (a) Should not donate blood

      (b) Close personal contacts, family members, and sexual contacts should be evaluated for active disease and may receive immune serum globulin for passive immunity (not useful once disease is clinically evident)

d. Follow-up

   (1) Follow weekly for the first 2 to 3 weeks; monthly thereafter if symptoms subside and liver function tests improving

   (2) Closer follow-up in those > 40 years of age

e. Complications

   (1) HBV infection tends to be longer and more severe than HAV

   (2) Carrier states and chronic hepatitis are associated with HBV and HCV, but not with HAV

   (3) Fulminant liver failure occurs in less than 1% of those with HAV and in about 5% of those with HBV

   (4) Chronic hepatitis can be associated with hepatic cancer

   (5) 50% of patients with Hepatitis C will develop chronic hepatitis

f. Prophylaxis—see Table 4

Table 4

Adult Prophylaxis for Viral Hepatitis

Time of Exposure	Agent	Dose	Time
PRE-EXPOSURE			
Hepatitis A			
Persons traveling to or working in endemic areas; men who have sex with men; drug users; those who work with non-human primates with HAV infection or in labs with HAV; persons with chronic liver disease; those with clotting factor disorders; and some food handlers.	HA vaccine (preferred over serum)	1 mL IM	2 doses separated by 6–12 months depending on brand; protection begins 4 weeks after first dose; both doses needed for long-term protection.
If travel or exposure expected in less than 4 weeks after 1st HA vaccine dose.	Immune serum globulin	0.02mL/kg once	
Hepatitis B			
Recommended for health care personnel especially laboratory personnel; surgeons; dialysis personnel. Also recommended for adolescents in areas with high incidence of HBV, drug abuse, STD, teen pregnancies and for homosexually active men	HB vaccine × 3	1 mL IM	Usually given in 3 doses; 2nd & 3rd given approximately 1 mo & 6 mo after the 1st dose; need all 3 doses for adequate protection
POST EXPOSURE			
Hepatitis A			
Close contacts; Family members; Sexual partners	Immune serum globulin	0.02 mL/kg	Once, not more than 2 weeks post exposure
Hepatitis B			
Percutaneious needle stick or mucosal exposure if unvaccinated and source HB_SAg +	HB immune globulin & HB vaccine × 3	0.06 mL/kg 1 mL IM	Within 24–48 hours of exposure; at same time as HBIg, then at 1 & 6 mo
Sexual exposure	Globulin & HB vaccine × 3	0.6 mL/kg 1 mL IM	Within 14 days of last sexual contact; at same time as HBIg, then at 1 & 6 mo

Contact Center for Disease Control Hotline for most current and more specific information (404) 332-4555 or URL http//www.cdc.gov

Acute Gastroenteritis

- Definition: Acute inflammation of the gastrointestinal mucosa

- Etiology/Incidence

    1. Commonly due to infectious agents—viruses, bacteria, and parasites (*Giardia,* amoebae)

        a. Exotoxins produced by some organisms, (e.g., staphylococcus) induce hypersecretion or increased peristalsis resulting in diarrhea or vomiting

    b.   Bacteria such as *E. coli* and salmonella penetrate and invade the gastric mucosa and lead to diarrhea accompanied by fever and fecal leukocytes

    c.   See Table 5 for characteristics of some etiologic agents in gastroenteritis

  2. Second leading cause of morbidity in the U.S.

    a.   Occurs universally in all age groups

    b.   Epidemic outbreaks of bacterial enteritis occur in groups of persons who have ingested contaminated food

    c.   Viral gastroenteritis occurs more frequently in the winter months

    d.   Primarily a self-limiting disease

    e.   The very young, elderly, and those with concomitant chronic debilitating disease are at higher risk for mortality

- Signs and Symptoms

  1. Abrupt onset of nausea, vomiting

  2. Explosive flatulence

  3. Crampy abdominal pain

Table 5

Characteristics of Select Etiologic Agents in Gastroenteritis

	Incubation or Onset	Fever	Fecal leukocytes	Other
E. coli	24–72 hr	+	+	Common cause of travelers' diarrhea; doxycycline, bismuth subsalicylate used preventively
Campylobacter	2–5 days	+	+	Erythromycin & tetracycline used in treatment
Staphylcoccus	1–6 hr	–	–	Grows in meats; dairy foods
Shigella/Salmonella	8–24 hr	+	+	Highly infectious
Botulism	12–36 hr	–	–	Neuro. signs—diplopia, vertigo, dysphagia; respiratory support may be needed
Giardia lamblia	7–21 days	–	–	Doxycycline, trimethoprim/sulfamethoxazole, and fluoroquinolones used in treatment; cause of travelers' diarrhea

4. Frequent, watery diarrhea

5. Myalgia

6. Headache

7. Fever

8. Generalized weakness/malaise

- Differential Diagnosis

  1. Acute appendicitis

  2. Cholecystitis

  3. Inflammatory bowel disease, e.g., colitis

  4. Fecal impaction with overflow

  5. Pelvic inflammatory disease

- Physical Findings

  1. General appearance—ill

  2. Vital signs—fever moderate to high 101 to 102° F in bacterial; up to 103° F in viral

  3. Abdomen—diffuse tenderness; no spasm or rebound tenderness except with salmonella infection; hyperactive bowel sounds; slight distention; absent or hypoactive bowel sounds common with botulism

  4. Neurological—dizziness, difficulty in swallowing and other neurological deficits are indication of botulism and require emergency intervention; with other etiologies findings are expected to be normal

- Diagnostic Tests/Findings

  1. CBC—normal indices

  2. Stool guaiac—usually negative in viral infections; positive with invasive bacterial infections

  3. Stool examination—if etiologic agent is an invasive bacteria, leukocytes will be present

  4. Stool culture—diagnostic for bacteria

     a. Done in suspected cases of bacterial infection, food poisoning, and if symptoms do not begin to abate in 48 hours

     b. Special cultures needed for suspected campylobacter, cholera

- Management/Treatment
  1. Immediately refer to a physician those with:
     a. Dehydration
     b. Rebound tenderness
     c. Severe abdominal pain
     d. Neurological symptoms
     e. Concomitant debilitating illness
  2. Most can be treated for 24 to 48 hours without laboratory testing with:
     a. Bedrest as needed progressing to regular activity
     b. NPO except for cracked ice while nausea and vomiting are present, then restriction to clear liquids for 24 hours; follow with addition of toast and crackers, proceeding to a bland then regular diet
     c. Antiemetics and antidiarrheals are usually not indicated and may prolong the problem; treatment of salmonella has been noted to prolong the carrier state
     d. Provide for parenteral administration of prescription medications if necessary
  3. General considerations
     a. Consult with physician if major symptoms do not abate in 48 hours; approach may include stool for ova and parasites, specialized stool cultures and proctosigmoidoscopy
     b. Report bacterial infections and food poisoning to the health department
     c. Patient education
        (1) Disease course and expected outcome; symptoms usually resolve in 24 to 48 hours but mild diarrhea may persist for a week or two
        (2) Explain proper food preparation and storage
        (3) Appropriate dosage and side effects of medications
        (4) Proper methods of hygiene including hand washing and disposal of stool and emesis

(5) Signs of dehydration; neurological involvement that require contacting health care professional

    d. Follow-up

        (1) Usually self-limiting; return visit warranted if symptoms (other than mild diarrhea) do not abate in 48 to 72 hours or worsen

        (2) Diarrhea may continue for 1 to 2 weeks with salmonella infection

Irritable Bowel Syndrome (IBS) (Functional Bowel Syndrome)

- Definition: Functional disturbance of intestinal motility marked by a common symptom complex which includes abdominal pain and alternating bouts of constipation and diarrhea

- Etiology/Incidence

    1. Disturbance in bowel motor activity thought to include a normal response to severe stress and learned visceral response to stress leading to:

        a. Nonpropulsive colonic contractions which lead to constipation

        b. Increased contraction in the small bowel and proximal colon with diminished activity in the distal colon leading to diarrhea

    2. Influenced by emotional factors

    3. Common GI disorder

        a. Accounts for about 50% of most GI complaints seen by health care professionals and a major cause of morbidity in the U.S.

        b. Onset usually occurs before age 35

        c. Women affected more often than men

- Signs and Symptoms

    1. Aching or cramping periumbilical or lower abdominal pain often precipitated by meals and relieved by defecation; does not awaken patient at night

    2. Pain may radiate to left chest or arm (gas in splenic flexure)

    3. Changes in bowel function

        a. Diarrhea

        (1)   4 to 6 movements/day

        (2)   Small watery stools with clear mucus

        (3)   Nocturnal diarrhea (rare)

    b. Constipation with irregular passage of small hard stools

    c. Alternating episodes of diarrhea and constipation

  4. Flatulence

  5. Exaggerated response to and preoccupation with bowel symptoms

  6. Bleeding, weight loss, and nocturnal diarrhea are not characteristic of IBS

- Differential Diagnosis

  1. Inflammatory bowel disorder, e.g., ulcerative colitis

  2. Viral or bacterial gastroenteritis

  3. GI neoplasms

  4. Parasitic infections

  5. Lactose deficiency

  6. Laxative abuse

  7. Side effects of drugs affecting bowel motility

  8. Rome criteria (Harris, 1997) for diagnosis require at least three months of continuous or recurrent symptoms that include:

    a. Abdominal pain relieved by defecation or pain with change in frequency or consistency of stool

    b. Disturbance in defecation at least 25% of time including at least two of the following

        (1)   Altered frequency

        (2)   Altered passage

        (3)   Altered consistency

        (4)   Passage of mucus

        (5)   Abdominal distention

- Physical Findings

  1. General appearance—"worried well," anxious, depressed

2. Vital signs—normal

3. Abdomen—mild abdominal tenderness, normal or mildly hyperactive bowel sounds

4. Rectal examination—normal

- Diagnostic Tests/Findings

  1. Stool examination—negative for blood, ova, parasite, pathogenic bacteria, and giardia specific antigen

  2. CBC, thyroid screen, chemical analysis—normal

  3. Barium enema—decreased motility, otherwise normal

  4. Proctosigmoidoscopy—normal

- Management/Treatment

  1. Confer with physician before ordering barium enema or proctosigmoidoscopy

  2. Provide emotional support, reassurance, information on stress reduction

  3. High fiber diet

  4. Pharmacologic agents

     a. Bulk laxatives—psyllium hydrophilic mucilloid

     b. Narcotics, depressants, and long term pharmaceutical use to be avoided

     c. Consult with physician regarding

        (1) Anticholinergics

            (a) Dicyclomine hydrochloride 20 to 40 mg orally q.i.d. or propantheline 15 mg orally q.i.d.

            (b) Usually given only after nonpharmacologic measures have failed

            (c) Side effects—dry mouth, tachycardia, orthostatic hypotension

            (d) Contraindicated if history of glaucoma, urinary retention, cardiac arrhythmia

   (2)   Loperamide or other opiate derived antidiarrheals are re-
         served for only very severe cases; potential for abuse in
         these patients is great

   (3)   Tricyclic antidepressants

5. Patient education

   a. Disease course and expected outcomes

   b. Rationale for treatment

   c. High fiber diet

6. Planned exercise (may help in stress reduction)

7. Need for annual rectal examination and sigmoidoscopy after age 40

8. Some patients may benefit from psychological counseling and/or relaxation techniques

Colorectal Cancer

- Definition: Malignancy of gastrointestinal tract primarily colon or rectum

- Etiology/Incidence

  1. Causes remain unclear

  2. Risk factors include history of colonic polyps, breast or female geni-
     tal tract cancer, chronic inflammatory bowel disorders, positive fam-
     ily history; high fat, low fiber, high-caloric diet

  3. Second most common cancer in western world, more common over
     the age of 50; peaks in the eighth decade

- Signs and Symptoms: Vary by location

  1. Right sided colon cancer

     a. Usually asymptomatic

     b. Vague or crampy, colicky abdominal pain

     c. Unexplained weight loss, fatigue, weakness

     d. Occult blood in stool

     e. Anemia

  2. Left sided colon cancer

     a. Alternating constipation with diarrhea

      b.   Change in stool caliber (narrow, ribbon-like)

      c.   Lower abdominal pain

      d.   Red blood in stool

      e.   Sensation of incomplete evacuation

  3. Rectal cancer

      a.   Tenesmus

      b.   Rectal bleeding (bright red)

      c.   Mucous discharge

- Differential Diagnosis

  1. Diverticular disease

  2. Lymphoma

  3. Irritable bowel syndrome

  4. Inflammatory bowel disease

- Physical Findings

  1. Palpable mass primarily in right colon

  2. Lymphadenopathy

  3. Rectal mass found on rectal examination

  4. Stools positive for occult blood

- Diagnostic Tests/Findings

  1. Barium enema radiograph—air contrast preferable to single contrast, may see an apple core lesion or mass

  2. Colonoscopy—may allow for biopsy of lesion found by barium enema

  3. Fiberoptic sigmoidoscope—may find distal tumors

  4. Testing of stools for occult blood—cancers detected with this technique are usually early stage and have a high cure rate

  5. Carcinoembryonic antigen (CEA) test—often performed, although not specific for colon cancer; normal level of CEA does not exclude possibility of malignancy

  6. CBC can demonstrate an anemia

    7. Chest radiograph may reveal metastases

- Management/Treatment

    1. Referral for surgical excision or resection depending upon the depth of invasion of tumors

    2. Patients with metastatic lesions, noted at the time of diagnosis, have a poor prognosis; palliative treatment is then indicated

    3. Patients with a resection often require a temporary colostomy

    4. General considerations

        a. Screening for colon cancer

            (1) Test stools for occult blood annually after age 50

            (2) Digital rectal examination annually after age 40

            (3) Sigmoidoscopy every 3 to 5 years after age 50

        b. Monitor for signs of dehydration during colon preps

        c. Instruct patient on possibility of a colostomy after procedure and begin patient teaching on care of colostomy preoperatively

        d. Encourage patient and family to ventilate feelings regarding the diagnosis

        e. Make referrals to pastoral care or mental health liaison as indicated

        f. Refer to community agencies for assistance after discharge, i.e., American Cancer Society, Ostomy Association

Questions
Select the best answer

1. Mr. P., 55-year-old of Irish decent, complains of pain in his chest and stomach for the past two weeks. He has been taking Alka Seltzer which seems to give him temporary relief. The pain is intermittent but has awakened him at night. The pain has a burning quality, and radiates up into his chest. He has hypertension which is controlled with diuretics.

   Which of the following would least likely be the cause of his pain?

   a. Coronary artery insufficiency
   b. Diverticulitis
   c. Duodenal ulcer
   d. Esophageal reflux

2. Your next step would be to:

   a. Start Mr. P. on antacids
   b. Discontinue his diuretic and switch to another class of antihypertensive
   c. Order an endoscopy
   d. Obtain additional medical history data

3. The fact that Mr. P.'s pain is not increased with activity and is unrelieved by rest makes it less likely that his problem is:

   a. Coronary artery insufficiency
   b. Gastric ulcer
   c. Duodenal ulcer
   d. Esophageal reflux

4. Which fact favors a diagnosis of gastric ulcer in this case?

   a. The patient's gender
   b. The patient's age
   c. The patient's ethnic origin
   d. The use of diuretics

5. Which of the following would be most beneficial in distinguishing a duodenal from a gastric ulcer in this patient?

   a. A history of a confirmed healed duodenal ulcer in the past year
   b. Reported unexplained weight loss in the past six months
   c. Pain aggravated by food intake

    d. An endoscopy or upper GI barium radiograph

6. Predisposing factors for duodenal ulcer include all of the following except:

    a. Genetic factors
    b. Stress
    c. Frequent laxative use
    d. Use of anti-inflammatory drugs

7. Bleeding from a duodenal ulcer:

    a. Usually causes increased pain
    b. In large amounts can cause diarrhea
    c. Is associated with constipation
    d. Indicates perforation

8. If Mr. P. has a peptic ulcer and his physical exam is unremarkable except for mild epigastric tenderness, it:

    a. Would not be unusual
    b. Indicates further diagnostic testing is unnecessary
    c. Is evidence that neoplastic disease is not present
    d. Rules out bleeding

9. A 55-year-old male with a peptic ulcer and mild anemia has a negative stool guaiac. You need to:

    a. Start iron supplementation
    b. Start H_2 antagonists and reschedule for return visit in 2 to 4 weeks
    c. Repeat the stool guaiac
    d. Refer for hematologic work up

10. After two weeks of treatment with omeprazole and clarithromycin all symptoms of a small non-bleeding duodenal ulcer have abated in your 35-year-old female. You:

    a. Need to confirm healing with an upper GI barium radiograph or endoscopy
    b. Instruct her to continue the omeprazole for two more weeks
    c. Instruct her to stop all medication and get a urea breath test
    d. Stop these medications and put her on H_2 antagonists

11. A major side effect of cimetidine that would be of special concern when prescribing for an elderly patient is:

    a. Confusion
    b. Decreased digoxin levels
    c. Hypophosphatemia
    d. Osteopenia

12. Mr. J. is an overweight 38 year old who has had intermittent heartburn for several months. He has been taking Tums which do provide temporary relief. During the past week he has been awakening during the night with a burning sensation in his chest. He is on no medication and has had no other major health problems.

    Which additional information would lead you to believe that gastroesophageal reflux is the cause of his pain?

    a. The pain seems better when he smokes to relieve his nerves
    b. Constipation has been a chronic problem and he uses over-the-counter laxatives at least weekly
    c. He often awakens at night with coughing and a bad taste in his mouth
    d. Coffee and fried foods never bother him

13. Mr. J. had no weight loss or dysphagia and his physical examination is unremarkable. Your next step would be to:

    a. Order an endoscopic exam
    b. Refer him to a gastroenterologist
    c. Start him on liquid antacids
    d. Tell him to eat a snack before bedtime

14. If you had decided his problem was esophageal reflux, you should tell him:

    a. He probably has a hiatal hernia causing the reflux
    b. He will probably require surgery
    c. He should avoid all fruit juices
    d. Smoking, alcohol, and caffeine can aggravate his problem

15. The most definitive test for LES incompetence and gastroesophageal reflux is:

    a. Stool guaiac
    b. Upper GI barium radiograph
    c. Cardiac and abdominal examination
    d. Bernstein test

16. Mary L. is 26 years old, slightly overweight, and 2 months post partum. She is complaining of heartburn, flatulence, and anorexia. During her pregnancy she had experienced similar symptoms but they have become more severe in the last week and she vomited twice. She has an intermittent pain in her right hypochondrium. She also thinks she pulled a shoulder muscle as she has an almost constant dull ache there. Your first step is to:

    a. Order liver function tests
    b. Obtain a more detailed history
    c. Refer her back to her obstetrician
    d. Refer her to a gastroenterologist

17. Mary's physical examination is unremarkable except for RUQ tenderness and a positive Murphy's sign. Which of the following could be excluded from your diagnosis at this point?

    a. Appendicitis
    b. Salpingitis
    c. Diverticulitis
    d. Cholecystitis

18. Which would be the most helpful diagnostic test at this point?

    a. CBC and liver function studies
    b. Ultrasound
    c. Liver scan
    d. Chest radiograph and ECG

19. On further testing Mary is diagnosed with cholecystitis and in consultation with a physician is put on a conservative treatment plan. Which of the following would be included in this plan?

    a. Encourage her to undertake a rapid weight reduction plan
    b. Put her on oral contraceptives if she isn't already on them
    c. Decrease fiber in her diet and eliminate all fats
    d. Direct her to contact a health provider if her pain increases or fever or chills develop

20. A 22-year-old male student comes to the student health service complaining of generalized abdominal pain and nausea. He had been out with a group of friends the night before and had been eating pizza and drinking beer. He awoke with generalized abdominal pain this morning and took some Alka Seltzer without much effect. The pain has gotten steadily worse throughout the day

and he now feels nauseated. He wonders if he might have food poisoning. Examination reveals hypoactive bowel sounds, and some tenderness in the RLQ. There is no guarding or rebound tenderness. His temperature is 100° F.

The absence of guarding and rebound tenderness:

    a. Suggests a psychogenic cause of his pain
    b. Rules out appendicitis
    c. Makes peritonitis unlikely
    d. Indicates irritable bowel syndrome

21. The next step you would take is:

    a. Refer to the physician
    b. Obtain a WBC and differential
    c. Obtain a stool culture
    d. Continue careful observation

22. Since he does not appear severely ill at this point, absence of vomiting and decreased bowel sounds and mild fever 15 hours after his last pizza and beer makes it highly unlikely that:

    a. Food poisoning is the problem
    b. He has appendicitis
    c. Perforation of the appendix can occur
    d. Surgery will be needed

23. In the meantime you:

    a. Encourage him to walk around to stimulate bowel activity
    b. Have him sip fluids to avoid dehydration
    c. Tell him you suspect appendicitis
    d. Give him an analgesic for pain relief

24. In elderly patients which of the following would not be an expected indication of appendicitis?

    a. Mild fever
    b. Abdominal distention with little pain
    c. Flatulence and hyperactive bowel sounds
    d. Shift to the left without leukocytosis

25. Ms. J is a 29-year-old accountant who comes in complaining of frequent

crampy abdominal pain after meals. She is often constipated and takes over-the-counter laxatives which are followed by a couple of days of diarrhea. She does feel better after having a bowel movement but only temporarily. She has also been embarrassed by flatulence and has noticed some abdominal distention. She has had no weight loss and has not noticed any blood in her stool. This problem has gone on for at least six months.

Your next step would be to:

  a. Obtain a complete history
  b. Order a barium enema
  c. Order a Bernstein test
  d. Suggest a trial of antispasmodics

26. Which of the following makes diverticulitis an unlikely diagnosis in this patient?

  a. Her age
  b. Frequent constipation
  c. Flatulence
  d. Crampy, intermittent pain

27. Which of the following might be expected to occur with irritable bowel syndrome?

  a. Rectal bleeding
  b. Nocturnal diarrhea
  c. Pain radiating to the left chest and arm
  d. Leukocytosis

28. Which of the following would be the reason for hospitalizing a patient with acute diverticulitis?

  a. LLQ tenderness
  b. Advanced age
  c. Leukocytosis
  d. Increased pain with defecation

29. Which of the following would not be considered conservative treatment of acute diverticulitis?

  a. Bedrest
  b. Liquid diet
  c. Antibiotics

  d. Colonic irrigations

30. A positive stool guaiac in a person suspected of having diverticulitis is:

  a. A common finding
  b. An ominous sign indicating need for hospitalization
  c. Requires immediate barium enema
  d. An indication of pending perforation

31. Bacturia in persons with acute diverticulosis may indicate:

  a. Abscess formation
  b. Bowel-bladder fistula
  c. Free perforation into the abdomen
  d. Reason for leukocytosis

32. Ms. S., a 19-year-old college freshman has just completed exam week. She comes in complaining of fatigue, headache, anorexia, and a runny nose. Symptoms began about two weeks ago. She has been taking vitamins and over-the-counter cold preparations but feels worse. ''Just the smell'' of food makes her nauseated. Her boyfriend had mono about a month ago and she wonders if she might have it. Physical examination reveals cervical lymphadenopathy, a slightly enlarged tender liver and enlarged spleen.

  Which laboratory tests in addition to a CBC, throat culture, and mono spot test would be most helpful in the differential diagnosis at this point?

  a. HAV IgG antibody test
  b. Anti-HB$_s$Ag
  c. Liver enzymes
  d. Stool culture

33. There is no indication in Ms. S's history to indicate IV drug abuse or exposure to blood products. Given the duration of her symptoms and a confirmed increase in her liver enzymes which test would be most helpful in confirming your diagnosis.

  a. IgM antibody to HAV
  b. IgG antibody to HAV
  c. Anti-HDV
  d. Anti-HB$_s$

34. A 30-year-old male with a history of acute hepatitis C over one year ago who

was treated with interferon still tests Anti-HCV positive. He should be considered:

    a. Infectious
    b. Incapable of transmitting the virus
    c. Fully recovered
    d. To have high serum viral levels

35. Infection with HDV requires antecedent or simultaneous infection with:

    a. HAV
    b. HBV
    c. HCV
    d. HGV

36. When jaundice occurs with hepatitis infection it:

    a. Indicates a more severe infection
    b. Increases the risk of acute liver failure
    c. Indicates development of chronic active hepatitis
    d. Usually resolves in 2 to 6 weeks

37. A normally healthy young adult diagnosed as having salmonella food poisoning should be told:

    a. To take doxycycline 100 mg t.i.d.
    b. That antidiarrheal drugs may decrease his diarrhea temporarily but may also prolong the problem
    c. That he should try to force fluids despite his nausea and vomiting to prevent dehydration
    d. The diarrhea should abate in about 24 hours

38. Which is the next laboratory test to obtain if diarrhea and vomiting persist for more than 48 hours?

    a. Stool guaiac
    b. Sigmoidoscopy
    c. Flat plate of the abdomen
    d. Stool culture and microscopic examination

39. Blurred vision and dizziness in a patient with suspected food poisoning requires:

    a. Gastroenterologic consult

    b. Antibiotic therapy

    c. Immediate hospitalization

    d. Follow-up in 24 hours

40. An 18-year-old previously healthy female presents with a case of a sudden onset of nausea, vomiting, generalized crampy abdominal pain followed by explosive diarrhea. The stools are uniformly thin and watery, without blood or pus. Physical exam reveals hyperactive bowel sounds and bilateral lower quadrant tenderness but no guarding or rebound. Rectal exam is negative and she is afebrile.

    The hypothesis that best explains these findings is:

    a. Acute appendicitis

    b. Acute salpingitis

    c. Acute gastroenteritis

    d. Ruptured ovarian cyst

Answers

1. b	14. d	28. b
2. d	15. d	29. d
3. a	16. b	30. a
4. b	17. c	31. b
5. d	18. b	32. c
6. c	19. d	33. a
7. b	20. c	34. a
8. a	21. a	35. b
9. c	22. a	36. d
10. b	23. c	37. b
11. a	24. c	38. d
12. c	25. a	39. c
13. c	26. a	40. c
	27. c	

37/40 92.5

Bibliography

Brady, W. M., & Ogorek, C. P. (1996). Gastroesophageal reflux disease. *Postgraduate Medicine, 100*(5), 76–89.

Bonagura, A. F., & Dabezies, M. A. (1996). *Helicobacter pylori* infection. *Postgraduate Medicine, 100*(5), 115–126.

Clinical Guidelines. (1997). Hepatitis B immunization/prophylaxis: Recommendations for adults/older adults. *Nurse practitioner, 21*(12), 64–78.

Cornell, S. (1997). New treatment for peptic ulcer disease. *ADVANCE for Nurse Practitioners, 5*(3), 57–59.

Damianos, A. J., & McGarrity, T. J. (1997). Treatment strategies for *Helicobacter pylori* infection. *American Family Physician, 55*, 2765–2774.

Friedman, L. S. (1998). Liver, biliary tract, and pancreas. In L. M. Tierney Jr., S. J. McPhee, & M. A. Papadakis (Eds.) *Current medical diagnosis and treatment* (37th ed., pp. 628–665). Stamford, CT: Appleton & Lange.

Harris, M. S. (1997). Irritable bowel syndrome. *Postgraduate Medicine. 101*, 215–226.

Hsu, H., Feinstone, S. M., & Hoffnagle, J. H. (1995). Acute viral hepatitis. In G. L. Mandell, J. E. Bennett, & R. Dolin (Eds.), *Principles and practice of infectious diseases* (pp. 1136–1151). New York: Churchill Livingstone.

King, R. R. (1997). Hepatitis C past, present and future issues. *ADVANCE for Nurse Practitioners, 5*(3), 51–52, 55–56.

Kowdley, K. V. (1996). Update on therapy for hepatobilliary diseases. *The Nurse Practitioner, 21*(7), 78–88.

Larson, R. R. (1997). Gastroesophageal reflux disease. *Postgraduate Medicine, 101*(2), 181–187.

Peek, R. M., & Blaser, M. J. (1996). Pathophysiology of *Helicobacter pylori*-induced gastritis and peptic ulcer disease. *The American Journal of Medicine, 102*, 200–207.

Stone, R. (1996). Primary care diagnosis of acute abdominal pain. *The Nurse Practitioner, 21*(12), 19–41.

Vail B. A. (1997). Management of chronic viral hepatitis. *American Family Physician, 55*, 2749–2756.

Endocrine Disorders

Sister Maria Salerno

Diabetes Mellitus

- Definition: Genetically influenced metabolic disorder of carbohydrate, fat, and protein metabolism characterized by abnormally high blood glucose levels due to inadequate or absent insulin production and/or impaired insulin action

- Etiology/Incidence

  1. Type 1—immune mediated (formerly insulin-dependent, [IDDM] type I, juvenile-onset, ketosis-prone)

     a. Genetic susceptibility (HLA-DR3 gene) with environmental exposure to virus or other infectious processes leading to abnormal autoimmune response and destruction of insulin producing pancreatic beta cells is suspected

        (1) Family history of autoimmune disorders

        (2) Islet cell antibodies

        (3) Insulin autoantibodies

        (4) Absence of C-peptide

     b. Occurs more often in those < 20 years of age; those with European ancestry

     c. 10% to 15% of diabetics are of this type

  2. Type 2 (formerly type II, non-insulin-dependent, [NIDDM] adult or maturity onset, ketosis-resistant)—may range from predominantly insulin resistant with relative insulin deficiency to predominantly insulin secretory defect with insulin resistance

     a. Strong genetic autosomal dominant familial pattern

        (1) Impaired insulin production response of beta cells to increased demands of obese state

        (2) Insulin resistance mediated by decreased insulin receptors in target cells

        (3) Post cell receptor defect impairing glucose transport into the cells

        (4) No specific HLA or islet cell antibodies

     b. Risk factors include:

        (1) Family history of diabetes

(2) Being previously identified as glucose intolerant

(3) African-American, Asian-American, Hispanic-American, Native-American, or Pacific Islander race

(4) Age ≥ 45

(5) Physical inactivity/obesity

(6) Having given birth to an infant weighing ≥ 9 lb.

(7) "Syndrome X"—a cluster of disorders which may include:

   (a) Hypertension

   (b) Abnormal lipid profile

      (1) HDL cholesterol ≤ 35 mg/dL

      (2) Triglycerides ≥ 250 mg/dL

   (c) Truncal obesity

   (d) Insulin resistance

   (e) Hyperinsulinism

3. Diabetes associated with certain conditions or syndromes

   a. Includes endocrinopathy, infection, drug/chemically induced

   b. Genetic syndromes

4. Impaired fasting glucose (IFG)

   a. Glucose levels fall between normal and overt diabetes

   b. May worsen over time, remain unchanged, or revert to normal

5. Gestational diabetes mellitus (GDM)

6. About 8 million diagnosed cases and estimated 8 million undiagnosed; after thyroid disease and obesity most common metabolic disorder encountered in primary care settings; third leading cause of death in U.S.

- Signs and Symptoms

   1. Type 1

      a. Usually sudden and severe in onset

      b. Early

        (1)   Polyuria

        (2)   Polydipsia

        (3)   Polyphagia

        (4)   Weight loss with normal or increased appetite

        (5)   Blurred vision

        (6)   Fatigue/weakness

        (7)   Nausea/vomiting

        (8)   Vaginal itching/infections

        (9)   Skin rashes

  c. With advanced disease and long-term complications

        (1)   Loss of appetite

        (2)   Bloating

        (3)   Dehydration

        (4)   Decreased level of consciousness

        (5)   Neurogenic and microvascular changes

            (a)   Paresthesias

            (b)   Progressive visual impairment

            (c)   Cold extremities

            (d)   Decreased or absent pedal pulses

            (e)   Constipation, nocturnal diarrhea

            (f)   Nocturia, neurogenic bladder, uremia, impotence

 2. Type 2

  a. Onset more insidious

  b. Early may not be noticed

        (1)   Polyuria

        (2)   Polyphagia

        (3)   Polydipsia

        (4)   Blurred vision

        (5)   Fatigue

      (6)   Sores that heal slowly

      (7)   Recurrent infections (vaginitis, especially candida; urinary tract, furuncules)

      (8)   Spontaneous abortion

   c.   With advanced disease and long term complications

      (1)   Similar to type 1, but macrovascular changes more prominent than microvascular

         (a)   Atherosclerosis

         (b)   Vascular insufficiency

         (c)   Coronary heart disease

      (2)   Hyperosmolar, hyperglycemic, nonketotic coma

- Differential Diagnosis
  1. Pancreatitis
  2. Cushing's syndrome
  3. Pheochromocytoma
  4. Acromegaly
  5. Cirrhosis
  6. Secondary effects of drug therapy
     a. Oral contraceptives
     b. Corticosteroids
     c. Thiazides
     d. Phenytoins
- Physical Findings
  1. Type 1
     a. Early
        (1) Thin, decreased weight
        (2) Ill appearance
        (3) Orthostatic hypotension
        (4) Skin infections

    b. With more advanced disease

        (1) Skin—ulcerations of feet and legs, "shin spots" over tibial bones; loss of hair over lower legs and toes

        (2) Eyes—retinopathy, including microaneurysms; yellow hard or fluffy "cotton wool" exudates; neovascularization, cataracts, glaucoma

        (3) Cardiovascular—diminished or absent pedal pulses; decreased capillary filling, pretibial edema, cool extremities

        (4) Neurologic—sensory loss, absent knee and ankle jerks, deficits in extraocular movements

  2. Type 2

    a. Early

        (1) Usually obese

        (2) Hypertension

    b. With advanced disease similar to type 1

- Diagnostic Tests/Findings

  1. Plasma blood sugar—criteria for confirmation

    a. Newer guidelines indicate the oral glucose tolerance test (OGTT) not be used but the diagnosis based on the fasting blood sugar (FBS)

    b. The diagnosis of diabetes will be made if FBS $\geq$ 126 mg/dL and is $\geq$ 126 mg/dL on repeat testing *or*

    c. A random non-fasting glucose level is $\geq$ 200 mg/dL and

        (1) Symptoms of polydipsia, polyuria, and weight loss are present *or*

        (2) On a subsequent day the FBS is $\geq$ 126 mg/dL or OGTT glucose level at 2 hours is $\geq$ 200 mg/dL

    d. It is advised that the OGTT not be used routinely

    e. If fasting glucose level are $\geq$ 110 mg/dL but < 126 mg/dL a diagnosis of "impaired fasting glucose" is made

    f. Pregnant women should be screened for gestational diabetes at 24 to 28 weeks gestation with a 50 g glucose load

(1) A 1 hour glucose level < 140 mg/dL is negative

(2) A 1 hour glucose level > 200 mg/dL is diagnostic

(3) A 1 hour glucose level between 140 mg/dL and 200 mg/dL requires confirmation by a 100 g OGTT—the diagnosis is confirmed if two of four values meet or exceed recommended cutoff points

    (a) Fasting 105 mg/dL

    (b) 1 hour 190 mg/dL

    (c) 2 hour 165 mg/dL

    (d) 3 hour 145 mg/dL

(4) Those with known risk factors such as race/ethnicity do not need the screening level 50 g exam but should receive the diagnostic 100 g exam at the 24 to 28 week point

2. Urinalysis—presence of glucose, acetone (in type 1), and in advanced stages protein

3. Blood urea nitrogen and urine creatinine—elevated in acute dehydration and with renal involvement

4. Serum cholesterol and triglyceride levels—often elevated especially in type 2

5. Electrocardiogram and chest radiography—for coronary and pulmonary pathology

6. Hemoglobin A_{1c}—predominately used as a measure of glycemic control; indicates average plasma glucose level for previous 60 to 90 days; tested every 3 to 6 months, 5.5 to 7% considered good control

7. Glycated serum protein (GSP)

    a. Index of glycemic status over past 1 to 2 weeks

    b. Clinical utility still under study

- Management/Treatment

1. Goals of therapy are to attain best possible metabolic control while avoiding potential side effects—see Table 1

Table 1

Glycemic Control for Diabetics

Glycemic Index	Target	Non-Diabetic	Therapeutic action suggested
Fasting and preprandial glucose (mg/dL)	80–120	< 115	< 80 > 140
Bedtime glucose (mg/dL)	100–140	< 120	> 160 < 100
HbA$_{1c}$ (%)	< 7	< 6	> 8

2. Unless acutely ill treatment can be instituted on an outpatient basis

3. Consult physician for:

   a. Newly diagnosed

   b. Anyone refractory to treatment

   c. Anyone with a blood sugar > 400 mg/dL

4. Give consideration to work schedule, life style, economic, social, and cultural aspects in management approach, e.g., persons who are homeless, persons working a night shift

5. Diet along with exercise is cornerstone of therapy

   a. Refer newly diagnosed to registered dietician and annually or semi-annually for follow-up

   b. Consistent dietary schedule; ideally 3 meals and 3 snacks; especially important for persons with type 1 diabetes and type 2 on insulin; teach use of exchange lists to those on insulin; for type 2, space meals 5 hours apart with few or no snacks

   c. Avoid refined carbohydrates and simple sugars

   d. Total carbohydrate intake should be 50% to 60% of total caloric intake

   e. Limit fats to 20% to 30% of total calories; saturated at < 8 to 9%

   f. Increase fiber to 25 g/1,000 calories

   g. Moderate protein intake, 0.8 g/kg/day or 20% of total caloric intake

   h. Total caloric intake to maintain or achieve ideal body weight (IBW)

    (1)   Calculation of IBW

        (a)   Females—allow 100 lb for first 5 feet of height plus 5 lb for each additional inch of height

        (b)   Males—allow 106 lb for first 5 feet of height and add 6 lb for each additional inch of height

        (c)   Small frame subtract 10%

        (d)   Large frame add 10%

    (2)   Caloric requirement

        (a)   Multiply IBW by 10 = baseline calories

        (b)   Add 3 × IBW if activity level is sedentary (most fall in this category); 5 × IBW if moderate; and 10 × IBW if strenuous

        (c)   IBW = 125 lb
125 × 10 = 1250 (baseline calories)
125 × 3 = 375 (activity calories)
1250 + 375 = 1625 (total calories needed per day)

        (d)   In type 2—obese, where weight reduction is primary treatment, subtract 500 calories from the total number needed per day

6. Exercise

    a.   Planned daily exercise is an essential component for all diabetics, at least 30 minutes every other day

    b.   Older persons with diabetes may be limited in types of exercise due to other concurrent problems such as arthritis, retinopathy

    c.   Diminishes need for insulin by enhancing oxidation of sugar and facilitating absorption of insulin from injection sites

    d.   Those on insulin should be instructed to inject insulin furthest from site of intensive exercise, e.g., abdomen rather than arms or thighs

    e.   Additional carbohydrate should be ingested prior to exercise

    f.   Contributes to weight and lipid control, reduces risks of CVD, improves insulin action

7. Oral pharmacologic agents

    a. Sulfonylureas—see Table 2

        (1) First generation potent with long duration of action, increased risk of hypoglycemia, especially in the elderly

        (2) Contraindicated in pregnancy, for those with sulfa allergy, gestational or type 1 diabetes, or in ketoacidosis

        (3) Few side effects, but special precautions in those with renal, liver, or cardiovascular disease

        (4) Risk of hypoglycemia and weight gain

    b. Insulin resistance reducers

        (1) Biguanide (Metformin) 1.5 to 2.5 g daily in divided doses

            (a) Causes moderate weight loss

            (b) Improved lipid profile regardless of glycemic effect

            (c) Low risk of hypoglycemia

            (d) Side effects of flatulence, diarrhea; metallic taste minimized by taking with meals and increasing doses more slowly

            (e) Contraindicated in renal, liver, or advanced cardiovascular disease

            (f) Rare incidence of lactic acidosis; check pharmacology reference for precautions

        (2) Thiazolidinedione (Troglitazone) 400 to 600 mg once a day

            (a) Used for type 2 diabetes when glucose control is inadequate with > 30 units insulin/day in divided doses with food

            (b) Start 200 mg and increase every 2 to 4 weeks

            (c) Reduce insulin when FBS < 120/dL

            (d) Increased risk of hypoglycemia

            (e) May induce postmenopausal ovulation/risk of unintended pregnancy

Table 2

Some Common Oral Hypoglycemics

Agent	Daily Dose mg	Doses/day	Onset hours	Duration hours	Metabolism
First Generation Sulfonylureas					
Tolbutamide (a) (Orinase)	500-3000	2-3	1	6-12	Hepatic
Acetohexamide (b) (Dymelor)	250-1500	1 or 2	1	10-14	Hepatic
Tolazamide (c) (Tolinase)	100-250	1 or more	4-6	10-14	Hepatic
Chlorpropamide (d) (Diabinese)	100-500	1	1	72	Renal
Second Generation Sulfonylureas					
Glyburide (e) (DiaBeta) (Micronase)	2.5-20	1 or 2	1.5	24	Hepatic
Glimepiride (Amaryl)	1-4	1	1	24	Hepatic
Glipizide (f) (Glucotrol)	2-40	1 or 2	1	12-18	Hepatic
(Glucotrol)	5-20	1	1	24	
(Glucotrol XL)	5-20	1	1	24	Hepatic

(a) Most benign, least potent, especially useful in renal disease
(b) Little advantage over tolbutamide; uricosuric effects
(c) Equipotent to tolbutamide with less severe side effects
(d) Potent; contraindicated for use in elderly and renal desease; disulfiram-like reaction with alcohol; may cause hyponatremia
(e) Take on empty stomach; low toxicity, NO disulfiram reaction; caution in elderly
(f) 50-200 times more potent than other hypoglycemics; no disulfiram-like reaction; low toxicity; caution in the elderly

    (f) Antagonized by cholestyramine—separate doses by at least 4 hours

    (g) Potential for multiple drug interactions

    (h) Asthenia, dizziness, GI disturbances

  c. Alpha-glucosidase inhibitor (Acarbose)

    (1) Lowers postprandial blood glucose levels

    (2) Low risk of hypoglycemia or weight gain

    (3) Somewhat less efficacious than sulfonylureas or biguanides

    (4) Flatulence, bloating, diarrhea frequent but abate with continued use

        d.   Administer angiotensin converting enzyme inhibitor (ACE) if not contraindicated

            (1)   Drug of choice to treat hypertension in those with D.M.

            (2)   Shown to prevent progression of nephropathy even in normotensives with type 2 D.M.

    8.   Insulin (see Table 3)

        a.   Indicated

            (1)   Confirmed or suspected type 1 or gestational diabetes

            (2)   Type 2 dietary and/or oral agent management fails to control glucose levels, or in times of stress

            (3)   For those for whom oral agents are contraindicated

        b.   Some may need more than three injections per day and or use an insulin pump to maintain control

        c.   Weight gain and need for frequent glucose monitoring can be problems

        d.   Purity

            (1)   Standard beef or pork— > 10 but < 25 parts per million (ppm) proinsulin (immunogenic agent)

            (2)   Purified beef or pork— < 10 ppm proinsulin

Table 3

Insulins

Type	Action	Onset (Hours) (a)	Peak (Hours)	Duration (Hours) (b)
Insulin analog (Lispro)	Very Rapid	0.25	1	3.5–4.5
Regular	Rapid	0.5–1	1–2	5–6
Semilente	Rapid	0.5–2	1–2	12–16
NPH	Intermediate	1–2	2–8	24–48
Lente (isophane)	Intermediate	1–2	2–8	24–48
NPH (70%) with Regular (30%) (Mixtard, Novolin 70/30)	Intermediate	0.5	4–8	24
PZI (protamine zinc)	Long	2–4	8–12	38
Ultralente	Long	2–4	8–12	36

NOTE: Pork, beef-pork, and human synthetic insulin available in rapid, intermediate, long-acting

Long-acting are not currently available in human insulin

(a) Onset depends on site of injection, dose size, brand

(b) Duration is proportional to dose size and is increased in renal failure

(3) Human synthetic < 10 ppm proinsulin

(4) Beef more antigenic than pork species; human insulin least antigenic of all

e. Initiation and adjustment of dosage

  (1) Exogenous insulin replacement begins with 10 to 30 units of intermediate acting insulin before breakfast each morning

    (a) Lower doses for thin patients and higher for obese (tend to have more insulin resistance)

    (b) Change dose no more than every 2 to 3 days

  (2) As long as plasma glucose is > 140 mg/dL before the evening meal, dose is increased by 2 to 5 units every 2 to 3 days

  (3) When afternoon postprandial plasma glucose is consistently < 140 mg/dL fasting plasma glucose is checked for sustained effect of single insulin dose; if fasting glucose is elevated, dose will be split with $\frac{2}{3}$ given before breakfast and $\frac{1}{3}$ before the evening meal; doses are adjusted until fasting plasma glucose is 120 to 140 mg/dL

  (4) Once afternoon and before breakfast regulation is achieved, late morning levels are assessed; if needed, regular insulin can be combined with morning injection to keep late morning plasma glucose levels < 140 mg/dL

    (a) THE AMOUNT OF REGULAR INSULIN NORMALLY SHOULD NOT EXCEED 50% OF THE INSULIN GIVEN AT ANY TIME

    (b) Do not mix lente or ultra lente with regular; zinc in lente precipitates regular, decreasing effective proportion of regular and increasing that of the lente

    (c) Do not mix lente with velosulin short acting (Nordisk)—phosphate buffer increases concentration of unmodified soluble insulin and diminishes effect of intermediate acting preparation

         (d)   Regular insulin should be drawn up first if mixing regular and NPH in the same syringe

    (5)   Once daily regimen is established, urine and self-monitored plasma glucose levels are tested 3 to 4 times a day as indicated by the insulin schedule and severity of the disease

         (a)   Daily dose requirement decreases with progressive renal failure

         (b)   Control is assessed at 3 to 6 month intervals; glycosylated Hgb which reflects average glucose levels of the preceding 8 to 12 weeks may be helpful

9.   Combination therapy usually instituted if failure of monotherapy in type 2

   a.   Most frequently used—sulfonylurea with insulin or biguanide or alpha-glucosidase inhibitor

   b.   Less frequently used—insulin with biguanide and a sulfonylurea; insulin with biguanide; insulin with alpha-glucosidase inhibitor; or biguanide with alpha-glucosidase inhibitor.

   c.   No evidence of significant adverse interactions

   d.   Increase complexity and cost of treatment regimen

   e.   Morning sulfonylurea and NPH-lente insulin in the evening for select persons with type 2 diabetes

    (1)   Helps control morning hyperglycemia without concomitant hypoglycemia seen with insulin alone

    (2)   May help patient avoid need for multiple insulin injections

    (3)   Seems to work best in those who are less than 150% of Ideal Body Weight and have had the disease for less than 15 years

10.   Patient education—should begin at time of diagnosis and will extend over several weeks

   a.   Cause and general management of diabetes

   b.   Importance of diet and weight control

   c.   Self-monitoring of blood and urine glucose

d. Administration of insulin, dosing, action, side effects, and site rotation

e. Administration of oral hypoglycemic agents, dosing, action and side effects

f. Potential alteration in glucose metabolism with acute illness, exercise, and emotional stress

g. Test for and significance of ketonuria

h. Recognition and treatment of hypoglycemia

i. Proper leg and foot care

j. Sick-day guidelines

k. Guidelines for economizing with repeated use of needles and splitting glucose test strips

11. Complications

    a. Hypoglycemia

        (1) Causes

            (a) Insulin overdosage

            (b) Omission or delay of meals

            (c) Heavy exercise

            (d) Errors in injection technique

            (e) Renal failure

            (f) Weight loss

            (g) Development of hepatitis, pituitary or adrenal insufficiency, or other conditions that cause hypoglycemia

            (h) Drugs that affect insulin metabolism/action; see Table 4

        (2) Symptoms

            (a) Weakness

            (b) Sweating

            (c) Shakiness

            (d) Tremors

(e) Nervousness

(f) Headache

(g) Dizziness

(h) Hunger

(i) Irritability

(j) Convulsions, confusion, coma

(k) Tachycardia, palpitations

b. Somogyi phenomenon

(1) Cause—morning rebound hyperglycemia; occurs in response to nocturnal hypoglycemia with excessive insulin administration

(2) Clues—erratic plasma glucose and urine ketone values; symptoms of nocturnal hypoglycemia (night sweats, nightmares, low serum glucose 2 to 3 a.m.), weight gain in presence of heavy glycosuria

(3) Treatment—reduce insulin dose 10% to 20%

(4) Distinguish from *Dawn Phenomenon* which is early morning fasting hyperglycemia without nocturnal hypoglycemia; thought to be related to circadian rhythm secretion of growth hormone and treated by evening or bedtime dose of insulin

c. Lipodystrophy

(1) Atrophy—subcutaneous fat atrophy at insulin injection sites

(a) Cause—impurities in the insulin, possible autoimmune mechanism

(b) Treatment—switch to purified insulin, inject directly into atrophic areas

(2) Hypertrophy—over-growth of subcutaneous tissue

(a) Cause—growth promoting effects of insulin; improper rotation of injection sites

(b) Treatment—prevent by proper rotation of injection sites

Table 4

Medication Effect On Insulin Metabolism/Action

Medication	Action
Alcohol	Decreased half-life of sulfonylureas in alcoholics, can cause severe hypoglycemia in those on hypoglycemics
Beta-adrenergic	Inhibit insulin secretion; block most hypoglycemia symptoms; prolong effect of insulin
Calcium channel blockers	Inhibit insulin secretion
Diazoxide	Inhibits insulin secretion
Glucocorticoids	Insulin antagonism
Nicotinic acid	Insulin resistance
Oral contraceptives	Insulin resistance
Phenytoin	Inhibits insulin secretion
Sympathomimetics	Insulin antagonism Inhibit insulin secretion
Thiazide diuretics	Inhibit insulin secretion
MAO inhibitors	Increase effects of antidiabetic agents
Salicylates	Increase effects of antidiabetic agents
Coumarin	Increase effects of sulfonylureas
Phenylbutazone	Increase effects of sulfonylureas

d. Insulin allergy

(1) Rare and usually localized

(2) Treatment—change to human synthetic insulin

(3) Localized allergies may be treated with antihistamines or corticosteroid; consultation required

e. Insulin resistance requiring more than 200 units per day

(1) Rare and even less common with increased use of human insulins

(2) Cause—over-production of insulin-binding immunoglobulins

(3) Treatment—change to less immunogenic pork or human synthetic insulins

(4) May require glucocorticoid treatment; consultation required

f. Diabetic ketoacidosis (DKA)—hyperglycemia with ketonuria and disruption of the fluid, electrolyte, and pH balance leading to coma and even death; marked by hyperglycemia, metabolic acidosis, and ketonemia; sometimes PRESENTING SIGN in undiagnosed type 1

    (1) Cause—infection, trauma, myocardial infarction, other severe stress, and noncompliance with therapeutic regimen

    (2) Treatment—emergency fluid replacement, insulin therapy, sodium bicarbonate therapy, and close monitoring of blood chemistries

  g. Hyperosmolar nonketotic syndrome—severe hyperglycemia, hyperosmolarity, and dehydration in the absence of ketoacidosis which may lead to coma; most often occurs in elderly on oral hypoglycemics and those with undiagnosed type 2

    (1) Precipitating factors—calcium channel blockers, corticosteroids, thiazide diuretics, propranolol, phenytoin

    (2) Treatment—similar to ketoacidosis, but need less insulin and more fluid replacement

    (3) Prognosis is poor in elderly, particularly those with concurrent renal disease, hypertension, or congestive heart failure

12. Follow-up

  a. Well controlled patients—minimum every 3 to 4 months

  b. Yearly ECG, chest radiograph, creatinine, urinalysis with microprotein analysis, lipid profile, physical examination including fundoscopic, full neurologic examination

  c. Annual ophthalmologic examination by ophthalmologist

  d. Skin inspection, feet inspection, fundoscopic, and evaluation of glycemic control by fasting or postprandial plasma glucose measurements at each visit

  e. Hemoglobin A_{1c} every 3 to 6 months

13. Referrals to local support groups and identification of local chapters of the American Diabetes Association for information, support, and publications

14. Routinely screen all ≥45 years of age, if negative repeat every three years or earlier if risk factors are present.

Hyperthyroidism (Thyrotoxicosis)

- Definition: Excessive secretory activity of the thyroid gland; symptoms produced by excess exogenous or endogenous thyroid hormone; called Graves' disease when associated with ocular signs or ocular disturbances and a diffuse goiter

- Etiology/Incidence

  1. Causes

     a. Autoimmune response (Graves' disease accounts for more than 85% of cases)

     b. Subacute thyroiditis

     c. Toxic multinodular goiter; toxic uninodular goiter (autonomous thyroid adenoma)

     d. Metastatic follicular thyroid carcinoma

     e. Thyrotoxicosis factitia

     f. TSH secreting pituitary tumor (secondary hyperthyroidism)

     g. hCG secreting tumors (choriocarcinoma, hydatiform mole)

     h. Testicular embryonal carcinoma

  2. One of the most common endocrine disorders

  3. Highest incidence in women between 20 and 40 years of age

- Signs and Symptoms

  1. Most frequent

     a. Anxiety

     b. Diaphoresis

     c. Fatigue

     d. Hypersensitivity to heat

     e. Nervousness

     f. Palpitations

     g. Weight loss

     h. Insomnia, nightmares

  2. Frequent

      a. Dyspnea

      b. Weakness

      c. Increased appetite

      d. Eye complaints, e.g., difficulty focusing

      e. Swelling of legs

      f. Hyperdefecation without diarrhea, hyperactive bowel sounds

      g. Diarrhea

      h. Oligomenorrhea or amenorrhea

      i. Tremors

      j. Angina

3. Infrequent

      a. Anorexia

      b. Constipation

      c. Weight gain

      d. Signs of pseudobulbar palsy

4. Elderly patients may present with few signs or symptoms noted in younger patients (apathetic hyperthyroidism); may present with cardiovascular problems unresponsive to digitalis, quinidine, or diuretics

      a. Atrial fibrillation

      b. Angina

      c. Congestive heart failure

- Differential Diagnosis

  1. Anxiety neurosis, especially in menopause

  2. Other diseases associated with hypermetabolism, e.g., pheochromocytoma and acromegaly

  3. Myasthenia gravis (causes the same ophthalmoplegic signs)

  4. Orbital tumors which can cause exophthalmos

  5. Psychosis

- Physical Findings

1. General—thin, muscle wasting may be evident; nervous; quick motions

2. Vital signs—tachycardia, irregular pulse, widened pulse pressure

3. Integumentary—skin moist, velvety, may show increased pigmentation or vitiligo; hair thin, fine; spider angiomas and gynecomastia may be evident

4. Eyes—prominent; appear to "stare;" lid lag; lack of accommodation, chemosis; proptosis (exophthalmos)

5. Neck—enlarged thyroid gland (goiter) smooth or nodular, symmetric or asymmetric; thyroid bruit or thrill; absence of signs does not rule out hyperthyroidism

6. Cardiovascular—paroxysmal atrial fibrillation, harsh pulmonary systolic murmur, congestive failure, possible enlargement

7. Neurologic—hyperactive reflexes; fine tremors of fingers, tongue; mental changes ranging from mild exhilaration to delirium; in elderly, apathy, lethargy and severe depression may be manifested

8. Lymphatic—lymphadenopathy and splenomegaly may be present

- Diagnostic Tests/Findings (see Table 5 for list of thyroid function tests)

1. TSH assay best text for thyroid dysfunction—decreased in hyperthyroidism

2. Free thyroxine index (FTI) usually elevated; if normal and clinical impression is strong for hyperthyroidism then do

3. T_3, radioimmunoassay (T_3, RIA)—elevated with a normal T_4 in early hyperthyroidism and T_3 toxicosis

4. T_4 level elevated in later stages

- Management/Treatment

1. Refer for hospitalization for suspected "thyroid storm"

   a. High fever

   b. Severe agitation

   c. Confusion

   d. Cardiovascular collapse

   e. Malignant exophthalmus

Table 5

THYROID ASSESSMENT TESTS

Thyroxine (T$_4$)	Major hormone secreted by the thyroid gland
T$_4$ (RIA-serum)	By radioimmunoassay (RIA); normal adult is 5 to 12 μg/dL
Free Thyroxine Index (FT$_4$I)	Unaffected by TBG and is a better reflection of the true index hormonal status; serum T$_4$ and T$_3$ resin uptake (T$_3$, RU) used to calculate this index; normal adults 0.9–2.2ng/dL
T$_3$ Resin Uptake (T$_3$RU)	Indirect measure of T$_4$ levels by assessing T$_4$ binding sites; may be thought of as the reciprocal of the T$_4$ RIA; in hyperthyroidism there is a high T$_3$ resin uptake; in hypothyroidism the T$_3$ is low; normal adult is 25 to 35%
T$_3$ RIA (Serum)	Direct measure of triiodothyronine (T$_3$) thyroid hormone; helpful in diagnosing thyrotoxicosis when T$_4$ is normal; in hypothyroidism T$_3$ often normal; T$_4$ more helpful; normal adult is 80 to 200ng/dL (RIA)
Thyroid Antibodies, Thyroglobulin	High titers suggest autoimmune disease, e.g., Hashimoto's thyroiditis; also elevated in carcinoma of the thyroid; normal adult is 1:20, 0–50 ng/mL (RIA)
Throid Stimulating Hormone (TSH)	Direct measure of TSH secreted from the anterior pituitary in response to thyroid-releasing hormone (TRH); normal adult is 2 to 5.4 μU/mL < 10 μU/mL (RIA)
TSH Immunoradiometric Assay (IRMA)	Newer assay replacing TSH (RIA); normal adult is 0.5 to 5.0 μU/mL; more sensitive to suppressed TSH in hyperthyroidism
Radioactive Iodine Uptake (RAIU)	Used primarily to detect hyperthyroidism etiology; radioactive iodine given orally or intravenously; the thyroid is scanned at 3 different intervals to determine iodine uptake of the thyroid gland; an elevated RAIU indicates hyperthyroidism; normal adult is 2 hr., 1 to 13%; 6 hr., 2 to 25%; 24 hr., 15 to 45%

      f.   Difficulty in breathing due to enlarged or tender thyroid gland

  2. Obtain physician consult for clients suspected of/or newly diagnosed with hyperthyroidism for treatment which may include:

      a.   Propranolol 10 to 60 mg orally every 6 hours to control symptoms

      b.   Radioactive iodine (^{131}I)

         (1)   Therapeutic dose is 80 to 120 mCi administered in doses of 5 to 15mCi based on estimated weight of the thyroid gland

         (2)   Most become euthyroid after 3 to 6 months

         (3)   Hypothyroidism is frequent and can occur anytime after radioactive iodine therapy

         (4)   Contraindicated in pregnancy

      c.   Antithyroid drugs—indicated for initial control of thyrotoxicosis especially in pregnant women, those not wanting to take

^{131}I, or in preparation for surgical removal; effective in patients with small goiters

    (1) Propylthiouracil (PTU)—usual dose 300 to 400 mg/day in divided doses

        (a) Preferred for use in pregnant women

        (b) During pregnancy dose kept < 200 mg/day

    (2) Methimazole (MMI)—15 to 60 mg/day orally in three divided doses

    (3) Side effects

        (a) Dermatitis

        (b) Nausea

        (c) Agranulocytosis (most serious)

        (d) Hypothyroidism which can cause a TSH stimulated increase in goiter size

3. Patient education:

    a. Medication is to be taken for about two years and not abruptly discontinued

    b. At first sign of infection or fever drug should be stopped and healthcare professional contacted

    c. Therapeutic effect of medication is not usually evident for about three weeks

4. Surgery

    a. Not used as frequently now

    b. Indicated for children, adolescents, pregnant women unable to tolerate PTU, adults nonresponsive to thiourea treatment who refuse RAI

    c. Usually rendered enthyroid with drugs preoperatively

5. General considerations

    a. Client education

        (1) Rationale for treatment; dosage and side effects of medications; takes at least three weeks before antithyroid medications become effective

(2) Instructions regarding nutritional needs: high carbohydrate, high caloric diet until medication takes effect; avoidance of stimulants such as caffeine

(3) Symptoms of "thyroid storm"

(4) Symptoms of hypothyroidism

    b. Follow-up

(1) Periodic examinations until euthyroid

(2) All patients who have been treated for hyperthyroidism should be periodically checked for hypothyroidism which may occur anytime during treatment

Adult Hypothyroidism (Myxedema)

- Definition: Decreased or deficient thyroid hormone—primary (glandular dysfunction) or secondary (pituitary insufficiency); occurs in all age groups

- Etiology/Incidence

    1. Major classifications

        a. Primary—caused by damage to the hormone producing capabilities of the thyroid gland itself

(1) Most common cause in adults is autoimmune thyroiditis (Hashimoto's, chronic lymphocytic)

(2) Can also be caused by ablation of the gland by surgery, medication, radiation, and goitrogens (thiocyanates, rutabagas, lithium carbonate)

(3) More common than secondary

        b. Secondary—often related to destructive lesions of the pituitary gland as with chromophobe adenoma or postpartum necrosis (Sheehan's syndrome); frequently associated with signs of adrenal and gonadal disorders

        c. Tertiary—TRH deficiency arising in the hypothalmus; sometimes grouped with secondary

    2. Occurs in all age groups; more prevalent in women and those

        a. With a history of thyroiditis

  b. With previously treated hyperthyroidism (all modalities)

  c. Being treated with lithium or para-aminosalicylic acid

  d. With coexistent autoimmune disorders (e.g., rheumatoid arthritis, lupus, pernicious anemia)

- Signs and Symptoms

  1. Most frequent

      a. Cold intolerance

      b. Coarse skin

      c. Decreased sweating

      d. Dry skin

      e. Lethargy

      f. Swelling of eye lids

  2. Frequent

      a. Anemia (normocytic, normochromic, microcytic, or macrocytic)

      b. Anorexia

      c. Coarse hair

      d. Cold skin

      e. Constipation

      f. Hair loss

      g. Hoarseness or aphonia, thick tongue

      h. Hyperlipidemia including hypercholesterolemia

      i. Leg edema

      j. Menorrhagia

      k. Memory impairment

      l. Swelling of face

      m. Paresthesias

      n. Weight change

- Differential Diagnosis
    1. Rule out coexisting autoimmune disease or secondary hypothyroidism
    2. Nephrotic syndrome
    3. Chronic renal disease
- Physical Findings
    1. Vital signs—bradycardia, mild hypotension, or diastolic hypertension
    2. Edema of hands, face, eyelids
    3. Integumentary—dry, scaly skin with carotenemic tone; brittle nails; alopecia; puffy eyelids; temporal thinning of the eye brows
    4. ENT—enlarged tongue, possible hearing decrease, thyroid often enlarged
    5. Cardiovascular—bradycardia, decreased intensity of heart tones, cardiac enlargement (myxedemic heart may be related to pericardial effusion)
    6. Respiratory—pleural effusion
    7. Abdominal—ascites, decreased bowel sounds
    8. Neuromuscular—slow or delayed deep tendon reflexes, cerebellar ataxia, dementia (myxedema madness, manifested with hallucinations, paranoid ideation, and hyperactive delirium), pseudomyotonia, carpal tunnel syndrome
- Diagnostic Tests/Findings
    1. Free thyroxine index (FTI) or T_4; if low a TSH is helpful in determining etiology
    2. TSH elevated in primary hypothyroidism
    3. If T_4 is normal and TSH is elevated, may be mild hypothyroidism
    4. Thyrotropin releasing hormone (TRH) stimulation done if low TSH with low T_4 or low FTI; may indicate secondary hypothyroidism
    5. CBC—may demonstrate anemia

- Management/Treatment

  1. Refer for immediate hospitalization any client suspected of developing myxedemic coma—severe hypothyroidism associated with hypothermia, decreased mentation, hypoventilation, respiratory acidosis, relative hypotension, hyponatremia, hypoglycemia

  2. Obtain physician consultation for clients with suspected or newly diagnosed hypothyroidism for further testing and/or initiation of treatment which would include administration of synthetic T_4 (levothyroxine); desiccated thyroid is no longer used due to variability in composition

     a. Average replacement dose of T_4 is thyroxine 0.125 mg/day in healthy, non-elderly adults and may range from 0.025 to 0.3 mg/day

     b. Dosage starts with 0.1 mg/day for those < 50 years of age, and 0.025 to 0.05 mg/day in those > 50 years of age or with known ischemic heart disease without angina

     c. Dosage is increased by 0.025 mg/day every two weeks until the patient is clinically euthyroid

     d. Patients with coexisting adrenal insufficiency, coronary insufficiency, or angina require particular care

     e. Initial effects of replacement not usually perceptible for at least two weeks after initiation of therapy and are initially demonstrated by decreased facial edema and increased urination

  3. On follow-up visits, after replacement therapy has been instituted:

     a. Check cardiopulmonary status; if pulse is > 100/minute consult with physician

     b. Monitor for symptoms or signs of too vigorous therapy, side effects, and toxic effects of replacement therapy; ask about dyspnea, orthopnea, angina, palpitations, nervousness, insomnia

     c. Be alert to concomitant use of opiates, barbiturates, other central nervous system depressants, digitalis, and insulin; persons with hypothyroidism are particularly sensitive to these agents; as they become euthyroid dosages may have to be increased

4. Monitor control of clinical symptoms and periodically monitor serum FTI and TSH; persistently high TSH or low FTI may indicate under-replacement; a high T_4 and low TSH with symptoms of hyperthyroidism usually indicates over replacement

5. Patient education

    a. Nature and chronicity of the disease and the need for life long treatment

    b. Rationale for treatment—dosage, side effects, and toxic effects of treatment

    c. Teach signs of hyperthyroidism

    d. Management of symptoms of hypothyroidism until abatement with replacement therapy

        (1) Fatigue

        (2) Dry skin

        (3) Constipation (increased fiber, fluids)

Thyroid Nodule

- Definition: Discrete enlargements within the thyroid gland
- Etiology unknown but nodules are common

    1. Palpable in 5 to 10% of U.S. population

    2. Majority are benign

    3. Risk of nodule malignancy less than 10% in most adults

        a. Men have a higher incidence than women

        b. Papillary and follicular carcinoma are most common types of malignancy

            (1) Papillary tends to spread within the thyroid gland or to cervical lymphatics

                (a) Twice as common in women as men

                (b) Accounts for 80% of thyroid malignancies in adults < 40

            (2) Follicular accounts for approximately 20% of all thyroid cancers

        (a)   Incidence somewhat higher in older individuals

        (b)   Usually slow growing but more aggressive than papillary; can spread rapidly to lymph nodes and to distant sites via the blood stream, often to lung, bone, brain, or liver

   c.   Medullary and anaplastic carcinoma are rarer but tend to metastasize very early; anaplastic carcinoma, because of high invasiveness and early metastasis, results in death in weeks or months regardless of treatment modality

   d.   Risk of carcinoma is increased with a history of radiation exposure, particularly during childhood, to the head or neck for acne, tonsils, adenoids; the risk is also increased in those with a family history of thyroid cancer—this is especially true for medullary carcinoma

- Signs and Symptoms

  1. Thyroid mass

  2. Expanding goiter or nodule which is hard and/or tender

  3. Hoarseness or dysphagia

- Differential Diagnosis: Distinguish from non-neoplastic enlargements, e.g., cystic nodules, multinodular goiters

- Physical Findings

  1. Single hard thyroid nodule (or multiple nodules) fixed to overlying tissue

  2. Regional lymphadenopathy

- Diagnostic Tests/Findings

  1. Free thyroxine index (FTI)—usually normal; if elevated chances of malignancy are decreased

  2. RAI scan—nonfunctioning (cold) nodule

  3. Ultrasonography—if cystic, rarely malignant

  4. Thyrocalcitonin—increased in medullary carcinoma

  5. Biopsy (open or needle)—positive cytology if malignant

- Management/Treatment

    1. Any individual with the signs and symptoms or physical findings previously described should be referred

    2. Treatment may include:

        a. Excision of the nodule (complete thyroidectomy in the case of medullary carcinoma) and regional lymph nodes

        b. Ablation of metastasis with large doses of radioactive iodine

        c. Suppression of thyroid function with L-thyroxine

        d. Chemotherapy for anaplastic carcinoma; (thyroid suppression and radioactive ablation of metastasis are not effective in medullary thyroid carcinoma)

    3. Client education related to diagnostic tests

    4. Follow-up for detection of metastasis, recurrence, and subsequent treatment is usually on an annual basis

Cushing's Syndrome

- Definition: A constellation of clinical abnormalities due to an excess of corticosteroids

- Etiology/Incidence

    1. Excessive or prolonged administration of glucocorticoids (most common)

    2. Excessive pituitary ACTH secretion (Cushing's disease)

    3. Secretion of ACTH by a non-pituitary tumor (ectopic tumor), e.g., carcinoma of the lung or other malignant growths

    4. Tumors within the adrenal cortex—adenomas or carcinoma

    5. Cushing's disease and primary adrenal tumors more common in females

    6. Ectopic corticotropin production more common in males

- Sign and Symptoms

    1. Central obesity with slender extremities

    2. Full face

    3. Muscular weakness

   4. Back pain

   5. Mental changes

   6. Thin fragile skin

   7. Poor wound healing

   8. Acne

   9. Menstrual disorders

- Differential Diagnosis

   1. Hypercortisolism due to alcoholism

   2. Hypercortisolism due to depression

- Physical Findings

   1. Moon face with facial plethora

   2. Hirsutism

   3. Skin—thin and atrophic

   4. Purplish-red striae on abdomen, breast or buttocks

   5. Truncal obesity with wasting of limbs

   6. Prominent supraclavicular and dorsal cervical fat pads ("buffalo hump")

   7. Hypertension

- Diagnostic Tests/Findings

   1. Plasma cortisol—evening cortisol levels and 24 hour total levels are elevated

   2. Urinary cortisol—elevated

   3. Dexamethasone test (most reliable for distinguishing among causes of Cushing's syndrome)

   4. MRI, CT and ultrasonographic imaging for identification of pituitary tumor, non-pituitary ACTH-producing neoplasms

   5. Blood glucose—increased

   6. Hypokalemia but not hypernatremia

- Management/Treatment

   1. Treatment of choice for Cushing's disease—surgery

2. Adrenal tumors or hyperplasia—removal

3. If surgery is contraindicated radiation and drug therapy (used to control cortisol excess) may be used which includes ketoconazole 400 to 500 mg b.i.d.; metyrapone 2 g per day; aminoglutethimide 1 g per day

4. For Cushing's syndrome due to prolonged administration of steroids

   a. Discontinuation of therapy gradually

   b. Reduction of steroid dose

   c. Changing to an alternate-day schedule

Addison's Disease (Primary adrenocortical insufficiency)

- Definition: An insidious, usually progressive disease due to destruction of the adrenal cortex

  1. Primary—due to destruction of adrenal cortex

  2. Secondary—lack of corticotropin stimulation

- Etiology/Incidence

  1. Idiopathic autoimmune destruction of adrenal tissue (over 80%); two to three times more common in females; usually diagnosed between ages 30 to 50 years

  2. Tuberculosis—second most frequent cause (common cause in under-developed countries)

  3. Acquired immunodeficiency syndrome (AIDS)—becoming a more frequent cause

  4. Less common—hemorrhage, fungal infections, antineoplastic chemotherapy, abrupt withdrawal of exogenous steroids

  5. Primarily a rare disease

- Signs and Symptoms

  1. Chronic primary adrenocortical insufficiency—develops gradually

     a. Weakness and fatigue, orthostatic hypotension may be early symptoms

     b. Anorexia, weight loss

     c. Tan appearance to the skin

     d.   Gastrointestinal symptoms

  2.   Acute adrenocortical insufficiency—seen more often in patients without previous diagnosis or those with a diagnosis who are exposed to stress with related increased requirement for glucocorticoids; symptoms of chronic are exaggerated especially profound hypotension

  3.   Most dangerous feature of Addison's disease is hypotension which may cause shock, especially during stress AND is nonresponsive to usual treatment; requires glucocorticoid replacement

- Differential Diagnosis

  1. ADH syndrome

  2. Salt-losing nephritis

  3. Hemochromatosis

- Physical Findings

  1. Hyperpigmentation of skin

  2. Hypotension

  3. Black freckles over forehead, face, neck, and shoulders

  4. Areas of vitiligo

  5. Bluish-black discolorations of the areolae and of the mucous membranes of the lips, mouth, rectum, vagina

- Diagnostic Tests/Findings

  1. Sodium levels—low (< 130 mEq/L; normal 135 to 145 mEq/L)

  2. Potassium levels—high (> 5 mEq/L; normal 3.5 to 5 mEq/L)

  3. BUN—elevated

  4. Plasma renin level—increased

  5. ACTH plasma levels—increased

  6. Ratio of serum sodium to potassium (< 30:1)

  7. Low fasting blood glucose (< 50 mg/dL; normal 60 to 115 mg/dL)

  8. Hematocrit—elevated

  9. WBC—low

  10. Eosinophils—increased

- Management/Treatment
  1. In acute crisis referral with hospitalization
  2. Chronic
     a. Lifetime of treatment
     b. Cortisol 15 to 20 mg orally every a.m.; 5 to 10 mg 4 to 6 p.m.
     c. Fludrocortisone acetate 0.05 to 0.3 mg daily or every other day if insufficient sodium retention with cortisol alone
     d. Monitor weight, blood pressure, and electrolytes
  3. General considerations
     a. Education regarding increasing cortisol during times of stress
     b. Education regarding carrying an identification bracelet or card
     c. Salt additives for excess heat or humidity
     d. Prognosis is excellent with continued substitution therapy

Questions
Select the best answer

Mrs. O. is a 46-year-old female whose hypertension has been controlled with hydrochlorothiazide 50 mg every day for the past three years. She is 5'8'' and weighs 220
lb. Although no other abnormal physical findings were noted, blood work done as
part of her routine annual physical examination reveals a fasting blood glucose of 300
mg/dL. Other abnormal laboratory tests included elevated serum cholesterol (250) and
triglyceride level (170), a K+ of 3.4, and 4+ glycosuria.

1. You should then:

    a. Discontinue her hydrochlorothiazide
    b. Order a glucose tolerance test
    c. Repeat a fasting glucose
    d. Start insulin therapy

2. Mrs. O. is about how many pounds over her ideal body weight?

    a. 80
    b. 105
    c. 140
    d. 154

3. Persons with type 2 diabetes:

    a. Are apt to develop ketosis
    b. Account for less than 10% of persons with diabetes
    c. Tend to be obese and hypertensive
    d. Often present with severe polydipsia, polyuria and polyphagia

4. Mrs. O. has led a fairly sedentary life style and asks if enrolling in an exercise club would help get her sugar down. You would tell her that:

    a. Exercise is an important part of control of her blood sugar
    b. She should start a virgorous exercise program as soon as possible
    c. Exercise at this point won't affect her blood sugar
    d. Exercise will probably increase her appetite

5. Given her sedentary life style and need to lose weight, how many calories/
day should Mrs. O. be consuming? Wt. 220 lb. Hgt. 5'8''

    a. 1,000
    b. 1,300

    c. 1,400
    d. 1,800

6. Mrs. O.'s second fasting blood sugar is 296 and she has been diagnosed with type 2 diabetes. Mrs. O. does not want to take insulin. You tell her:

    a. Most type 2 diabetics never have to take insulin
    b. It is usual to try dietary modification and exercise first
    c. It would be a lot easier if she started insulin as soon possible
    d. The value of using insulin to control type 2 diabetes is not clear

7. Dietary recommendations for persons with diabetes do not include:

    a. Strict carbohydrate restriction
    b. Limiting fats and cholesterol
    c. Limiting protein intake
    d. Eating meals at regular intervals

8. Indications for starting a person with diabetes on oral hypoglycemics include:

    a. Allergy to sulfa drugs
    b. Pregnancy in a type 2 diabetes controlled by diet
    c. Diagnosis of type 2 diabetes
    d. Failure to control hyperglycemia with diet in a client with diabetes type 2

9. A person with type 2 diabetes has had good control of his blood glucose with oral hypoglycemics. He is in for a routine three month check. He had a complete work up 6 months ago. Which of the following is LEAST likely to be done at this visit?

    a. Urinalysis.
    b. Blood glucose.
    c. Fundoscopic examination
    d. ECG

10. Mr. P. is on 30 units of NPH and 5 units of regular insulin each morning and 15 units of NPH each evening to control his type 1 diabetes. His blood glucose levels for the past three days have been:

Fasting	Before Lunch	Before Supper	At hs
200–250	95–110	110–120	95–130

He should be instructed to:

a. Add 2 units of NPH to his p.m. dose
b. Add 2 units NPH before breakfast
c. Add 2 units of regular insulin to his pm dose
d. Do nothing

11. Hemoglobin A_{lc} gives an indication of glucose control over the past:

a. Week
b. Four to six weeks
c. Month
d. 60 to 90 days

12. When treating diabetes the goal for hemoglobin A_{lc} (normal 4% to 6%) should be:

a. < 6%
b. < 7%
c. < 8%
d. < 10%

13. Which of the following is an adverse effect of sulfonylureas?

a. Increased blood pressure
b. Weight loss
c. Gastrointestinal distress
d. Hypoglycemia

14. In addition to controlling glucose levels metformin also:

a. Causes weight loss
b. Increases total cholesterol levels
c. Increases triglyceride levels
d. Is likely to cause hypoglycemia

15. Synthetic human insulin:

a. Causes more antibody formation
b. Contains more impurities than purified pork insulin
c. Is least antigenic of all insulins
d. Has a more rapid action onset than pork counterparts

16. Mr. J. is a 50-year-old person with type 2 diabetes who has been on insulin for the past six months. He reports that his fasting blood glucose levels have been

running above two hundred but they have been great during the rest of the day. His evening dose of NPH insulin has been increased three times in the last two weeks with no improvement in the fasting values. Currently he is on 30 units NPH/4 units regular in the morning and 18 Units NPH/4 units regular before supper. This is his most recent glucose pattern

B	L	S	hs
250–280	130–144	120–132	100–120

If he has fairly good dietary compliance, you should instruct him to:

a. Increase the evening NPH by 2 more units
b. Check his blood glucose between 2 and 3 a.m. for the next 2 days
c. Increase the morning dose of regular insulin by 2 units
d. Increase the morning dose of NPH insulin by 2 units

17. High fasting glucose after a nocturnal hypoglycemia in a person with diabetes otherwise in good control with insulin would indicate:

a. Dawn phenomenon
b. Somogyi effect
c. Insulin allergy
d. Lipodystrophy

18. Which action would counteract this problem?

a. Increase his morning dose of NPH
b. Have him use human insulin instead of pork insulin
c. Decrease his evening NPH insulin dose
d. Increase his morning dose of regular insulin

19. Mrs. J. is a person with type 2 diabetes who has been on pork insulin for the past two years and she has begun to develop hard lumpy raised areas in her right thigh where she has been placing injections. The only action that will prevent further development of such areas would be to:

a. Switch to human synthetic insulin
b. Inject insulin directly into the lumpy areas
c. Rotate the injection sites
d. Switch to oral hypoglycemics

20. Ms. W. is a 34-year-old who is seeking care because of increased irritability, weight loss "despite a great appetite" and diarrhea (not watery but 2 to 3

stools a day). She feels exhausted but can't seem to sleep and states she "feels like I could jump out of my skin."

If excess thyroid hormone is the problem which of the following might be noted?

   a. Yellowing skin
   b. Fine tremor
   c. Delayed tendon reflex
   d. Sinus bradycardia

21. Graves' disease is caused by:

   a. Viral infection
   b. Use of lithium
   c. An autoimmune response
   d. Excessive ingestion of thyroid hormone

22. In Graves disease you would expect:

   a. TSH to be decreased
   b. T_3 to be decreased
   c. T_3 resin uptake to be decreased
   d. T_4 to be decreased

23. If Ms. W. is diagnosed with Graves' disease and placed on antithyroid medication you will include which of the following in your initial patient teaching?

   a. The need of life long use of antithyroid medications
   b. Initial signs of the effectiveness of treatment will be increased urination
   c. The possibility of developing myxedemic coma
   d. Signs of hypothyroidism

24. The most serious side effect of both PTU and methimazole is:

   a. Skin rash
   b. Diarrhea
   c. Agranulocytosis
   d. Hepatitis

25. The best guide to adequacy of the dosage of antithyroid medication in thyrotoxicosis is:

   a. Thyroid antibodies
   b. T_3 (RIA)

  c. TSH

  d. T_4

26. Sally G. is a 44-year-old who thinks she is beginning menopause because her menstrual periods have become irregular. Her major complaint is a lack of energy and weight gain. Physical examination reveals dry skin, thinning hair, a puffy facial appearance, and an enlarged, nontender thyroid. Her BP is 130/92 with a heart rate of 60. These findings are consistent with:

  a. Graves disease

  b. Hypothyroidism

  c. Plummer's disease

  d. Thyrotoxicosis

27. Which of the following findings would be consistent with a hypothyroid state?

  a. Hyperactive bowel sounds

  b. Lid lag

  c. Insomnia

  d. Parethesias

28. Ms. H. is diagnosed with hypothyroidism and placed on levothyroxine 0.1 mg per day. After a week she calls to tell you she hasn't seen any improvement and wants to discontinue her medication. Your best response would be to:

  a. Add propranolol to her regimen

  b. Change to desiccated thyroid

  c. Increase her dosage 0.125 mg/day

  d. Encourage her to take this dose for at least another week

29. Ms. L. is a 50-year-old female who has been diagnosed as having primary myxedema. An initial dose of 0.15 mg/day of levothyroxine has been prescribed. Patient education would include which of the following?

  a. Discussion of the chronicity of the disease and the life-long medication use

  b. That it will take six months to a year for her fatigue to disappear

  c. Avoidance of foods causing increased peristalsis

  d. Explanation that after two years of therapy this medication may not be needed

30. Your 57-year-old patient has been on prednisone for her rheumatoid arthritis.

She has the typical ''moon face,'' excess weight in her torso area, and is complaining that she bruises easily when she bumps herself. As her primary care provider the best action would be to:

   a. Discontinue her prednisone immediately
   b. Add a NSAID to her treatment regimen
   c. Convert to an alternate-day schedule
   d. Discontinue prednisone immediately and start on naproxen 250 mg b.i.d.

31. Skin changes in Addison's disease include:

   a. Circumoral pallor
   b. Maculopapular eruptions associated with stress
   c. Hyperpigmentation
   d. Facial plethora and hirsutism

Answers:

1. c	11. d	21. c
2. a	12. b	22. a
3. c	13. d	23. d
4. a	14. a	24. c
5. b	15. c	25. c
6. b	16. b	26. b
7. a	17. b	27. d
8. d	18. c	28. d
9. d	19. c	29. a
10. a	20. b	30. c
		31. c

28/31 90%

Bibliography

Bell, D. S., & Alele, J. (1997). Diabetic ketoacidosis: Why early detection and aggressive treatment are crucial. *Postgraduate Medicine, 101*(4), 193–198, 201– 204.

Bohannon, N. J. (1997). Benefits of lispro insulin. *Postgraduate Medicine, 101*(2), 73–80.

Davidson, M. B., & Peters, A. L. (1997). An overview of metformin in the treatment of Type II diabetes mellitus. *The American Journal of Medicine, 102*(3), 99–110.

Drass, J. A., & Peterson, A. (1996). Type II diabetes exploring treatment options. *American Journal of Nursing, 96*(11), 45–50.

Fitzgerald, P. A. (1998). Endocrinology. In L. M. Tierney, S. J. McPhee, & M. A. Papadakin (Eds.), *Current medical diagnosis and treatment* (37th ed., pp. 1031–1094). Stamford, CT: Appleton & Lange.

Flick, M., & Schumann, L. (1997) Continuing education forum. Non-insulin-dependent diabetes mellitus. *Journal of the American Academy of Nurse Practitioners, 9*, 337–343.

Minchoff, L. E., & Grandin, J. A. (1996). Syndrome X recognition and management of this metabolic disorder in primary care. *Nurse Practitioner, 21*(6), 74–75, 79–80, 83–86.

Mudlair, S. R. (1997). Strategies for preventing type II diabetes. *Postgraduate Medicine, 101*(1), 181–189.

Schilling, J. S. (1997). Hyperthyroidism: Diagnosis and management of Graves' disease. *The Nurse Practitioner, 22*(6), 72, 74–75, 78, 83, 87–90.

Singer, P. A., Cooper, D. S., Levey, E. G., Ladenson, P. W., Braverman, L. E., Daniels, D., Greenspan, F. S., McDougall, I. R., & Nikolai, T. F. (1995). Treatment guidelines for patients with hyperthyroidism and hypothyroidism. *Journal of the American Medical Association, 273*(10), 808–12.

Skyler, J. S. (1997). Insulin therapy in type II diabetes. *Postgraduate Medicine. 101*(2), 85–90, 92–94, 96.

The Expert Committee on the Diagnosis and Classification of Diabetes. (1997). Report of the Expert Committee on the Diagnosis and Classification of Diabetes. *Diabetic Care, 20*, 1183–1197

Thyroid Guidelines Task Force (1996). *AACE clinical practice guidelines for the evaluation and management of hyperthyroidism and hypothyroidism.* Washington DC: American Association of Clinical Endocrinologists.

White, J. R., & Campbell, R. K. (1997). Insulin analogues new agents for improving glycemic control. *Postgraduate Medicine, 101*(2), 58–60, 63–70.

Genitourinary and Gynecologic Disorders

Pamela A. Shuler
Mary D. Knudtson

Acquired Immunodeficiency Syndrome (AIDS)

- Definition: Secondary immunodeficiency syndrome resulting from Human Immunodeficiency Virus (HIV) infection and characterized by opportunistic infections, neurologic dysfunction, malignancies, systemic wasting and a variety of other disorders

- Etiology/Incidence
  1. HIV invades, multiplies within one or more types of susceptible cells; circulating $CD4^+$ lymphocytes, macrophages and monocytes are most commonly affected, destroying the host's immune system
  2. Median time from HIV infection to AIDS is 10 years
  3. Estimated 1.5 million Americans are infected with HIV, half are unaware they are infected
  4. 40,000 to 80,000 new infections diagnosed each year
  5. Most diagnoses are made in persons 20 to 49 years old; women aged 15 to 44 constitute one of the fastest growing segments of the U.S. epidemic
  6. HIV is transmitted through direct contact with bodily fluids (blood, semen, vaginal secretions)
  7. Major routes of HIV transmission
     a. Sexual intercourse (homosexual and heterosexual)
     b. Needle sharing (IV drug users)
     c. Transfusions of blood and blood products
     d. Needle stick, open wound and mucous membrane exposure to health care workers (0.4% incidence according to the Centers for Disease Control and Prevention [CDC])
     e. Injection with previously used unsterilized needle (acupuncture, tattooing, medical injection)
     f. Pregnancy (mother to unborn fetus)
     g. Breastfeeding (mother to infant)
  8. Trends
     a. Plateau in number of newly infected homosexual males since 1991

b. African-Americans and Hispanics are disproportionately repre-sented

c. One in four new HIV infections occur in people younger than 20

d. Sexual contact leading mode of transmission for women

- Signs and Symptoms—CDC Classification

1. Asymptomatic HIV infection (may last > 10 years)—inoculation to seroconversion 90% by three months and 98% by six months

2. Acute HIV infection

a. Two to eight weeks after infection 30 to 40% may have acute viremia symptoms

(1) High fever, lymphadenopathy, rash, aseptic meningitis

(2) Usually mistaken for flu or mononucleosis

b. Months to years before AIDS—may have chronic fatigue, weight loss, nightsweats, persistent dermatitis, shingles, persistent diarrhea, oral candidiasis, hairy leukoplakia, chronic vaginal candidiasis, tuberculosis, cognitive changes

3. Persistent generalized lymphadenopathy (PGL)

a. Palpable lymph node enlargement (2 sites other than inguinal)

b. No concurrent illness to explain lymphadenopathy

4. HIV diseases that contribute to progression of AIDS

a. *Pneumocystis carinii* pneumonia, Kaposi's sarcoma, cytomegalovirus and/or other opportunistic infections/cancers

b. Encephalopathy

c. Wasting syndrome (involuntary weight loss greater than 10% of baseline body weight, plus either chronic diarrhea or chronic weakness and documented fever)

- Differential Diagnosis:

1. Cancer

2. Tuberculosis

3. Enterocolitis

4. Endocrine diseases

- Physical Findings: Variable, depending upon infection stage
- Diagnostic Tests/Findings
  1. Initial blood test for antibody detection
     a. Enzyme-linked immunosorbent assay (ELISA) (screening test)
     b. Western blot assay—confirmatory blood tests for HIV specific antibody profile
     c. Some individuals may not generate an antibody response for up to 36 months
  2. Detection/quantification of HIV
     a. HIV-1 p24 antigen used to diagnose infection before antibodies measurable
     b. Qualitative polymerase chain reaction (PCR) circulating cells or plasma—can use in early disease instead of p24
     c. Quantitative viral RNA levels—used to decide when to initiate treatment, as a prognostic indicator, and as a basis for evaluating response to treatment
     d. CD4$^+$ count used to assess magnitude of disease and to monitor effectiveness of treatment
- Management/Treatment
  (All STD treatment regimens throughout this chapter based on *1998 Sexually transmitted treatment guidelines*, published by CDC)
  1. No cure or vaccination for HIV infection at present
  2. New treatment regimens are constantly evolving
  3. Treatment of HIV and opportunistic infections, malignancies and prophylaxis against opportunistic infections continue to evolve rapidly; basic guidelines include:
     a. Therapy for opportunistic infections and malignancies
        (1) Conditions include *P. carinii* pneumonia, toxoplasmosis, cryptococcus, lymphoma, cytomegalovirus, esophageal candidiasis, Herpes simplex and zoster, Kaposi's sarcoma
        (2) Medications include antibiotics, antifungals and corticosteroids

b. Antiretroviral treatment (CDC, 1998); treatment of HIV changes very rapidly, please refer to most recent CDC guidelines

   (1) Initial use of combination therapy is recommended; monotherapy is no longer standard

   (2) Antiretroviral therapy should be started:

      (a) Option 1—in any patient with CD4$^+$ count < 500 or viral RNA levels > 5000; general consensus regarding need to initiate treatment in these patients

      (b) Option 2—treat any patient with detectable plasma viral RNA > 500 regardless of CD4$^+$ count or clinical stage

      (c) Option 3—treat all patients who are HIV positive even if viral RNA levels are negative and CD4$^+$ counts > 500

      (d) Therapy should be initiated in all patients with symptomatic HIV, e.g., night sweats, recurrent candidiasis

   (3) Medications:

      (a) Currently 13 FDA approved drugs available for use against HIV; new drugs and treatments continually evolving

      (b) Nucleoside reverse transcriptase inhibitors (NRT)

         (i) Zidovudine (AZT) 200 mg t.i.d. or 300 mg b.i.d.—major adverse effects include anemia, headache, nausea, myositis

         (ii) Stavudine (d4T) 40 mg b.i.d. for > 60 kg; 30 mg b.i.d. for < 60 kg—major adverse effects include peripheral neuropathy

         (iii) Didanosine (ddl) 200 mg b.i.d. on empty stomach for > 60 kg; 125 mg b.i.d. < 60 kg—major adverse effects include pancreatitis, diarrhea, peripheral neuropathy

(iv)   Zalcitabine (ddC) 0.75 mg t.i.d.—major adverse effects include oral ulcers, peripheral neuropathy, pancreatitis

(v)   Lamivudine (3TC) 150 mg b.i.d.—major adverse effects nausea, headache

(vi)   Lamivudine 150 mg/zidovudine 300 mg combination (Combivir)—increases sensitivity in patients resistant to zidovudine

(c)   Non-nucleoside reverse transcriptase inhibitors (NNRTI)

(i)   Nevirapine 200 mg daily for 2 weeks, then 200 mg b.i.d.—major adverse effect is rash

(ii)   Delavirdine 400 mg t.i.d.—major adverse effect is rash

(d)   Protease inhibitors (PI)

(i)   Saquinavir 600 mg t.i.d. with food—major adverse effects include diarrhea, nausea, headache

(ii)   Saquinavir 1200 mg t.i.d.—improved formulation of Saquinavir with greater bioavailability

(iii)   Indinavir 800 mg every 8 hr on empty stomach or with light food—major adverse effects include nephrolitiasis, hyperbilirubinemia

(iv)   Ritonavir 300 mg b.i.d. with food then escalate over 2 weeks to 600 mg b.i.d.—major adverse effects include significant drug interactions, bitter after taste

(v)   Nelfinavir 750 mg t.i.d.—major adverse effects include diarrhea, elevated liver function tests (LFT)

(e)   Viral load monitoring—measure viral RNA every 3 to 6 months, more frequently if:

(i)   Non-compliance suspected

(ii)   CD4$^+$ count drops

(iii) Clinical symptoms appear

(iv)   Drug adjustments are made (measure at 2 to 4 weeks then again at 8 to 12 weeks to document drug effect)

(f)   Initial therapy regimens—important to determine if patient can be compliant with regimen; complicated schedules are extremely difficult to adhere to; viral replication accelerates immediately with non-compliance

    (i)   AZT 300 mg b.i.d. + 3TC 150 mg b.i.d. + PI (indinavir 800 mg every 8 hr or ritonavir 300 mg b.i.d.) with 2 week dose escalation to 600 mg b.i.d.

    (ii) d4T 40 mg bid + ddl 200 mg b.i.d. or 3TC 150 mg b.i.d. + PI (indinavir or ritonavir or nelfinavir 750 mg t.i.d.)

    (iii) d4T + ddL + PI not previously used

    (iv) d4T + 3TC + PI

(g)   Acute retroviral syndrome—AZT + 3TC + indinavir for two years

c.   Prophylaxis of opportunistic infections

(1)   *P. carinii* pneumonia (begin when CD4$^+$ count < 200)

    (a)   Trimethoprim-sulfamethoxazole (TMP/SMX) one double-strength tablet daily or three times a week

    (b)   Dapsone 100 mg per day or aerosolized pentamidine 300 mg monthly if unable to tolerate TMP/SMX

(2)   *Mycobacterium tuberculosis*

    (a)   Isoniazid—10 mg/kg/day up to 300 mg daily for one year

    (b)   All patients with positive PPD reaction (5 mm of induration or greater) without positive chest radiography should receive prophylactic treatment

(3) Toxoplasmosis begin when CD4+ count < 100)—trimethoprim-sulfamethoxazole (TMP/SMX) one double strength tablet orally three times per week or daily

(4) *Mycobacterium avium* complex (begin when CD4$^+$ count < 50)

   (a) Clarithromycin 500 mg orally b.i.d. or

   (b) Azithromycin 500 mg orally three times a week or

   (c) Rifabutin 150 mg orally b.i.d.

d. Recommended immunizations for HIV infected persons

   (1) Pneumococcal vaccination

   (2) Annual influenza vaccination

   (3) Three-dose schedule of hepatitis B vaccine for those who lack immunity

   (4) Tetanus-diptheria booster

   (5) Inactivated polio virus vaccine (IPV)

   (6) Measles, mumps, rubella vaccine

4. Discuss therapeutic and diagnostic plans

5. Educate regarding prevention, transmission and treatment of the disease

6. Emphasize importance of behavioral measures to protect and enhance the immune system

   a. No tobacco, street drugs, alcohol use

   b. Nutritious diet

   c. Stress management, imagery

   d. Exercise as tolerated

   e. Decrease exposure to infectious agents since HIV virus is spread when immune system is activated

7. Encourage continued "safer sex" practices and/or abstinence

8. Assist patient, as appropriate, in meeting physical, psychological, social, cultural, environmental and spiritual needs

9. Report AIDS cases to local health department

Gonorrhea (Uncomplicated Gonococcal Infections)

- Definition: A sexually transmitted bacterial infection that produces urethritis in men and cervicitis in women

- Etiology/Incidence

    1. Causative organism is *Neisseria gonorrhoeae*, a gram-negative diplococcus

    2. Approximately 600,000 infectious new cases annually

    3. Greatest incidence in the 15 to 29 year old age group

    4. Incubation period usually 3 to 10 days

    5. Spectrum of infection—cervicitis, urethritis, salpingitis, proctitis, P.I.D., pharyngitis, conjunctivitis, arthritis

    6. A leading cause of infertility among U.S. females

- Signs and Symptoms

    1. Female

        a. Often asymptomatic

        b. Dysuria, urinary frequency, urgency with a purulent urethral discharge

        c. Vaginal discharge

        d. Pelvic pain

        e. Intermenstrual bleeding

        f. Pharyngitis

        g. Septic arthritis

        h. Rash—petechial or pustular skin lesions

    2. Male

        a. One quarter are asymptomatic

        b. Dysuria (urethra most common site in male), frequency

      c. Copious penile discharge (serous/milky to yellow with blood-tinge)

      d. Testicular pain

      e. Pharyngitis

      f. Septic arthritis

      g. Rash—petechial or pustular skin lesions

- Differential Diagnosis
    1. Nongonococcal cervicitis, vaginitis or urethritis
    2. Reiter's syndrome (chlamydia)
    3. Pelvic inflammatory disease (PID)
    4. Proctitis (other origin)
    5. Nongonococcal pharyngitis or arthritis

- Physical Findings
    1. Female
        - a. Purulent discharge from cervix (primary site in reproductive age women)
        - b. Inflammation of Bartholin's glands
        - c. Evidence of P.I.D. (untreated infection)
    2. Male
        - a. Evidence of urethritis, prostatitis
        - b. Evidence of epididymitis (with untreated infection)
        - c. Copious purulent discharge

- Diagnostic Tests/Findings
    1. Female tests
        - a. Gram stain of endocervical canal discharge shows WBC with gram negative intracellular diplococci; sensitivity only 40 to 70% in women; greater than 90% in men
        - b. Wet prep of purulent cervical discharge may show polymorphonuclear leukocytes (WBC) > 10/HPF

    c. Culture material from endocervix and other suspect sites on to Thayer-Martin or Transgrow media to confirm diagnosis

    d. DNA probe—sensitivity comparable to culture, two hour turn around time, only one specimen needed for chlamydia and *N. gonorrhoea*

  2. Male tests

    a. Gram stain of urethral discharge smear shows gram-negative diplococci and WBC

    b. Culture of urethra and other suspect sites

    c. DNA Probe

  3. Test for concomitant infection from other STD including HIV, syphilis, and chlamydia

  4. Test partners

- Management/Treatment

  1. Treat all contacts

  2. First choice—ceftriaxone 125 mg IM once, or ciprofloxacin 500 mg orally once, or cefixime 400 mg orally once, or ofloxacin 400 mg orally once, *plus* doxycycline 100 mg orally b.i.d. for 7 days, or erythromycin base or stearate 500 mg orally q.i.d. for seven days if the patient is pregnant; or azithromycin 1 g orally in a single dose (may use if pregnant and over 16 years of age); high incidence of co-existing chlamydia

  3. Alternative regimens—spectinomycin 2 g IM once or ceftizoxime 500 mg IM once, or cefotaxime 500 mg IM once, or cefotetan 1 g IM once, or cefoxitin 2g IM once, with probenecid 1 g orally, enoxacin 400 mg orally once, or lomefloxacin 400 mg orally once, or norfloxacin 800 mg orally once, *plus* doxycycline as above

  4. Test of cure not essential; rescreening one to two months after treatment recommended, or sooner for repeat culture if symptoms persist or recur

  5. Discuss therapeutic and diagnostic plans

  6. Emphasize importance of complete treatment

  7. Avoid sexual intercourse until patient and partner(s) cured

8. Educate regarding prevention, transmission and treatment of the disease; encourage continued use of condoms

9. Report cases to health department

10. Can cause disseminated infection, acute arthritis

Genital Chlamydial Infection

- Definition: A sexually transmitted disease that produces urethritis in men and cervicitis in women

- Etiology/Incidence

   1. Causative organism is *Chlamydia trachomatis*

   2. Approximately 4 million new cases occur annually

   3. The most common bacterial sexually transmitted disease in the U.S.

   4. A leading cause of female infertility and ectopic pregnancy in U.S.

   5. Incubation period 7 to 21 days

   6. Screening for high risk individuals recommended—sexually active adolescents, multiple partners, history of previous or current STD

- Signs and Symptoms

   1. Female

      a. Often asymptomatic

      b. Dysuria

      c. Vaginal discharge/spotting

      d. Lower abdominal/pelvic pain

      e. Dyspareunia

      f. Dysmenorrhea, menstrual irregularity

      g. Infertility

      h. Enlarged, tender inguinal lymph nodes

   2. Male

      a. Often asymptomatic

      b. Urethral discharge (any color)

      c. Dysuria

      d.   Testicular pain/swelling

      e.   Enlarged, tender inguinal lymph nodes

      f.   Rectal pain, bleeding and diarrhea

- Differential Diagnosis

  1. Gonococcal cervicitis
  2. Urethritis
  3. Proctitis
  4. P.I.D.
  5. Urinary tract infection
  6. Epididymitis
  7. Prostatitis from other infective agent
  8. Vaginitis

- Physical Findings

  1. Female

     a. Mucopurulent urethral and/or cervical discharge

     b. Hypertropic, eroded and friable cervix (maybe)

     c. Evidence of P.I.D. (advanced infection)

  2. Male

     a. Mucopurulent urethral discharge

     b. Evidence of prostatitis

     c. Evidence of epididymitis (untreated infection)

- Diagnostic Tests/Findings

  1. Female

     a. Wet prep or gram stain shows WBC > 10/HPF

     b. Most common tests—enzyme immunoassay (EIA) and direct fluorescence assay (DFA) *or* lipase chain reaction (LCR) for confirmation

     c. Other tests include tissue culture, DNA hybridization and polymerase chain reaction (PCR)

2. Male

   a. Gram stain or wet prep shows WBC > 10/HPF

   b. Same indirect antigen-detection tests

3. Test for concomitant infection from other STD in patient (HIV, gonorrhea, syphilis, trichomonas)

4. Test partners

- Management/Treatment

   1. Treat all contacts

   2. First choice—doxycycline, 100 mg orally b.i.d. for 7 days or azithromycin one g orally once (may be used in pregnancy if > 16 years of age)

   3. Ofloxacin 300 mg orally b.i.d. for 7 days, or erythromycin base 500 mg orally q.i.d. for 7 days, or erythromycin ethylsuccinate 800 mg orally q.i.d. for 7 days

   4. During pregnancy—erythromycin base or stearate, 500 mg orally q.i.d. for 7 days or erythromycin base 250 mg orally q.i.d. for 14 days, erythromycin ethylsuccinate 800 mg orally q.i.d. for 7 days or erythromycin ethylsuccinate 400 mg orally q.i.d. for 14 days, or amoxicillin, 500 mg orally t.i.d. for 7 days or azithromycin 1 g orally once if > 16 years of age

   5. No test-of-cure after treatment unless symptoms persist or re-infection suspected (wait more than three weeks after treatment to determine if test-of-cure needed)

   6. Discuss therapeutic and diagnostic plans

   7. Emphasize importance of complete treatment

   8. Avoid sexual intercourse until patient and partner(s) complete treatment

   9. Educate regarding prevention, transmission and treatment of the disease; encourage continued use of condoms

   10. Report cases to health department

Syphilis

- Definition: A complex infectious disease that can affect almost any organ or tissue in the body and mimics many diseases

- Etiology/Incidence
    1. Causative organism is *Treponema pallidum*, a spirochete
    2. Transmission primarily occurs through minor skin or mucosal lesions during sexual encounters; genital and extragenital areas may be inoculated
    3. Can be transmitted via placenta (after 10th week) from mother to fetus (congenital rate—1 in 10,000 pregnancies)
    4. Incidence has steadily increased since 1985; approximately 80,000 cases (primary and secondary types) reported in U.S. annually
    5. Risk of contraction—30 to 50% (partner-primary syphilis)
- Signs and Symptoms
    1. Primary
        a. Painless chancre
        b. Regional lymphadenopathy
    2. Secondary
        a. Skin rash—especially palmar, plantar and oral mucosa
        b. Malaise, anorexia
        c. Alopecia
        d. Arthralgias/myalgias/flu-like symptoms
        e. Other symptoms depending on affected organs
        f. Generalized lymphadenopathy
    3. Latent
        a. May be asymptomatic
        b. Integumentary, ocular, cardiovascular, gastrointestinal, respiratory or neurological manifestations may be present
    4. Neurosyphilis
        a. May occur during any stage of syphilis
        b. Optic, auditory, cranial nerve and/or meningeal symptoms are most common
- Differential Diagnosis

1. Primary
   a. Herpes genitalis
   b. Chancroid
   c. Neoplasm
   d. Lymphogranuloma venereum (LGV)
   e. Superficial fungal infections
2. Secondary
   a. Conditions associated with rash or other presenting symptoms, e.g., flu, mononucleosis, pityriasis rosea, drug eruptions
   b. Infectious hepatitis
3. Latent
   a. Neoplasms of skin, liver, lung, stomach or brain
   b. Other forms
      (1) Meningitis
      (2) Cardiovascular disorders
      (3) CNS disorders
      (4) Arthritis
      (5) Primary neurologic lesions

- Physical Findings
  1. Neurological signs may be present at any stage
  2. Primary
     a. Indurated ulcer (chancre) on:
        (1) Genitals
        (2) Mouth
        (3) Rectum
        (4) Nipple
     b. Regional lymphadenopathy
  3. Secondary
     a. Low-grade fever

   b. Highly variable skin rash (including palms and soles)

   c. Mucous patches

   d. Evidence or manifestations of condyloma latum

   e. Generalized lymphadenopathy

   f. Evidence of meningitis, iritis, hepatitis, glomerulonephritis

4. Latent

   a. May have no clinical signs of infection

   b. Granulomatous lesions (gummas)—skin, mucous membranes, bone

   c. Leukoplakia

   d. Evidence of periostitis, osteitis or arthritis

   e. Gummatous infiltrates in larynx, trachea, pulmonary parenchyma, stomach and/or liver

   f. Diminished coronary circulation

   g. Acute myocardial infarction

   h. Cardiac insufficiency

   i. Aortic aneurysm

   j. Meningitis

   k. Hemiparesis

   l. Hemiplegia

   m. Tabes dorsalis

   n. General paresis

- Diagnostic Tests/Findings

1. Early syphilis—primary, secondary or latent syphilis of less than one year's duration

   a. Definitive methods

     (1) Darkfield microscopy

     (2) Direct fluorescent antibody tests of lesion exudate or tissue

b. Presumptive methods (neither test alone is sufficient for diagnosis)

(1) Treponemal serologic tests

(a) Fluorescent treponemal antibody absorption (FTA-ABs) test

(b) Microhemagglutination assay for antibody to *T. pallidum* (MHA-TP)

(c) Tests/titers should be reported as positive or negative and used to confirm nontreponemal tests

(d) FTA-ABs or MHA-TP confirmation tests positive in 85% to 95% of primary and in 100% of secondary cases

(2) Nontreponemal serologic tests

(a) Veneral Disease Research Laboratory (VDRL)

(b) Rapid Plasma Reagin (RPR)

2. Latent syphilis of more than one year's duration and cardiovascular syphilis

a. VDRL or RPR test (+ in 75% of cases)

b. FTA-ABs or MHA-TP confirmation test (+ in 98% cases)

c. Lumbar puncture with tests on cerebrospinal fluid (CSF)

3. Neurosyphilis (occurs at any stage)

a. Treponemal and nontreponemal serologic tests results dependent upon stage of disease

b. CSF examinations as above

4. Test for concomitant infection from other STD in patient and contacts

a. HIV

b. Gonorrhea

c. Chlamydia

5. Test partners

• Management/Treatment

1. Pregnant patients allergic to penicillin should be treated with penicillin after desensitization for all stages

2. Penicillin alternative treatment for all stages of syphilis except neurosyphilis

3. Early syphilis and persons exposed within last 90 days

    a. Treat all partners

    b. First choice—benzathine penicillin G, 2.4 million units IM once

    c. Penicillin allergy—doxycycline 100 mg orally b.i.d. for 2 weeks or tetracycline 500 mg orally q.i.d. for 2 weeks

4. Late latent cases and cardiovascular syphilis (normal CSF examination)

    a. First choice—benzathine penicillin G, 2.4 million units IM weekly for 3 weeks

    b. Penicillin allergy—doxycycline 100 mg orally b.i.d. for 4 weeks or tetracycline 500 mg orally q.i.d. for 4 weeks

5. Neurosyphilis

    a. First choice—18 to 24 million units aqueous crystalline penicillin G daily, administered as 3 to 4 million units IV every 4 hours for 10 to 14 days

    b. Alternate regimen if compliance assured—2.4 million units procaine penicillin IM daily, plus probenecid 500 mg orally q.i.d., both for 10 to 14 days

6. Post-treatment follow-up

    a. Primary and secondary baseline RPR or VDRL at time of treatment and repeated every 3 months; titer should fall fourfold in 3 months, eightfold in 6 months and become negative within 2 years (MHA-TP and FTA-AB$_s$ will be positive for lifetime)

    b. Latent—RPR or VDRL repeated at 6 month and 12 month intervals; titer should fall fourfold in 12 to 24 months

    c. Neurosyphilis—CSF examination every 6 months until normal

7. Discuss therapeutic and diagnostic plans

8. Emphasize importance of complete treatment

9. Avoid sexual intercourse until patient and partner(s) cured

10. Educate regarding prevention, transmission and treatment of the disease; encourage continued use of condoms

11. Report cases to health department

Herpes Genitalis

- Definition: A viral STD that produces recurrent, painful genital lesions and has no cure

- Etiology/Incidence

    1. Caused by herpes simplex virus (HSV) types 1 (5% to 15%) and 2 (85 to 95%)

    2. Initial (primary) and recurrent infections affect approximately 270,000 and 30 million persons respectively annually

    3. Duration of initial infection—10 to 14 days; recurrent 7 to 10 days; viral shedding (without clinical symptoms) occurs during latency (interval between outbreaks)

    4. Virus resides in presacral ganglia during latency

    5. Can lead to neuralgia, meningitis, ascending myelitis, urethral strictures, and lymphatic suppuration

    6. Infection during pregnancy can lead to spontaneous abortion or fetal morbidity/mortality; risk for transmission to neonate appears highest among women with first episode near time of delivery

    7. Incubation period 2 to 21 days after exposure

- Signs and Symptoms

    1. First clinical episode

        a. Fever/chills

        b. Malaise

        c. Headache

        d. Dysuria

        e. Vaginal discharge, abnormal bleeding

        f. Dyspareunia

g. Pruritic/burning genital vesicles that rupture and become painful ulcers—mean duration 12 days

2. Recurrent episodes—pruritic/burning vesicles that rupture into less painful ulcers; mean duration 4.5 days

- Differential Diagnosis

1. Syphilis

2. Lymphogranuloma venereum

3. Gonorrhea

4. Chlamydia

5. Chancroid

6. Vaginitis

7. Herpes zoster

8. Condyloma latum

9. Erythema multiforme

10. Neoplasm (especially cervical)

- Physical Findings

1. Fever—first episode

2. Single or multiple vesicles surrounded by inflammation/edema on external genitalia, penis, scrotum, anus, vagina or cervix (75%); vesicles spontaneously rupture and form painful, erythematous ulcers, scab over and heal

3. Cervix may appear diffusely inflamed, edematous with large punched-out ulcers or a granulomatous-appearing tumor-like mass covered with gray exudate

4. Profuse, watery vaginal discharge often present and may be only sign

- Diagnostic Tests/Findings

1. Papanicolaou or other histochemical stain—identification of multinucleated giant cells with intranuclear inclusions in a cytologic smear

2. Identification of HSV virus(es) from tissue (vulvar, vaginal, cervical) cultures or antigen test

3. Serologic tests for HSV types 1 and 2 antibodies are also available

4. Test for concomitant infection of other STD in patient and contacts

   a. HIV

   b. Syphilis

   c. Condylomata acuminata

   d. Gonorrhea

   e. Chlamydia

   f. Chancroid

- Management/Treatment

  1. Symptomatic treatment—drying and antipruritic agents and topical anesthetic agents

  2. Chemotherapeutic agents—acyclovir (available in topical, oral and intravenous formulation), famciclovir, or valacyclovir

     a. Topical therapy—minimal benefit except may be useful for immunocompromised patients, use is discouraged

     b. Oral therapy

        (1) Recurrent herpes simplex infections

            (a) Famciclovir 125 mg b.i.d. for 5 days

            (b) Valacyclovir 500 mg b.i.d. for 5 days

            (c) Acyclovir 400 mg t.i.d. for 5 days or 200 mg 5 times per day for 5 days or 800 mg b.i.d. for 5 days

        (2) Uncomplicated primary herpes simplex infections

            (a) Acyclovir 200 mg 5 times per day for 7 to 10 days or 400 mg t.i.d. for 7 to 10 days

            (b) Famciclovir 250 mg t.i.d. for 7 to 10 days

            (c) Valacyclovir 1 g b.i.d. for 7 to 10 days

        (3) Prophylactic or suppressive therapy (if 6 or more outbreaks per year)

            (a) Acyclovir 400 mg b.i.d. or 800 mg daily

            (b) Famciclovir 250 mg b.i.d.

           (c)   Valacyclovir 250 mg b.i.d. or 500 mg daily or 1000 mg daily

      c.   Intravenous therapy

          (1)   Used in severe disease and when complications necessitate hospitalization

          (2)   Acyclovir 5 to 10 mg/kg IV every 8 hours for 5 to 7 days

      d.   Acyclovir is eliminated by the kidneys; hydration is particularly important

      e.   Safety of systemic treatment has not been established during pregnancy

3. Discuss therapeutic and diagnostic plans

4. Avoid sexual intercourse when lesions present; encourage continued use of condoms

5. Educate regarding prevention, transmission and treatment of the disease and dangers during pregnancy

6. Up to 80% may have viral shedding during asymptomatic periods

Genital Warts (Condylomata acuminata)

- Definition: Sexually transmitted warty growths appearing on any part of the genitalia

- Etiology/Incidence

  1. More than 20 types of human papillomavirus (HPV) cause genital warts; types 16, 18, 31, 33, and 35, are predominately detected in high-grade neoplastic lesions

  2. HPV increases risk of penile, vulvar and cervical cancers

  3. Greatest incidence in the 15 to 25 year old age group; correlated with multiple sex partners, early coitus and lack of contraceptive barrier methods

  4. Approximately 3 million cases diagnosed annually

  5. The most common symptomatic viral STD in the U.S.; highly contagious

- Signs and Symptoms

1. Painless, pruritic or burning warts on external genitalia (male and female)

2. Possibly—dyspareunia, dysuria, bleeding

- Differential Diagnosis

    1. Condyloma latum

    2. Neoplasm

    3. Granuloma inguinale

    4. Moles

- Physical Findings

    1. Single or multiple soft, fleshy, papillary or sessile, painless keratinized growths (may be multilobulated papules and quite large) around anus, vulvovaginal area, penis, urethra, perineum or oral cavity

    2. In women, similar lesions may appear in vagina/on cervix; vaginal discharge from co-existing infection(s) may be present; men may have lesions in urethra

    3. May have no signs since flat warts often difficult to visualize

- Diagnostic Tests/Findings

    1. Tissue sample (biopsy) for detection of viral DNA is widely available, but clinical utility is questionable

    2. Application of 5% acetic acid and colposcopy aids in diagnosis— turns lesions white; biopsies may be taken to rule out dysplasia and carcinoma

    3. Pap smear may indicate koilocytosis (indicative of HPV infection) on cervix

    4. Test for concomitant infection of other STD

        a. HIV

        b. Gonorrhea

        c. Syphilis—RPR or VDRL to rule out Condyloma latum

        d. Chlamydia

- Management/Treatment

1. New treatment regimens are evolving to ameliorate symptoms; no current methods are curative

   a. Small vulvar and perianal warts

      (1) Self-treatment with podofilox 0.5% solution or gel—apply with cotton tip applicator b.i.d. for 3 days followed by no treatment for 4 days; cycle can be repeated 4 times

      (2) 80 to 90% solution of trichloroacetic acid (TCA) or tincture of podophyllin weekly for 6 weeks (patient must wash off podophyllin in four hrs); protect surrounding skin with petroleum jelly

      (3) TCA is preferred since it is more effective, not absorbed and can be used during pregnancy and on penis; treatment may be slightly more painful than podophyllin; immediate application of sodium bicarbonate paste following treatment will decrease pain

      (4) Imiquimod 5% cream applied at bedtime 3 times a week for 16 weeks; wash off 6 to 10 hours after application

      (5) Surgical removal with tangential scissor or shave excision, curretage or electrosurgery

      (6) Intralesional interferon

   b. Large warts (> 2 cm), vulvar/vaginal warts

      (1) CO_2 laser

      (2) Electrodesiccation, electrocautery, cryocautery, Leep

2. NO MORE THAN 1/3 OF LESION ENCIRCLING AN ORIFICE SHOULD BE TREATED AT SINGLE VISIT

3. Cervical warts—see section on dysplasia

4. Discuss therapeutic and diagnostic plans

5. Educate regarding prevention, transmission and treatment of the disease; encourage continued use of condoms

6. Emphasize importance of follow-up particularly if Pap abnormal

7. Discuss possible chronicity

   a. Treatment may not be successful

      b.   High recurrence rate due to dormant and asymptomatic viral shedding

      c.   Individuals who smoke have more difficulty with recurrence

      d.   Smoking is HPV co-factor for cervical cancer

Pelvic Inflammatory Disease (P.I.D.)

- Definition: Infection of the upper genital tract, including the endometrium, oviducts, ovaries, uterine wall/serosa, broad ligaments and pelvic peritoneum

- Etiology/Incidence

  1. A disease of polymicrobial infection caused by a variety of aerobic and anaerobic bacteria including *N. gonorrhoeae*, chlamydia, group β streptococcus, *Escherichia coli*, bacteroides bacterial vaginosis organisms, *Mycoplasma hominis* and *Ureaplasma urealyticum*

  2. Clinical P.I.D. is usually a polymicrobial infection

  3. More than 1 million episodes occur annually

  4. Most prevalent serious infection for women 16 to 25 years of age

  5. After initial infection, women more susceptible to reinfection, ectopic pregnancy and infertility

  6. Oral contraceptives and barrier methods with spermicide provide significant protection

  7. Depo-medroxyprogesterone acetate and Norplant cause changes in cervical mucosa which provide some protection from P.I.D.

  8. Annual costs of P.I.D. and its sequelae is $4.2 billion

- Signs and Symptoms

  1. Often symptoms are mild, atypical, subtle or absent

  2. Fever/chills

  3. Nausea/vomiting

  4. Dysuria

  5. Vaginal discharge

  6. Dysmenorrhea

  7. Menstrual irregularity

8. Lower abdominal/pelvic pain (usually < 1 week duration)

9. Dyspareunia

10. Infertility

- Differential Diagnosis

    1. Appendicitis

    2. Ectopic pregnancy

    3. Septic abortion

    4. Hemorrhagic or ruptured ovarian cysts or tumors

    5. Twisted ovarian cyst

    6. Degeneration of a myoma

    7. Enteritis

- Physical Findings and Diagnostic Tests/Findings (clinical criteria for diagnosing P.I.D.)

    1. Minimum criteria—empiric treatment required if all three present

        a. Lower abdominal tenderness

        b. Cervical motion tenderness

        c. Adnexal tenderness

    2. Additional criteria to increase specificity of diagnosis

        a. Laboratory documentation of cervical infection with *C. trachomatis* or *N. gonorrhoeae*

        b. Fever > 38.3° C or 101° F

        c. Abnormal cervical or vaginal discharge

        d. Elevated erythrocyte sedimentation rate and/or C-reactive protein

    3. Elaborate criteria for diagnosis

        a. Histopathologic evidence of endometritis on endometrial biopsy

        b. Tubo-ovarian abscess on sonography or other radiologic tests

        c. Laparoscopic abnormalities consistent with P.I.D.

- Management/Treatment

1. Resolution of symptoms and preservation of tubal function are the primary goals in management of P.I.D.; ideally all patients are hospitalized; however, for economic and practical reasons many are treated as outpatients

2. Hospitalization is highly recommended if:

   a. Diagnosis is uncertain and surgical emergencies cannot be excluded

   b. Pelvic abscess is suspected

   c. Patient is pregnant, an adolescent or HIV infected

   d. Severe illness, e.g., nausea and vomiting precludes outpatient treatment

   e. Patient unable to follow or tolerate outpatient regimen

   f. Patient has failed to clinically respond to outpatient treatment

   g. Clinical follow-up within 72 hours of starting antibiotic therapy cannot be arranged

3. Outpatient treatment

   a. First choice—ofloxacin 400 mg orally b.i.d. for 14 days plus clindamycin 450 mg orally q.i.d. or metronidazole 500 mg orally b.i.d. for 14 days

   b. Cefoxitin 2g IM plus probenecid, 1 g orally once or ceftriaxone 250 mg IM or other parenteral third-generation cephalosporins plus doxycycline 100 mg orally twice daily for 14 days

4. Follow-up appointment in 72 hours, then tests-of-cure conducted 7 to 10 days and 4 to 6 weeks post-treatment

5. Test and treat partners

6. Discuss therapeutic and diagnostic plans

7. Emphasize importance of complete treatment

8. Avoid sexual intercourse until patient and partner(s) cured

9. Education regarding prevention, transmission and treatment of the disease; encourage continued use of condoms

10. Discuss fertility issues as appropriate

Vulvovaginitis

- Definition: Inflammation and infection of the vulva/vagina
- Etiology/Incidence
    1. Commonly caused by *Trichomonas vaginalis* (a motile protozoan), bacterial vaginosis (a polymicrobial bacterial vaginal infection) or *Candida albicans* (a fungi or yeast)
    2. Trichomonas—transmitted through intercourse and also infects the lower urinary tract in men as well as women
    3. Bacterial vaginosis (BV)—the most frequently diagnosed symptomatic vaginitis in the U.S.; not necessarily sexually acquired
    4. Candida vaginitis—occurs in close to 30% of women; is not considered to be a STD; is predisposed by pregnancy, diabetes, use of broad-spectrum antibiotics or corticosteroids; heat, moisture and occlusive clothing also increase risk
    5. Several types of vaginitis may co-exist
- Signs and Symptoms
    1. Trichomoniasis
        a. Malodorous yellow-green discharge with pruritus
        b. Dyspareunia
        c. Dysuria (male partners may also have dysuria)
    2. Bacterial vaginosis
        a. Malodorous, white (''fishy'') discharge
        b. Spotting
    3. Candida vaginitis
        a. Thick discharge with pruritus
        b. Erythema of vagina and vulva
- Differential Diagnosis
    1. Chlamydia
    2. Gonorrhea
    3. Herpes genitalis
    4. Condylomata acuminata

    5.   Allergy, contact dermatitis

    6.   Atrophic vaginitis

- Physical Findings

    1.   Trichomoniasis

        a.   Diffuse vaginal erythema

        b.   Intensely inflamed lesions on cervix and vaginal mucosa—"strawberry patches"

        c.   Discharge

            (1)   Ranges from white/watery to green, thick and frothy

            (2)   Vaginal pH—higher than 4.5

    2.   Bacterial vaginosis

        a.   Watery, grayish homogenous discharge

        b.   Discharge slightly adherent to vaginal walls

    3.   Candida vaginitis

        a.   White, "cottage-cheese" discharge

        b.   Marked vulvovaginal erythema/edema with intense pruritus

- Diagnostic Tests/Findings

    1.   Wet prep microscopic examination of vaginal secretions viewed on low or high power

        a.   Trichomoniasis—discharge mixed with saline will show motile trichomonas on microscopic examination

        b.   Bacterial vaginosis—discharge mixed with saline will show clue cells on microscopic examination; amine-like odor present when discharge alkalinized with 10 to 20% potassium hydroxide (KOH) "whiff test"; vaginal pH of 4 to 5 or more

        c.   Candida vaginitis—discharge mixed with 10% KOH will show branched and budding pseudohyphae on microscopic examination

    2.   Test for concomitant infection from other STD

        a.   HIV

        b.   Syphilis

    c. Condylomata acuminata

    d. Gonorrhea

    e. Chlamydia

- Management/Treatment

  1. Trichomoniasis—recommended treatment is metronidazole 2 g orally as a single dose, alternative treatment metronidazole 500 mg b.i.d. for 7 days; treat partner

  2. Bacterial vaginosis

    a. Drugs of choice

      (1) Clindamycin cream 2%, one full applicator 5 g intravaginally at bedtime for 7 days

      (2) Metronidazole 500 mg orally b.i.d. for 7 days or

      (3) Metronidazole gel, 0.75%, one full applicator (5 g) intravaginally b.i.d. for 5 days

    b. Alternative regimens

      (1) Clindamycin, 300 mg orally b.i.d. for 7 to 10 days (safe during pregnancy)

      (2) Metronidazole 2 g orally in a single dose

  3. Candida vaginitis—many different preparations and treatment regimens exist; the following are commonly prescribed

    a. Miconazole 2% or clotrimazole 1% cream, 5 g intravaginally at bedtime for seven days

    b. Terconazole 80 mg suppository, 1 suppository intravaginally at bedtime for three days

    c. Resistant cases may need partner treatment

    d. Fluconazole 150 mg orally once

  4. Discuss therapeutic and diagnostic plans

  5. Avoid sexual intercourse until patient and partner(s) cured

  6. Education regarding prevention, transmission and treatment of the disease; encourage continued use of condoms

7. Education regarding dangers of douching and incidence of infection

8. Education regarding P.I.D.; association with bacterial vaginosis

Urinary Tract Infection (UTI, Cystitis: Acute, Uncomplicated)

- Definition: Inflammation and infection of the urinary bladder; urethra may be involved

- Etiology/Incidence

    1. Most common causative organisms—*Escherichia coli*, (women) and *Proteus species* (men)

    2. More common in women than men; urological evaluation required for men with UTI

    3. 30 to 40% of women will experience at least 1 UTI

    4. Contributing factors in women

        a. Sexual intercourse; diaphragm use

        b. Pregnancy

        c. Diabetes

        d. Catheterization

        e. Instrumentation

        f. Retaining urine in bladder despite urge to void

    5. Contributing factors in men

        a. Residual urine (prostatic enlargement)

        b. Neuropathic bladder

        c. Calculi

        d. Prostatitis

        e. Catheterization

        f. Instrumentation

- Signs and Symptoms

    1. Dysuria, frequency, urgency

    2. Suprapubic discomfort

    3. Foul smelling urine

- Differential Diagnosis
  1. Vaginitis (females)
  2. Prostatitis (males)
  3. Gonorrhea
  4. Chlamydia infection
  5. Renal calculi
  6. Pyelonephritis
- Physical Findings
  1. Urinary meatus may be erythematous/edematous
  2. Negative costovertebral angle tenderness
  3. Negative pelvic or prostate examination
  4. May have suprapubic tenderness on palpation
- Diagnostic Tests/Findings
  1. Pyuria—> 10 WBC/HPF (may not be present)
  2. Complete urinalysis (clean catch) with culture and sensitivity testing
     a. Bacteria count over 100,000 organisms per mL in fresh "clean catch" midstream specimen is reliable indicator of active urinary tract infection; women with acute cystitis may have more than 10^3 but less than 10^5 per mL in midstream urine cultures
     b. Leukocyte esterase dipstick test—positive
     c. Urine dipstick positive for protein, blood, nitrites suggestive of UTI
- Management/Treatment
  1. Single-dose regimens—due to higher than expected relapse rates, three day course is recommended
  2. Three-day regimens (uncomplicated lower tract infection)—trimethoprim/sulfamethoxazole (TMP/SMX) double-strength tablet orally b.i.d. for three days, or ciprofloxacin 500 mg orally b.i.d. for three days, or amoxicillin/clavulanate 500 mg orally t.i.d. for three days
  3. Standard oral regimens—sulfisoxazole 2 g orally then 1 to 2 g orally q.i.d. for 10 days or nitrofurantoin 50 mg orally q.i.d. for 7 to

10 days or cephalexin 500 mg orally q.i.d. for 7 to 10 days or tri-methoprim/sulfa methoxazole double-strength tablet orally b.i.d. for 7 to 10 days or ciprofloxacin 250 mg orally b.i.d. for 7 to 10 days

4. Treatment during pregnancy—ampicillin 500 mg orally q.i.d. for 7 to 14 days or amoxicillin 500 mg orally t.i.d. for 7 to 14 days; cephalosporin 500 mg q.i.d. for 7 to 14 days

5. Consider adding phenazopyridine hydrochloride 200 mg orally t.i.d. for two days for discomfort associated with urinary tract irritation (caution patient of orange/red tinge to urine)

6. Increase water and decrease carbonated drink intake

7. Repeat urinalysis with culture and sensitivity after medication regimen completed

8. Discuss therapeutic and diagnostic plans

9. Advise return appointment if symptoms increase or no improvement

10. Emphasize importance of complete treatment and follow-up for repeat urinalysis

Acute Pyelonephritis (Upper UTI)

- Definition: An acute bacterial infection of the upper urinary tract (kidney and renal pelvis); usually results from an ascending infection

- Etiology/Incidence

  1. *Escherichia coli* (gram negative) accounts for 80% of infections; *Staphylococcus saprophyticus* and *Streptococcus faecalis* (gram positive) account for 5 to 10%

  2. If urologic abnormalities or calculi present, the following organisms may cause infection—Enterobacter, Proteus, Klebsiella, Serratia and Pseudomonas

  3. Majority of infections occur in young women; rare occurrence in men under age 50 years

  4. Most commonly occurs in patients who are pregnant or have disruptive urinary flow, neurogenic bladder dysfunction or vesicoureteral reflux

- Signs and Symptoms—usually develop rapidly over a few hours

  1. Shaking chills

2. Malaise, generalized muscle tenderness

3. Nausea, vomiting and diarrhea

4. Flank/back pain (unilateral or bilateral)

5. Abdominal pain

6. Dysuria, frequency or urgency (may be absent)

- Differential Diagnosis

    1. Cystitis

    2. Prostatitis

    3. Musculoskeletal back pain

    4. Appendicitis

    5. Diverticulitis

    6. Pelvic inflammatory disease

    7. Ectopic pregnancy

- Physical Findings

    1. Fever, tachycardia

    2. Costovertebral angle pain (unilateral or bilateral) upon percussion

    3. Peritoneal signs are usually absent

    4. Patient appears very ill

- Diagnostic Tests/Findings

    1. Microscopic urinalysis

        a. 5 to 10 WBC/HPF

        b. Occasional erythrocytes

        c. White cell casts may be present

        d. Mild proteinuria

    2. Urine culture—> 100,000 bacteria per mL of urine; sensitivity testing should be done

    3. Gram stain of uncentrifuged urine—one bacterium per oil-immersion correlates with 100,000 bacteria per mL of urine or more

    4. Complete blood count (CBC)—leukocytosis with left shift

5. Elevated ESR

6. BUN and creatinine are usually normal

7. Electrolytes may be abnormal if dehydrated

- Management/Treatment

    1. M.D. referral or consult is required

    2. Inpatient therapy

        a. Patients who are pregnant, have underlying illness, have decreased renal reserve, very toxic (high fever, hypotensive, etc) or unable to tolerate oral therapy should be hospitalized for parenteral antibiotics

        b. IV antimicrobial therapy is based upon culture and sensitivity report

        c. IV hydration is also required

    3. Outpatient therapy—if compliant/reliable and have immediate access to health care services if condition worsens

        a. Antibiotics may include trimethoprim-sulfamethoxazole (if gram stain indicates gram negative organism), norfloxacin, ciprofloxacin, or amoxicillin/clavulanate for 14 days

        b. Resistance to ampicillin is 30%, therefore should not be used as sole therapy

        c. Follow-up within 24 hours

        d. Hydration measures

    4. Repeat urine culture two weeks after completed course of antibiotics

    5. Discuss therapeutic and diagnostic plans

    6. Emphasize importance of complete treatment and follow-up appointments

    7. Instructions regarding no sexual intercourse until treatment completed

    8. Education regarding emergency signs and symptoms if managed as outpatient

    9. Second episode of acute pyelonephritis requires urologic consultation or work-up

Acute Bacterial Prostatitis

- Definition: Inflammation/infection of the prostate gland
- Etiology/Incidence
    1. *Escherichia coli* or other gram-negative bacteria are common causative agents
    2. Occasionally acute urinary retention develops, requiring urgent hospitalization; suprapubic drainage may be necessary; URINARY CATHETERIZATION SHOULD BE AVOIDED
    3. Absence of zinc in prostatic fluid can predispose patient to infection
    4. Young adult men may be more prone to nonbacterial prostatitis or prostatosis
        a. WBC are present in expressed prostatic secretions, but no organisms are cultured
        b. Causative agents include mycoplasma, ureaplasma, gardnerella and chlamydia
- Signs and Symptoms
    1. Fever/chills, malaise, myalgias
    2. Low back pain
    3. Dysuria, urgency, nocturia, frequency
    4. Perineal pain increased with defecation
- Differential Diagnosis
    1. Acute/chronic bacterial cystitis (urinary retention)
    2. Chronic prostatitis
    3. Nonbacterial prostatosis
    4. Prostatodynia
    5. Prostatic or seminal vesicle abscesses
    6. Benign prostatic hypertrophy
    7. Prostatic cancer
    8. Epididymitis
- Physical Findings

1. Fever

2. Prostate—edematous, firm or "boggy," warm and tender; AVOID VIGOROUS MASSAGE, CAN LEAD TO BACTEREMIA

- Diagnostic Tests/Findings

    1. Urine cultures—positive

    2. Prostatic secretions—expressed prostatic secretions (EPS), WBC > 20 cells/HPF is abnormal

    3. Diagnosis is best made by performing simultaneous quantitative bacterial cultures of urethral urine, bladder urine, and EPS

    4. Patient often treated based only on physical findings and urine culture

- Management/Treatment

    1. Patients who appear septic and/or have urinary retention should be hospitalized

    2. Outpatient treatment

        a. First choice if age > 35 years is trimethoprim/sulfamethoxazole double-strength tablet b.i.d. for 2 to 4 weeks; if age < 35 years doxycycline 100 mg orally b.i.d. for 10 days

        b. Alternative choices are carbenicillin 2 tablets orally q.i.d. for 2 to 4 weeks or ciprofloxacin 250 to 500 mg orally b.i.d. for 2 to 4 weeks

    3. Bed rest

    4. Sitz bath t.i.d. for 30 minutes

    5. Follow-up appointment 48 to 72 hours

    6. Discuss therapeutic and diagnostic plans

    7. Avoid sexual intercourse until acute phase resolved; encourage continued use of condoms if multiple partners

    8. Education regarding signs/symptoms of urinary retention and epididymitis

    9. Emphasize importance of follow-up appointments

Chronic Bacterial Prostatitis

- Definition: Chronic inflammation/infection of prostate gland

- Etiology/Incidence

  1. Causative organisms are *Escherichia coli*; enterobacter organisms, *Proteus species*, *Chlamydia trachomatis*

  2. Often associated with urethritis or infection of lower urinary tract

  3. One of the most common causes of recurrent urinary tract infection in men

- Signs and Symptoms

  1. Symptoms similar to, but milder than acute bacterial prostatitis

  2. Hallmark of disease is relapsing UTI due to same pathogen found in prostatic secretions

  3. Urinary frequency, dysuria, decreased flow, hesitancy, dribbling

  4. Vague lower abdominal pain

  5. Lumbar and perineal pain

  6. Fever and urethral discharge uncommon

  7. May experience swelling and severe tenderness of scrotum

- Differential Diagnosis: Same as acute bacterial prostatitis

- Physical Findings

  1. May involve scrotal contents, producing intense local discomfort, swelling, erythema, and severe tenderness to palpation

  2. Prostate may be tender, irregularly indurated, or boggy

- Diagnostic Tests/Findings: Diagnosis made by examination of EPS and quantitative bacterial cultures

  1. EPS—abnormal if greater than 10 WBC/HPF

  2. More than 1 or 2 lipid-laden macrophages/HPF—abnormal

- Management/Treatment

  1. Often difficult to treat

  2. Usual antibiotics—trimethoprim/sulfamethoxazole, carbenicillin, ciprofloxacin, norfloxacin for 4 to 12 weeks

  3. Sitz baths, prostatic massage, intercourse, masturbation

  4. Avoid over-the-counter decongestants if urinary outlet symptoms

Epididymitis

- Definition: An acute intrascrotal infection
- Etiology/Incidence
    1. Caused by infection from bladder urine, the prostate, or an ascending urethral infection
    2. Common affliction of men 35 years and younger; chlamydia usual causative organism for this population (*Neisseria gonorrhoeae* far less common)
    3. Infection in men > 35 years usually arises from bladder bacteriuria secondary to coliform organisms or following instrumentation, catheterization or surgery (prostatectomy)
    4. "Sterile" epididymitis associated with vigorous physical activity is caused by vasal reflux of sterile urine which leads to a chemical inflammation of the epididymis
    5. Epididymitis in boys may indicate underlying congenital anatomic abnormalities (i.e., ectopic ureter, posterior urethral valve)
    6. Condition is usually unilateral
    7. Epididymitis may be complicated by development of testicular necrosis, testicular atrophy or infertility
- Signs and Symptoms
    1. Painful, scrotal swelling (pain may radiate up the spermatic cord into the lower abdomen)
    2. Sensation of scrotal heaviness
    3. Symptoms of prostatitis or UTI may be present
    4. Systemic symptoms may develop—fever, chills and malaise
- Differential Diagnosis
    1. Mumps
    2. Testicular torsion
    3. Testicular abscess
    4. Tumor of testicle with or without hemorrhage
    5. Hydrocele
    6. Trauma

- Physical Findings
    1. Enlarged, tender indurated epididymis
    2. Urethral discharge may be present
    3. Massaging prostate may exacerbate epididymitis
- Diagnostic Tests/Findings
    1. Men
        a. STD testing (chlamydia, gonorrhea and syphilis)
        b. Culture and gram-stained smear of uncentrifuged urine
        c. Scrotal ultrasonography if condition initially severe or if fever continues while on antibiotics (rule out abscess)
        d. CBC—may show increased white blood cell count with left shift
    2. Boys—require more extensive work-up
        a. Intravenous urography
        b. Cystourethroscopy
        c. Voiding cystourethrography
        d. Scrotal ultrasonography (with or without Doppler imaging)
        e. Radionuclide scanning
        f. Surgical exploration may be required
- Management/Treatment
    1. M.D. referral or consult required if:
        a. Patient is a child
        b. Systemic symptoms of infection (leukocytosis, fever) present in adults; patient should be hospitalized for parenteral antibiotics
        c. Surveillance for possible torsion of testes
    2. Outpatient therapy
        a. Antibiotic therapy based on patient's age and symptoms
            (1) Adult < 35 years of age—first choice is ceftriaxone 250 mg IM in a single dose plus doxycycline 100 mg orally

b.i.d.; alternative choice for men 17 years of age or older is ofloxacin 200 to 400 mg orally b.i.d. for 10 days

  (2) Adult > 35 years of age—trimethoprim/sulfamethoxazole one double-strength tablet orally b.i.d. or ciprofloxacin 250 mg orally b.i.d. for 10 days; treat for 4 weeks if underlying prostatitis present

 b. Scrotal elevation, support and bed rest

 c. Analgesics—nonsteroidal anti-inflammatory agents

 d. Ice (early), heat (late)

 e. Spermatic cord block with lidocaine may be used

3. Follow-up within 48 hours if symptoms persist or worsen

4. Discuss therapeutic and diagnostic plans

5. Emphasize importance of complete treatment

6. Avoid sexual intercourse until course of antibiotics completed

7. Inform patient that swelling and discomfort may persist for weeks or months after eradication of infecting organism; epididymis may remain enlarged or indurated indefinitely

8. Educate regarding prevention, transmission and treatment of sexually transmitted disease (if causative agent); encourage continued use of condoms

9. Encourage patient to discuss concerns and/or fears

Benign Prostatic Hypertrophy (BPH)

- Definition: Progressive, benign hyperplasia of prostate gland tissue

- Etiology/Incidence

 1. Cause is uncertain

 2. Approximately 50% of men have BPH by age 60; incidence increases to 90% by age 85

 3. The most common cause of bladder outlet obstruction in males > 50 years

 4. Symptoms are attributed to mechanical obstruction of the urethra by the hyperplastic prostate gland

- Signs and Symptoms
    1. Frequency, urgency, urge incontinence
    2. Nocturia, dysuria
    3. Weak urinary stream, dribbling, hesitancy
    4. Sensation of full bladder immediately after voiding
    5. Retention
- Differential Diagnosis
    1. Urethral stricture
    2. Prostate or bladder cancer
    3. Neurogenic bladder
    4. Bladder calculus
    5. Acute or chronic prostatitis
    6. Bladder neck contracture
    7. Medications that affect micturition
- Physical Findings
    1. Abdomen—may have distended bladder secondary to retention
    2. Prostate (patient should void prior to examination)
        a. Nontender with asymmetrical or symmetrical enlargement; gross enlargement atypical
        b. Consistency is smooth and rubbery (consistency of a pencil eraser)
        c. Distinct nodules (spheroids) may be present
            (1) M.D. referral/consultation required
            (2) Differentiation between BPH nodules and cancerous ones is based on induration or hardness of gland
            (3) Urology referral and biopsy may be required
- Diagnostic Tests/Findings
    1. Urinalysis—NO hematuria, urinary tract infection
    2. Urinary flow rate—voided volume and peak urinary flow rate (uroflowmetry) tests prostatic obstruction

3. Abdominal ultrasound—rules out associated upper tract pathology

4. Serum creatinine and BUN—normal

5. Prostate-specific antigen (PSA) levels may be elevated between 4 to 10 ng/mL; levels > 10 ng/mL may be indicative of carcinoma

- Management/Treatment

   1. Observation

   2. Urology consult required for pharmacologic, mechanical, or surgical treatments

   3. Pharmacologic—drugs selected that reduce bulk and/or tone of gland

      a. Terazosin—1 mg orally at bedtime, increase up to 10 mg at bedtime

      b. Prazosin—1 mg orally b.i.d. to t.i.d.; increase up to 6 to 15 mg per day

      c. Doxazosin—1 mg orally every day up to 16 mg if required

      d. Finasteride 5 mg orally daily

   4. Mechanical—balloon dilation of prostatic urethra

   5. Surgery—indications

      a. Acute urinary retention (urgent urology referral)

      b. Gross hematuria

      c. Epididymitis (especially if recurrent)

      d. Recurrent urinary tract infections

      e. Renal failure from obstruction

      f. Intolerable chronic symptoms

   6. Discuss therapeutic and diagnostic plans

   7. Educate regarding signs/symptoms of urinary retention, renal failure and epididymitis

   8. Emphasize importance of follow-up appointments

   9. Avoid caffeine and alcohol to decrease bladder irritation

   10. Avoid decongestants, antihistamines, tricyclic antidepressants, anti-cholinergics

Prostate Cancer

- Definition: A malignant neoplasm of the prostate gland
- Etiology/Incidence
  1. Etiology is unknown; environmental factors may be involved; adeno-carcinoma is most common type
  2. Second most common malignancy in American men and second most common cause of cancer deaths in men over 55
  3. The relative survival rates have improved over the past 30 years (due to increased awareness and early detection, rather than improved therapy)
  4. May be associated with high-fat diet
  5. Risk factors—family history, age, African-American
- Signs and Symptoms
  1. Many patients are asymptomatic
  2. Symptoms may mimic BPH with frequency, dribbling, nocturia
  3. Occasionally bone pain from metastases (advanced stage)
  4. Occasionally symptoms of uremia due to urethral obstructions (advanced stage)
- Differential Diagnosis
  1. BPH, urethral stricture
  2. Bladder cancer
  3. Neurogenic bladder
  4. Bladder calculus
  5. Acute/chronic prostatitis
  6. Bladder neck contracture
  7. Medications that affect micturition
- Physical Findings
  1. May present with lymphadenopathy, signs of uremia, or urinary retention with distended bladder
  2. More common physical findings are confined to prostate—on rectal

examination prostate feels harder than normal and normal boundaries of gland may be obscured; nodules may be present

3. Prostate may have asymmetric enlargement

- Diagnostic Tests/Findings (performed by consultant M.D.)

1. Transperineal or transrectal needle biopsy of prostate—diagnostic accuracy rate > 90%

2. PSA levels between 4 to 10 ng/mL may indicate BPH, levels > 10 ng/mL are suggestive of carcinoma; false negatives occur

3. Transrectal ultrasound can aid in identification of solid nodules and is used to guide biopsy

4. Other tests such as bone scans may be conducted

- Management/Treatment

1. Consult/referral required

2. Treatment predicated largely on stage of tumor; accurate staging is therefore essential

3. Methods of treatment include surgery, radiation, hormonal therapy

4. Assistance as appropriate in meeting physical, psychological, social, cultural, environmental and spiritual needs

5. Emphasize importance of follow-up appointments

Fibrocystic Breast Changes

- Definition: Benign breast condition characterized by increased growth of fibrous tissue, proliferation of the ductal epithelial lining and/or formation of cysts

- Etiology/Incidence

1. Cause is unknown, estrogen dependency is suspected; condition occurs clinically in 50% and histologically in 90% of women

2. Three types of fibrocystic changes have been identified

   a. Nonproliferative lesions

   b. Proliferative lesions without atypia

   c. Atypical hyperplasia

3. Presence of atypical hyperplasia is associated with an increased risk of breast cancer

4. May be related to dietary intake of methylxanthines, e.g. coffee, chocolate (inconclusive)

- Signs and Symptoms (more pronounced premenstrually)

    1. Cyclic breast tenderness, engorgement, increased density, increased nodularity, enlargement of cystic lump(s)

    2. Nipple discharge may be present

    3. Symptoms of discomfort decrease after menopause

- Differential Diagnosis

    1. Fibroadenosis

    2. Fat necrosis

    3. Fibroadenoma

    4. Carcinoma (especially in women > 40 years)

    5. Breast cysts

- Physical Findings

    1. Skin and contour usually normal

    2. Mass or thickened area present

        a. Location—upper outer quadrant or any area

        b. Size—varies

        c. Shape—round, oval or nodular

        d. Mobility—mobile

        e. Consistency—soft to firm (depends on tension of fluid within cysts)

        f. Number—solitary or multiple (may give impression of "beads on a string")

        g. Nipple—clear/serous discharge may be present (rare)

- Diagnostic Tests/Findings

    1. Fine needle aspiration (FNA)—fluid should return

    2. Excisional biopsy (most definitive test)—no cancer cells

3. Mammography—negative (for women > 35 years)

4. Ultrasound—distinguishes cyst vs. solid mass

- Management/Treatment

  1. Warm compresses applied t.i.d.; supportive brassiere

  2. Low-salt diet; diuretics may also be given premenstrually

  3. Elimination of dietary methylxanthines (coffee, tea, colas, chocolate) (inconclusive)

  4. Vitamin E—400 to 600 international units orally daily

  5. Vitamin B_6—50 to 100 mg daily

  6. Hormonal and anti-hormonal therapy are controversial; the following agents may be used in severe cases

     a. Oral contraceptives—low estrogen with relatively high progesterone

     b. Danazol

     c. Bromocriptine

     d. Tamoxifen

  7. Surgical excision is controversial

  8. Discussion of diagnostic and therapeutic plans

  9. Reassurance of low risk for malignancy

  10. Instruction and demonstration of breast self-examination

  11. Encouragement to report any new mass that does not resolve following menstruation

  12. At follow-up, assess for progression of condition and/or concurrent malignancy

Breast Cancer

- Definition: A malignant neoplasm of the breast

- Etiology/Incidence

  1. Most common cancer in women; second leading cause of death from cancer in women

  2. Frequency increases steadily after age 35

3. 12% of women will develop breast cancer in the U.S.

4. Family history increases a woman's risk twofold to threefold

5. Approximately 182,000 new cases occur annually

6. Risk factors include:

   a. Increasing age

   b. Positive family history (premenopausal more significant); prior personal history of breast cancer

   c. Nulliparity

   d. Late first pregnancy (over age 30)

   e. Early menarche and late menopause after age 55

   f. Fibrocystic changes associated with atypical hyperplasia

   g. Previous unilateral breast or endometrial cancer

   h. Alcohol intake

   i. High fat diet

   j. Obesity

7. Whites have higher incidence than non-whites

- Signs and Symptoms

  1. Often asymptomatic

  2. Single, firm, nontender, painless mass is usual presenting sign

  3. Later manifestations

     a. Skin erythema, dimpling, ulceration

     b. Breast pain

     c. Nipple retraction, eczema, or ulceration

     d. Nipple discharge

- Differential Diagnosis

  1. Fibrocystic breast changes

  2. Fibroadenoma

  3. Intraductal papilloma

  4. Lipoma

5. Fat necrosis

6. Mastitis

7. Dermatitis (Paget's disease)

- Physical Findings

    1. Most common manifestation is single, firm, nontender, ill-defined lump in breast; associated findings may include:

        a. Diffuse nodularity

        b. Skin dimpling

        c. Nipple retraction, discharge (usually bloody)

        d. Lymphadenopathy

        e. Ulcerated/fungating mass (rare)

        f. Palpable supraclavicular and/or axillary lymph nodes

    2. Inflammatory cancer—skin erythema/edema, pain

    3. Paget's disease

        a. Associated with about 5% of mammary carcinomas

        b. Nipple erosion, crusting, bloody discharge

        c. Eczema-like change in skin

- Diagnostic Tests/Findings

    1. Mammography—mass or calcifications indicated; may be negative since 10% of palpable masses are missed on mammogram

    2. Ultrasound—distinguishes cyst vs. solid mass

    3. FNA cytology—fluid vs solid mass, 10% false-negative

    4. Large-needle (core needle) biopsy—histological examination reveals cancer cells (problems with sampling occur)

    5. Excisional biopsy—most reliable diagnostic test where staging of the tumor is done

    6. Determination of hormone receptor tumor cells

    7. Various tests may be conducted if metastasis is suspected including bone and organ scans

- Management/Treatment

1. Referral to an oncology team is required

2. Dependent upon tumor stage, presence of hormone receptors and patient's symptoms/preferences

3. May include surgery, chemotherapy, radiation therapy and/or hormonal therapy

4. Discussion of diagnostic and therapeutic plans

5. Encouragement to express concerns and fears

6. Education and demonstration of breast self-examination to patient and family members, especially daughters

7. Encouragement to report new mass or changes

8. Assistance, as appropriate, in meeting physical, psychological, sexual, social, cultural, environmental and spiritual needs

9. Emphasis on importance of maintaining follow-up with specialists and primary care providers

Dysfunctional Uterine Bleeding (DUB)

- Definition: Excessive, abnormal uterine bleeding, that occurs at irregular intervals, with no demonstrable organic cause

- Etiology/Incidence

  1. Usually results from irregular sloughing of endometrium during anovulatory cycles (90% of cases); but occasionally occurs with poor quality ovulatory cycles

  2. Most frequently due to abnormalities of endocrine function

  3. Estrogen withdrawal or estrogen breakthrough bleeding

  4. Progesterone breakthrough bleeding—continuous low-dose contraceptives

  5. Heaviest bleeding due to high sustained levels of estrogen and seen with:

     a. Polycystic ovarian disease

     b. Obesity

     c. Immaturity of the hypothalamic-pituitary-ovarian axis (postmenarchal teenagers)

     d. Late ovulations (perimenopausal women)

   e. Unopposed estrogen replacement therapy

  6. Not related to oral contraceptive use

- Signs and Symptoms

  1. A carefully obtained history and character of bleeding pattern is critical to assist in ruling-out other conditions

  2. Bleeding is usually characterized by one or more of the following

   a. Persistent or intermittent uterine bleeding

   b. Episodes of extremely heavy bleeding

   c. Oligomenorrhea

  3. DUB bleeding patterns

   a. Intermenstrual bleeding—variable amounts of bleeding that occur between regular menstrual periods

   b. Menometrorrhagia—prolonged, frequent, excessive uterine bleeding that occurs at irregular intervals

   c. Menorrhagia (hypermenorrhea)—prolonged (> 7 days) and excessive (> 80 mL) uterine bleeding occurring at regular intervals

   d. Metrorrhagia—uterine bleeding between normal cycle

   e. Polymenorrhea—frequent, irregular bleeding < 18 day intervals

   f. Oligomenorrhea—infrequent, irregular uterine bleeding that occurs at intervals > 40 days

- Differential Diagnosis

  1. *Inappropriate* to assume that abnormal uterine bleeding is endocrine in origin; other conditions must be ruled-out according to reproductive age

  2. Adolescents

   a. Vaginal trauma secondary to athletics or early sexual exposure

   b. Hypothalamic-pituitary dysfunction secondary to exercise

   c. Pregnancy

   d. Genital infection

     e.   Oral contraceptive use/misuse

     f.   Blood dyscrasias

  3. Women in reproductive years

     a.   Previously noted causes

     b.   Endocrine-related anovulatory abnormal uterine bleeding, common with exercise

     c.   Organic pathology

        (1)   Uterine fibroids

        (2)   Endometrial polyps

        (3)   Chronic systemic illness, e.g., liver cirrhosis, renal failure

     d.   Neoplasia

     e.   Secondary to stress

     f.   Excessive weight change

  4. Perimenopausal women

     a.   Previously listed causes

     b.   Follicular dysfunction (predominant cause)

  5. Postmenopausal women

     a.   Previously noted causes

     b.   Hormone replacement therapy

     c.   Cancer

- Physical Findings

  1. A thorough general and pelvic examination should be performed to assist in ruling out conditions included in the differential diagnosis; source of bleeding must be determined

  2. For DUB, the examination may be essentially negative, or an adnexal mass may indicate polycystic ovaries

- Diagnostic Tests/Findings

  1. Of secondary importance and usually only substantiates a diagnosis already determined by history and physical examination findings

2. Three most important initial tests

   a. Pregnancy test (quantitative Beta hCG)

   b. Prolactin determination (hyperprolactinemia may initially present as ovulatory dysfunction or anovulation and abnormal uterine bleeding)—may be elevated after breast examination

   c. Thyroid stimulating hormone (TSH)

3. Additional initial tests should include:

   a. Follicle stimulating hormone (FSH) and luteinizing hormone (LH)

   b. Complete blood count, blood smear, platelet count, prothrombin time, bleeding time

   c. Cervical Pap smear

   d. STD screening tests

4. Additional tests may be done to rule out other conditions as indicated by the history and physical examination, such as:

   a. Coagulation profile

   b. Serum iron studies

   c. Pelvic ultrasound

5. Tests more important in older women

   a. Endometrial biopsy

   b. Endometrial aspiration

   c. D & C

- Management/Treatment

  1. Should be considered according to amount of blood loss and with an age-related perspective

  2. Medical consult is usually required

  3. Arrest of heavy acute or prolonged bleeding may require intravenous conjugated estrogens followed by combined oral contraceptives or medroxyprogesterone acetate to prevent recurrence

  4. Induction of ovulation is reserved for those desiring pregnancy (use of clomiphene citrate)

5. Iron supplementation if indicated

6. Patient should maintain a basal body temperature chart and record symptoms during cycles

7. Instruction regarding basal body temperature monitoring

8. Discussion of therapeutic and diagnostic plans

9. Review of emergency instructions for acute, heavy bleeding

10. Review of nutritional requirements and encourage intake of iron-rich foods

11. Encouragement of expression of concerns and fears

12. Emphasis on importance of maintaining follow-up

Endometriosis

- Definition: Presence of endometrial glands and stroma outside the endometrial cavity and uterine musculature

- Etiology/Incidence

  1. Etiology is unknown, theories include:

      a. Familial tendency, seven fold increase if first degree female relative

      b. Retrograde menstruation

      c. Metaplastic transformation of epithelium to endometrial tissue at extrapelvic sites

      d. Spread of endometrial tissue through lymphatic and vascular channels

  2. Estimated to affect 5 to 20% of all women of reproductive age

  3. Median age at diagnosis 29 years

- Signs and Symptoms

  1. Presence and severity of symptoms correlate poorly with degree of disease

  2. Pain (most common complaint)

      a. Cyclic pelvic pain due to blood and menstrual debris in surrounding tissues

      b. Constant pain with secondary dysmenorrhea

    c. Pelvic heaviness

    d. Chronic pelvic pain

  3. Dysmenorrhea, primary or secondary

  4. Dyspareunia from fixed uterine retroversion

  5. Infertility

  6. Menstrual irregularities, especially premenstrual spotting

- Differential Diagnosis

  1. Chronic pelvic inflammatory disease

  2. Pelvic adhesions

  3. Ovarian cyst or tumors

- Physical Findings

  1. Uterosacral ligament nodularity and/or tenderness

  2. Fixed uterine retroversion

  3. Adnexal enlargement and/or tenderness

  4. Endometrioma

  5. Tenderness in vaginal cul de sac or cervical motion tenderness

- Diagnostic Tests

  1. Visualization of disease by laparoscope gold standard "powder burn lesions"

  2. Ultrasound—detection of endometrioma (cannot be used as specific test of endometriosis)

  3. Cancer antigen-125 (CA-125)—chemical marker and noninvasive test; of limited value in following course of disease and response to treatment (Mishell, Stenchever, Droëgemueller and Herbst, 1997)

- Management/Treatment

  1. Medication:

    a. Combined low-estrogen monophasic oral contraceptive pills taken continuously to produce amenorrhea

    b. Non-steroidal anti-inflammatory medications for pain relief

    c. Medroxyprogesterone acetate (MPA)—30 mg orally daily causes atrophy of endometrial tissue

    d. Depot MPA—100 to 400 mg intramuscularly monthly causes atrophy of endometrial tissue

    e. Danazol—200 to 400 mg orally twice a day creates anovulation and amenorrhea

    f. GnRH agonists—leuprolide acetate 1 mg subcutaneously daily or 3.75 mg (depot) intramuscularly monthly or nafarelin acetate 200 μg intranasally twice a day creates anovulation and amenorrhea

2. Surgery:

    a. Ablation of endometrial implants laser or electrocautery

    b. Hysterectomy with salpingo-oopherectomy is curative 90%

3. Optimal treatment depends on goal, pain relief or fertility

4. Complications—infertility

Dysplasia—Abnormal Papanicolaou (Pap) Smear Management

- Definition: Squamous intraepithelial lesions (SIL) refers to precancerous cellular development of the cervix (includes mild, moderate and severe dysplasia) and carcinoma in situ of the cervix

- Etiology/Incidence

1. Etiology is most likely related to a sexually transmitted factor; the human papillomavirus (HPV) is suspected to be an initiator of malignant transformation

2. Suspected HPV co-factors include cigarette smoking and folate deficiency

3. Major risk factors for cervical cancer

    a. Sexual intercourse prior to age 20

    b. More than three sexual partners in a lifetime

    c. Intercourse with a male who has had multiple sexual partners

    d. Smoking or history of smoking

    e. Presence or history of HPV (types 16, 18, 31, 33, 35, 45 and

56) more commonly associated with high-grade lesions—see section on Genital Warts or Condylomata acuminata

    f.   Intercourse with man who has HPV

  4.   Approximately 90% are squamous cell carcinomas

  5.   Globally, carcinoma of the cervix is the most common female malignancy; in the U.S. it ranks as the third most common gynecologic malignancy (behind endometrial and ovarian cancer)

- Cervical Cancer Screening

  1.   The Papanicolaou (Pap) smear has reduced disease-related mortality in the U.S. by 50% in the past 40 years

  2.   Screening has also increased detection of preinvasive cervical neoplasms including dysplasia and carcinoma in situ (CIS)

  3.   30% of Pap smears may have false-negative results

  4.   Risk of invasive cervical cancer significantly increases when screening exceeds 3 year intervals

  5.   Recommended screening criteria (U.S. Preventive Task Force)

    a.   Initiate at age 18 or at the age of first intercourse

    b.   Between the ages of 18 and 65, Pap smears should be repeated every one to three years depending upon patient's risk factors for cervical cancer

    c.   After age 65

       (1)   Routine screening may be discontinued if findings are normal on two consecutive Pap smears

       (2)   If abnormal Pap smear, annual screening should occur until two consecutive Pap smears are normal

- Pap smear interpretation: The Bethesda Classification System is most commonly used

  1.   Statement on specimen adequacy

    a.   Satisfactory for interpretation

    b.   Less than optimal

    c.   Unsatisfactory

  2.   General categorization

a. Within normal limits

b. Other

    (1) Infection

    (2) Reactive or reparative changes

    (3) Squamous cell abnormalities

        (a) Atypical—undetermined significance

        (b) Low grade squamous intraepithelial lesion (SIL)—associated with HPV and/or mild dysplasia (cervical intraepithelial neoplasia 1 (CIN 1)

        (c) High grade squamous intraepithelial lesion (SIL)—moderate dysplasia (CIN 2), severe dysplasia (CIN 3) or carcinoma in situ (CIS)

        (d) Squamous cell carcinoma

    (4) Glandular cell abnormalities

        (a) Presence of endometrial cells—menstruating or postmenopausal women

        (b) Atypical—undetermined significance (endometrial or endocervical)

        (c) Adenocarcinoma

    (5) Nonepithelial malignant neoplasm

    (6) Hormonal evaluation (vaginal smears only, i.e., hysterectomy)

- Management of Pap smear results

    1. Within normal limits—repeat annually or as indicated according to cervical cancer risk factors and age

    2. Infection

        a. Treat based on agent causing inflammation

        b. Repeat Pap smear in one year

    3. Reactive or reparative changes

        a. Treat if infectious agent present

      b. May be related to contraceptive mechanical devices (IUD), atrophic changes, chemotherapy and/or radiotherapy etc.

      c. Repeat Pap in one year

   4. Atypical squamous cells of undetermined significance

      a. Indicates abnormality, cause unclear but often an infection

      b. Repeat Pap smear 3 months after appropriate treatment

      c. Colposcopy and cervical biopsies with ECC if atypia persists

   5. Low and high grade SIL

      a. Colposcopy and cervical biopsies with ECC if atypia persists

      b. Low-grade lesions may be monitored with Pap smears every 6 months if ECC is negative

      c. Common treatments include cryotherapy, large loop excision of transformation zone (LLETZ), laser vaporization

      d. Referral to M.D. specialist if carcinoma in situ present

   6. Squamous cell carcinoma, adenocarcinoma and other epithelial or nonepithelial malignant neoplasm—refer to M.D. specialist

   7. Hormonal evaluation—treat atrophic changes if present (see Pregnancy, Contraception, Menopause chapter)

   8. Discuss therapeutic and diagnostic plans

   9. Emphasize importance of regular screening

   10. Review patient's individual risk factors as appropriate

   11. Educate regarding recommended management and treatment as appropriate

   12. Encourage patient to discuss concerns and/or fears

Amenorrhea

- Definition

   1. Primary amenorrhea—absence of normal spontaneous menstrual period by age 16

   2. Secondary amenorrhea—cessation of menses after a variable period of normal function, usually 3 to 6 consecutive cycles

- Etiology—potential underlying conditions

1. Primary amenorrhea

    a. Hypergonadotropic hypogonadism

    b. Turner's syndrome (gonadal dysgenesis)

    c. Severe malnutrition

    d. Pituitary tumors

    e. Head trauma

    f. Encephalitis

    g. Uterine malformations, congenital absence of uterus

    h. Imperforate hymen

    i. Androgen insensitivity

    j. Polycystic ovaries

2. Secondary amenorrhea

    a. Pregnancy (most common cause)

    b. Oral contraceptives

    c. Menopause

    d. Emotional stress

    e. Malnutrition

    f. Excessive exercise

    g. Lactation

    h. Hyperprolactinemia (pituitary tumor)

    i. Anorexia/obesity

    j. Drug use

    k. Polycystic ovaries

    l. Hypothalamic suppression

    m. Hyper and hypothyroidism

    n. Addison's disease

    o. Anovulation

- Signs and Symptoms

    1. Primary amenorrhea

    a.   Absence of menarche

    b.   Failure to develop pubic hair and other secondary sex characteristics

    c.   Abnormal growth and development may be present

    d.   Normal breast development may or may not occur

    e.   Patient symptoms are dependent upon the etiology of the amenorrheic condition

2. Secondary amenorrhea

    a.   Absence of menses at expected time intervals

    b.   Previous regular menses

- Differential Diagnosis

1. First, rule out pregnancy

2. All the potential underlying conditions listed under etiology should be considered in the differential diagnosis

3. A thorough and complete history/physical examination, with supplemental diagnostic/laboratory testing will assist in ruling out unrelated etiologies

- Physical Findings

1. A thorough general and pelvic examination should be performed, partially directed by the history

2. Findings will be related to the underlying etiology

3. The examination may be essentially negative if the amenorrhea is secondary to such conditions as oral contraceptive use or unreported emotional stress

- Diagnostic Tests/Findings

1. Primary amenorrhea—refer to endocrinologist if suspected

2. Secondary amenorrhea

    a.   Pregnancy test (quantitative Beta hCG)—initial test

    b.   Prolactin (if negative pregnancy test), FSH, LH

    c.   Progestin challenge test

    d.   TSH

(1) Elevated TSH—hypothyroid

(2) Normal TSH—rule out pituitary adenoma

   e. Cervical Pap smear

   f. STD screening tests

   g. Urinalysis

3. Additional tests may be done to rule out other conditions as indicated by the history and physical examination

- Management/Treatment

1. Dependent upon underlying etiology

2. Medical consult is often required

3. Discuss therapeutic and diagnostic plans

4. Encourage expression of concerns and fears

5. Emphasize importance of maintaining follow-up

Dysmenorrhea

- Definition: Crampy pain that occurs prior to or during menses, often with a constellation of other symptoms

1. Primary—usually begins in women under 20 years; no other pelvic disease identified

2. Secondary—usually occurs after age 20 in women with pelvic pathology

- Etiology/Incidence

1. Primary—probably the result of excessive uterine prostaglandin production; usually appears shortly after onset of ovulatory cycles; affects approximately 50% or more of all menstruating females

2. Secondary—usually occurs in the presence of organic disease, e.g., endometriosis, pelvic adhesions, adenomyosis, cervical stenosis, uterine fibroids, chronic pelvic infection

- Signs and Symptoms

1. Primary

   a. Pain usually crampy in nature, may radiate to back, thighs and lower abdomen

b. May also have other symptoms, e.g., nausea, vomiting, diarrhea, headache, fatigue

c. Usually begins at onset of menstruation or several hours before; duration is usually 48 to 72 hours

2. Secondary

a. Signs and symptoms associated with organic disease listed under Etiology/Incidence

b. Pain occurs at any point in cycle

- Differential Diagnosis

1. Differentiation between primary and secondary dysmenorrhea

2. Rule out secondary pathologic conditions as noted under Etiology/Incidence

- Physical Findings

1. Primary—usually no significant physical findings; uterine corpus may be tender during menstruation; no pelvic masses or uterine fixation

2. Secondary—findings associated with organic disease

- Diagnostic Tests/Findings

1. Primary—prostaglandin F_{2x} elevated

2. Secondary—tests related to suspected organic pathology

- Management/Treatment

1. Primary

a. Prostaglandin synthetase inhibitors (PGSI), e.g., naproxen, indomethacin, mefenamic acid, ibuprofen

b. Oral contraceptives for sexually active individuals

c. Moderate exercise on a regular basis

d. Diet high in whole grains, beans, vegetables, fruit

e. Elimination of or decreased salt, sugar, caffeine

2. Secondary—treatment related to organic pathology

Premenstrual Syndrome (PMS)

- Definition: A group of somatic and affective symptoms occurring during the luteal phase of the menstrual cycle, decreasing shortly after onset of menstruation

- Etiology/Incidence

  1. Exact cause unknown

  2. Postulated etiologic factors include insufficient progesterone, fluid retention, nutritional problems, glucose metabolism disorders, vitamin deficiencies, ovarian infections, altered serotonin, endorphin levels; elevated prolactin levels

  3. Peak prevalence in the thirties with a decline noted in the forties

  4. Incidence ranges from 5% to 95%; generally agreed about 40% of women are significantly affected at one time or another; only 2% to 3% of women of childbearing age suffer severe symptoms

  5. Most women experience some physical and emotional changes before onset of menstrual flow

- Signs and Symptoms

  1. Bloated feeling, feeling of weight increase

  2. Breast pain or tenderness

  3. Skin disorders

  4. Hot flushes

  5. Headache

  6. Pelvic pain

  7. Change in bowel habits

  8. Irritability, aggression, tension, anxiety, depression, crying, lethargy

  9. Insomnia

  10. Change in appetite, thirst

  11. Change in libido

  12. Loss of concentration

  13. Poor coordination, clumsiness, accidents

- Differential Diagnosis

1. Depression
2. Anxiety disorders
3. Marital discord
4. Substance abuse

- Physical Findings
    1. Because etiology is still unknown, diagnosis is made by history
    2. Complete history and physical examination should be conducted to rule out any medical problems that could be influencing symptomatology

- Diagnostic Tests/Findings: No laboratory tests are available to make diagnosis

- Management/Treatment
    1. Exercise 3 to 4 times per week, especially during luteal phase
    2. Appropriate diet with reasonable amounts of protein (from fish and poultry rather than red meats), vegetables, and fruit
    3. Elimination of tobacco, alcohol, caffeine
    4. Pyridoxine
    5. Diuretics, if fluid retention predominates
    6. Progesterone is controversial; in several studies no more effective than placebo
    7. Prostaglandin inhibitors, e.g., mefenamic acid, naproxen sodium
    8. Oral contraceptives
    9. Danazol
    10. Bromocriptine
    11. PMS support group referral
    12. Fluoxetine hydrochloride

Questions
Select the best answer

1. Which of the following statements regarding AIDS is incorrect?

   a. Most diagnoses are made in persons 20 to 49 years old
   b. Over 1.5 million Americans are infected with HIV
   c. HIV is transmitted through casual kissing
   d. The ELISA is a screening test

2. During the acute phase of HIV infection (first 2 to 8 weeks) which of the following symptoms may be present?

   a. Rash
   b. Shingles
   c. Persistant dermatitis
   d. Pulmonary symptoms

3. Which of the following is not considered in a HIV treatment program?

   a. Zidovudine (AZT)
   b. Didanosine (ddI)
   c. Nutritious diet and stress management
   d. Acyclovir

4. Which of the following may not develop with AIDS?

   a. Kaposi's sarcoma
   b. Cytomegalovirus
   c. Wasting syndrome
   d. Prostatic hypertrophy

5. Which of the following is a diagnostic test for gonorrhea?

   a. Western blot assay
   b. VDRL
   c. Wet prep with WBC
   d. Culture of endocervix on Thayer-Martin media

6. Which of the following is not a correct statement regarding *Neisseria gonorrhoeae?*

   a. One of the leading causes of infertility among U.S. females
   b. The majority of male patients are asymptomatic

    c. P.I.D. is a possible complication

    d. Fever may indicate systemic complications

7. Which of the following is not recommended for the treatment of gonorrhea?

    a. Ceftriaxone

    b. Ciprofloxacin

    c. Acyclovir

    d. Ofloxacin

8. The most common serious gonococcal complication that occurs in women is:

    a. PID

    b. Cervicitis

    c. Arthritis

    d. Conjunctivitis

9. The most common sexually transmitted disease in the U.S. is:

    a. Gonorrhea

    b. Syphilis

    c. Chlamydia

    d. Herpes

10. The causative organism of chlamydia is:

    a. *Chlamydia coli*

    b. *Chlamydia megalovirus*

    c. *Chlamydia trachomotis*

    d. *Chlamydia hominos*

11. A 20-year-old female presents to your clinic with dysuria, dyspareunia, mucopurulent discharge. She reports that her boyfriend was recently treated for nongonococcal urethritis, what STD has she most probably been exposed to?

    a. Gonorrhea

    b. HPV

    c. Chlamydia

    d. Trichomonas

12. Which of the following is a diagnostic test for chlamydia?

    a. Culture of endocervical smear on Thayer-Martin

    b. Tissue culture

c. RPR

d. VDRL

13. Which of the following does not apply to syphilis?

   a. It cannot be transmitted via the placenta
   b. Incidence has steadily increased since the mid-1980s
   c. Risk of contraction through sexual intercourse approaches 50%
   d. It can affect any organ or tissue in the body

14. Which of the following is not a characteristic of secondary syphilis?

   a. Skin rash
   b. Arthralgias
   c. Chancre
   d. Malaise

15. The treatment of choice for a 32-year-old male with early syphilis who is allergic to penicillin is:

   a. Ciprofloxacin
   b. Doxycycline
   c. Erythromycin
   d. Amoxicillin/clavulanate

16. A 38-year-old female presents to your clinic with meningeal symptoms; what stage of syphilis must you rule-out?

   a. Primary
   b. Secondary
   c. Latent
   d. Any stage

17. One of the definitive methods of diagnosis of early syphilis is:

   a. FTA-ABs
   b. Darkfield microscopy
   c. VDRL
   d. MHA-TP

18. A 24-year-old female seen in your clinic has been diagnosed with urethral strictures. What STD is probably included in her past history?

   a. Chlamydia

  b. Herpes genitalis
  c. Syphilis
  d. HPV

19. Which of the following statements regarding herpes genitalis is not true?

  a. Causative agent is a virus
  b. Genital lesions are painless
  c. Infection during pregnancy can lead to spontaneous abortion
  d. Treatment focuses on relieving symptoms

20. The most common symptomatic STD in the U.S. is:

  a. Gonorrhea
  b. Chlamydia
  c. Genital warts (HPV)
  d. Herpes genitalis

21. Which of the following statements regarding genital warts is incorrect?

  a. More than 20 types of HPV cause warts
  b. Increased risk of developing cervical, penile and vulvar cancer
  c. Lesions on the vulva, cervix and penis are treated with TCA
  d. RPR aids in diagnosing cervical lesions

22. All of the following conditions are included in the differential diagnosis for PID except:

  a. Enteritis
  b. Appendicitis
  c. Degeneration of a myoma
  d. Cholecystitis

23. After an initial case of PID, a woman is more susceptible to experience:

  a. Multiple births
  b. Dysmenorrhea
  c. Twisted ovarian cysts
  d. Infertility

24. Which of the following is not found in P.I.D.?

  a. Direct abdominal tenderness
  b. Cervical motion tenderness

    c. Vulvovaginal tenderness

    d. Adnexal tenderness

25. A 22-year-old female seen in your clinic has the following signs and symptoms—malodorous, greenish discharge, perineal itching, red macular cervical lesions, and a vaginal pH of 5.0 to 7.0. What type of vulvovaginitis does she probably have?

    a. Candidiasis

    b. Gardnerella

    c. Bacterial vaginosis

    d. Trichomoniasis

26. Which of the following is not related to bacterial vaginosis?

    a. Multiple bacterial causative agents

    b. "Curdy" white discharge

    c. Positive "whiff test"

    d. Metronidazole is a treatment of choice

27. A classic description of the discharge associated with candida vaginitis is:

    a. "Cottage-cheese"

    b. "Fishy" odor

    c. Green, frothy

    d. Nonpruritic

28. One of the most common causative organisms of UTI in women is:

    a. Klebsiella

    b. Beta-hemolytic streptococci

    c. Chlamydia

    d. *E. coli*

29. Which of the following statements regarding UTI are not relevant?

    a. 30 to 40% of women will experience at least 1 UTI in life-time

    b. Men with UTI should be referred to a urologist

    c. Condom use by sex partner is a contributing factor in women

    d. Prostatitis is a contributing factor in men

30. Which of the following is not a characteristic sign or symptom associated with a UTI:

    a. Fever
    b. Pyuria
    c. Urgency
    d. Negative CVA tenderness

31. Which of the following activities is contraindicated in a patient with suspected acute bacterial prostatitis?

    a. Ejaculation
    b. Urinary catheterization
    c. Prostate examination
    d. Masturbation

32. The drug of choice for a 40-year-old, monogamous male with prostatitis is:

    a. Ciprofloxacin
    b. Doxycycline
    c. TMP/SMX
    d. Carbenicillin

33. Which of the following statements regarding BPH is incorrect?

    a. 90% of men by 85 years of age have BPH
    b. BPH often leads to bladder outlet obstruction
    c. Drugs to reduce bulk of gland may be prescribed
    d. Upon palpation, the prostate surface is roughened

34. The most common type of prostate cancer is:

    a. Adenocarcinoma
    b. Squamous cell
    c. Lymphoma
    d. Sarcoma

35. What is the most common physical finding associated with prostate cancer?

    a. Boggy prostate
    b. Tender prostate
    c. Enlarged, smooth prostate
    d. Hard, nodular prostate

36. Which of the following statements regarding prostate cancer is incorrect?

    a. The largest cancer mortality rate in men 55 to 74 years of age

b. Relative survival rates have improved over the past 30 years

c. Prostate-specific antigen is used as a laboratory marker

d. Bladder calculus is considered in the differential diagnosis

37. The type of fibrocystic breast change that has been associated with malignancy is:

a. Proliferative changes without atypia

b. Nonproliferative changes

c. Atypical hyperplasia

d. Dysplasia

38. What diagnostic test is most definitive in diagnosing fibrocystic changes?

a. Mammography

b. Fine needle aspiration

c. Excisional biopsy

d. Ultrasound

39. A 30-year-old woman is diagnosed with fibrocystic breast changes in your office. All of the following components may be included in the treatment plan except:

a. Yearly mammograms starting now

b. Low-salt diet

c. Limited consumption of caffeine

d. Oral contraceptives

40. The most common cancer in women is:

a. Cervical

b. Breast

c. Ovarian

d. Endometrial

41. Which of the following is not considered a risk factor for breast cancer?

a. Nulliparity

b. Alcohol intake

c. Positive family history

d. Late menarche and early menopause

42. Which description is most characteristic of breast cancer?

a. Single, firm, non-tender, ill-defined breast lump
b. Multiple, firm, non-tender, ill-defined breast lumps
c. Single, firm, tender, circumscribed breast lump
d. Single, rubbery, non-tender, circumscribed breast lump

43. Which of the following does not apply to breast cancer?

    a. 10% of palpable masses are missed on mammography
    b. Excisional biopsy is the most reliable diagnostic test
    c. Paget's disease affects the nipple
    d. Inflammatory breast cancer may be painful

44. Dysfunctional uterine bleeding is most often (90%) associated with:

    a. Polycystic ovaries
    b. Ovulatory cycles
    c. Anovulatory cycles
    d. Late ovulation

45. Menorrhagia refers to:

    a. Uterine bleeding that occurs at regular intervals < 21 days apart
    b. Prolonged and excessive uterine bleeding occurring at regular intervals
    c. Infrequent uterine bleeding that occurs at intervals > 40 days apart
    d. Uterine bleeding that occurs at irregular but frequent intervals

46. Which of the following is least likely to be included in the differential diagnosis of dysfunctional uterine bleeding for a perimenopausal women?

    a. Neoplasia
    b. Blood dyscrasias
    c. Pregnancy
    d. Vaginal trauma

47. Which one of the following characteristics is not associated with primary amenorrhea?

    a. Irregular menses
    b. Absence of menarche
    c. Lack of pubic hair
    d. Abnormal growth and development

48. The most common cause of secondary amenorrhea is:

a. Oral contraceptives
b. Polycystic ovaries
c. Pregnancy
d. Anovulation

49. What is the first test that should be ordered in a woman who presents with secondary amenorrhea?

a. Thyroid profile
b. Prolactin
c. Pregnancy test
d. Progestin challenge

50. Which of the following findings suggest the diagnosis of endometriosis?

a. Retroversion of the uterus
b. Nodularity of the uterosacral ligament
c. Ovarian cyst
d. Amenorrhea

51. Medical treatment options for endometriosis include:

a. DES
b. Triphasic oral contraceptives
c. Methyltestosterone
d. Medroxyprogesterone acetate

52. Endometriosis:

a. Is the development and deposition of endometrial tissue in the myometrium
b. Is not a significant factor in infertility
c. Is common in postmenopausal women
d. Is a common cause of pelvic pain

Answers

-1. c	- 18. b	35. d
2. a	- 19. b	36. a
3. d	20. c	37. c
4. d	- 21. d	38. c
5. d	- 22. d	39. a
- 6. b	23. d	40. b
7. c	24. c	41. d
8. a	25. d	42. a
9. c	26. b	- 43. b
10. c	27. a	44. c
11. c	28. d	45. b
- 12. b	29. c	- 46. d
- 13. a	30. a	47. a
14. c	31. b	- 48. c
15. b	32. c	49. c
16. d	33. d	- 50. b
- 17. b	34. a	- 51. d
		- 52. d

Bibliography

Centers for Disease Control and Prevention. (1998). "1998 Sexually transmitted diseases treatment guidelines" *Morbidity and Mortality Weekly Report.* January 23, (47) RRI

Conn, R. B., Borer, W. Z., & Snyder, J. W. (1997). *Current Diagnosis 9.* Philadelphia: W. B. Saunders.

Cunningham, F. G., MacDonald, P. C., Gant, N. F., Leveno, K. J., & Gilstrap, L. C. (1997). *Williams obstetrics* (20th ed.). Norwalk, CT: Appleton & Lange.

Fanning, M. M. (1997). *HIV infection: A clinical approach* (2nd ed.). Philadelphia: W. B. Saunders.

Gompel, C., & Silverberg, S. G. (Eds.). (1994). *Pathology in gynecology and obstetrics* (4th ed.). Philadelphia: J. B. Lippincott.

Harris, J. R., Hellman, S., Henderson, I. C., & Kinne, D. W. (Eds.). (1996). *Breast diseases.* Philadelphia: J. B. Lippincott.

Hatcher, R. A., Trussell, J., Stewart, F., Cates Jr. W., Stewart, G. K., Guest, F., & Kowall, D. (1998). *Contraceptive technology* (17th rev. ed.). NY: Ardent Media.

Mishell, D. R., Stenchever, M. A., Droëgemueller, W., & Herbst, A. L. (1997). *Comprehensive gynecology* (3rd ed.). St. Louis: Mosby.

Rakel, R. E. (Ed.). (1997). *Conn's current therapy.* Philadelphia: W. B. Saunders.

Rakel, R. E. (Ed.). (1997). *Textbook of family practice.* Philadelphia: W. B. Saunders.

Sanfilippo, J. S., Muram, D., Dewhurst, J., & Lee, P. A. (Eds.). (1998). *Pediatric and adolescent gynecology.* Philadelphia: W. B. Saunders.

Scott, J. R., DiSaia, P. J., Hammond, C. B. & Spellacy, W. N. (1994). *Danforth's obstetrics and gynecology.* Philadelphia: J. B. Lippincott.

Stenchever, M. A. (Ed.). (1996). *Office gynecology.* St. Louis: Mosby Year Book.

Pregnancy, Contraception and Menopause

Susan B. Moskosky

Pregnancy

- Definition: The condition of having a developing embryo or fetus within the female body (usually within the uterus)

- Incidence

  1. Birth rate, or number of births per 1,000 total population, in the U.S. for the year ending 1996 was 14.8—same rate as 1995

  2. Birth rate for teenagers during 1996 was 54.7 per 1,000 women aged 15 to 19 years, down 4 percent compared with 1995; teenage birth rate has declined by 12 percent since 1991

  3. Fertility rate, or number of births per 1,000 women of childbearing age (15 to 44 years), for the year ending 1996 was 65.7

  4. Pregnancy rate, or number of pregnancies per 1,000 women of childbearing age (15 to 44 years), for the year ending 1992 was 109.9

- Preconception Care Improves Pregnancy Outcome

  1. Goal is to maximize health of mother and infant

  2. Includes history-taking, physical examination and laboratory/diagnostic testing

  3. Preconception counseling

     a. Menstrual record—record first day of last normal menstrual period (LNMP)

     b. Exercise and nutrition

        (1) 0.4 mg of folic acid per day recommended to reduce risk of neural tube defects

        (2) Encourage attainment of ideal weight prior to conception

        (3) Begin exercise program to improve cardiovascular status, assist with weight loss, and lessen potential for hypertension and diabetes in pregnancy

        (4) Avoid teratogens—environmental and medications

        (5) Identify genetic risks

        (6) Affirm readiness for parenthood

(7) Appropriate vaccinations/immunizations (e.g., rubella, tetanus, hepatitis)

- Early Diagnosis of Pregnancy is Essential

    1. Begin prenatal care; physical examination; laboratory tests; risk assessment; discontinue use of tobacco, alcohol, street drugs and/or teratogenic medications; provide educational materials

    2. If pregnancy is unintended, make timely decision regarding pregnancy options (e.g., continuation, termination, adoption)

- Signs and Symptoms of Pregnancy

    1. Presumptive—subjective; frequently reported with pregnancy, but not conclusive for pregnancy

        a. Nausea with or without vomiting

        b. Urinary frequency

        c. Fatigue

        d. Perception of fetal movement by mother (quickening); with pregnancy, usually occurs 16 to 20 weeks

        e. Amenorrhea

        f. Breast changes

        g. Vaginal mucosa discoloration (Chadwick's sign)

        h. Increased skin pigmentation and abdominal striae

    2. Probable—more objective; often noted on physical examination or with laboratory testing

        a. Enlargement of abdomen and uterus

        b. Uterine changes in size, shape, consistency; softening of lower uterine segment at 6 to 8 weeks gestation (Hegar's sign)

        c. Softening of cervix at 6 to 8 weeks gestation (Goodell's sign)

        d. Braxton-Hicks contractions

        e. Ballottement

        f. Outlining of fetus by examiner

        g. Pregnancy tests—endocrine tests that detect human chorionic gonadotropin (hCG) in maternal blood or urine

3. Positive—noted with absolute confirmation of pregnancy

    a. Detection of fetal heartbeat—auscultation with fetoscope at 17 to 20 weeks gestation; auscultation with doppler by 10 to 12 weeks gestation

    b. Perception of fetal movement by examiner

    c. Visualization of fetus by ultrasonography

- Differential Diagnosis

    1. Myomas, hematometra, adenomyosis

    2. Ovarian tumor or extrauterine mass

    3. Amenorrhea/irregular menses of other origin

    4. Urinary tract infection

    5. Gastrointestinal problem

    6. Gestational trophoblastic disease

- Physiologic Changes (Maternal)

    1. Cardiovascular/Respiratory

        a. Blood volume increased by 30 to 50% at term

        b. Increased cardiac output

        c. Heart displaced by uterus upward and to left

        d. Pulse rate increased by 10 to 15 beats per minute

        e. Dependent edema of feet and hands by third trimester

        f. Exaggerated heart sounds; functional systolic murmurs common

        g. Physiologic anemia common due to unequal expansion of red cell volume (30%) and plasma volume (50%)

        h. Increased respiratory tidal volume

        i. Dyspnea common during early pregnancy; progressive elevation of diaphragm later in pregnancy

    2. Gastrointestinal

        a. Decreased smooth muscle tone and decreased motility due to progesterone resulting in:

          (1)   Decreased intestinal peristalsis

          (2)   Gastric reflux and heartburn

  b. Abdominal distention secondary to increased uterine size and flatus

  c. Hypertrophy and bleeding of gums due to estrogen

3. Musculoskeletal

  a. Progesterone-induced relaxation of pelvic structures and joints (may cause discomfort)

  b. Center of gravity shifts causing lordosis and posture changes; lower back pain common

  c. Diastasis recti possible (separation of rectus abdominis muscles)

4. Integumentary

  a. Cutaneous vascular changes—spider angiomas, palmar erythema

  b. Increased pigmentation of face (chloasma), areolae, abdomen (linea nigra), and genitalia

  c. Striae gravidarum

  d. Increased sebaceous and sweat gland activity

5. Endocrine

  a. Diffuse thyroid gland enlargement

  b. Insulin needs increase due to action of human placental lactogen (hPL)

6. Breasts

  a. Early tenderness and tingling

  b. Increase in size and nodularity; striae may develop

  c. Veins prominent

  d. Nipples erectile; arealoe darken

  e. Montgomery follicles hypertrophy

  f. Colostrum after first few months

7. Genitalia/reproductive

a. External genitalia

    (1) Increased pigmentation

    (2) Pelvic congestion; swelling of labia majora near term

    (3) Vulvar varicosities possible

b. Vagina

    (1) Increased vascularity causing bluish/purple color (Chadwick's sign)

    (2) Rugations of vaginal mucosa prominent

    (3) Increased secretions (leukorrhea)

c. Cervix

    (1) Pronounced softening and cyanosis (early)

    (2) Proliferation of endocervical glands (cervical "erosion")

    (3) Mucus plug blocks endocervical canal

d. Uterus

    (1) Increases in size and weight

    (2) Softening of lower uterine segment (Hegar's sign)

    (3) Blood supply increased

e. Ovaries

    (1) Corpus luteum—continues for first 10 to 12 weeks of pregnancy; produces progesterone until placenta develops

    (2) Ovarian function ceases during pregnancy

f. Urinary

    (1) Dilation of ureters and kidneys (especially on right), decreased bladder tone—increased risk for urinary stasis and infection

    (2) Urinary frequency common early and late in pregnancy

    (3) Incontinence common, particularly with multiparity

- Prenatal Care

  1. Initial visit

     a. Laboratory confirmation of pregnancy—urine and serum tests available, all test for hCG

        (1) Agglutination inhibition test—urine test, reliable 14 to 21 days post-conception

        (2) Enzyme-linked immunosorbent assay (ELISA); immunometric test (urine or serum) reliable 7 to 10 days post-conception

        (3) Beta subunit radioimmunoassay (RIA)—serum test, reliable 7 days post-conception

     b. Expected date of birth (EDB)—Nagele's rule subtract 3 months from LNMP and add 7 days

     c. History—emphasize factors that may affect maternal or fetal outcome

        (1) Menstrual history—extremely important for estimating gestational age

        (2) Contraceptive history

        (3) Maternal history—attention to acute or chronic health problems

        (4) Family history—multiple gestation, congenital anomalies, inherited diseases, maternal family history of diabetes or hypertension

        (5) Medication history

        (6) Substance use—tobacco, alcohol or other drugs

        (7) Exposure to environmental or occupational toxins or hazards

        (8) History of domestic violence

        (9) Reproductive/obstetric history

            (a) Each previous pregnancy including outcome—e.g., **T**erm birth, **P**reterm birth, **A**bortion (spontaneous or induced) and number of **L**iving children (T-P-A-L)

        (b)   Complications during previous pregnancy/delivery/postpartum—e.g., gestational diabetes, pregnancy induced hypertension (PIH), preterm labor (PTL) and/or preterm birth, postpartum hemorrhage, postpartum depression

        (c)   Previous pregnancy loss including gestational age and related factors

        (d)   Method of delivery for previous pregnancies—vaginal or cesarean

  d. Physical examination

    (1) Vital signs and complete head-to-toe examination—attention to ruling out pre-existing medical conditions

    (2) Assess uterine size to confirm pregnancy and determine gestational age—most accurately assessed by bimanual examination up to 14 weeks

        (a)   8 weeks—approximately 9 cm

        (b)   10 weeks—approximately 10 cm

        (c)   12 weeks—uterine fundus at symphysis pubis

        (d)   16 weeks—fundus midway between symphysis pubis and umbilicus

        (e)   20 weeks—fundus at umbilicus

        (f)   20 weeks to term—abdominal measurement of fundal height

            (i)   Measure from top of symphysis pubis to top of uterine fundus

            (ii) Between 18 and 32 weeks gestation, good correlation between gestational age in weeks and measurement of fundal height in centimeters

    (3) Evaluate pelvic dimensions (pelvimetry)

    (4) Obtain Pap smear and cervical cultures

    (5) Auscultation of fetal heart by doppler (usually audible by 10 to 12 weeks with doppler) or fetoscope (usually audible by 17 to 20 weeks)

e. Laboratory testing (routine)

    (1) ABO blood group/Rh factor determination

    (2) Complete blood cell count (CBC) with indices

    (3) Antibody screen and titer

    (4) Rubella titer—titer of > 1:10 indicates immunity

    (5) Syphilis screening—Venereal Disease Research Laboratories test (VDRL), rapid plasma reagin (RPR)

    (6) Hepatitis B surface antigen screening

    (7) Urinalysis; urine culture if indicated

    (8) Chlamydia/gonorrhea screening

    (9) Offer human immunodeficiency virus (HIV) antibody testing

    (10) Other tests indicated by individual risk status or general patient population, e.g., postprandial 50 g glucose screen, sickle cell screen, tuberculin testing

f. Risk assessment

    (1) Referral for genetic counseling if indicated

        (a) Maternal age of 35 or older by delivery

        (b) Family history of genetic anomaly—e.g., Down syndrome, other chromosomal abnormality, hemophilia, muscular dystrophy, cystic fibrosis

        (c) History of three or more spontaneous abortions

        (d) Previous unexplained pregnancy loss

        (e) Parents possible carriers of sickle cell, thalassemia, or Tay-Sachs disease

    (2) PTL risk assessment

        (a) Medical/obstetrical factors—multiple gestation, diethylstilbestrol (DES) exposure, hydramnios, uterine anomaly, cervical effacement or dilatation at 32 weeks gestation, previous history of PTL and/or preterm delivery, history of cone biopsy, uterine irritability, febrile illness, history of pyelonephritis

(b) Behavioral factors—smoking, substance use/abuse, malnutrition

g. Education

(1) Nutrition

(a) Dietary assessment

(b) Ideal weight gain during pregnancy is 25 to 35 pounds for woman of normal weight; obese (> 120% of ideal body weight) 15 to 25 pounds; underweight (< 90% of ideal body weight) 28 to 40 pounds

(i) First trimester—2 to 5 pounds

(ii) Second and third trimesters—0.8 to 1 pound per week

(c) Discourage weight loss during pregnancy

(d) Nutritional requirements

(i) Calories—1800 to 2400 kilocalories per day (increase by 300 over normal consumption)

(ii) Protein—75 to 100 grams per day

(iii) Calcium—1200 mg per day

(iv) Iron—30 to 60 mg supplement per day

(v) Folic acid—0.4 mg per day

(vi) Other vitamin and mineral needs can usually be met from a balanced diet; encourage fiber and fluids

(2) Encourage good hygiene; douching not recommended

(3) Exercise

(a) Regular exercise recommended throughout pregnancy

(b) May continue with pre-pregnancy exercise routine, but should not begin new strenuous exercise program

(c) Walking and swimming are ideal during pregnancy

       (d)   Avoid excessive fatigue and excessive overheating

  (4)   Sexual activity

       (a)   Coitus not contraindicated during normal pregnancy

       (b)   Changes in position may be required as pregnancy progresses

       (c)   Sexual intercourse contraindicated during pregnancy with undiagnosed vaginal bleeding, rupture of membranes, preterm labor, threatened abortion

  (5)   Warning signs—patient should contact provider promptly

       (a)   Signs of ectopic pregnancy or threatened abortion

           (i)   Abdominal pain

           (ii)   Vaginal bleeding

           (iii)   Passage of tissue

           (iv)   Syncope

       (b)   Hyperemesis—severe nausea and vomiting; unable to retain food or fluids

       (c)   Signs of pyelonephritis

           (i)   Fever above 100.6° F

           (ii)   Dysuria, flank pain

       (d)   Signs of PIH

           (i)   Severe headache, dizziness

           (ii)   Scotomata, blurring of vision

           (iii)   Swelling of face; severe dependent edema that does not respond to rest/elevation

           (iv)   Epigastric pain

       (e)   Signs of PTL

           (i)   Loss of fluid from vagina

           (ii)   Lower back pain or lower abdominal cramping

          (iii) Frequent, palpable uterine contractions with or without pain

          (iv) Heaviness or pressure

          (v) Increased vaginal discharge, especially if blood-tinged, mucoid or watery

    (f) Decreased or absent fetal movement

(6) Signs and symptoms of labor

    (a) True labor

          (i) Contractions—timed from beginning of one contraction to beginning of the next

              a) Occur at regular intervals which gradually shorten

              b) Initially felt in back, then radiate to lower abdomen

              c) Duration and strength of contractions increase

              d) Intensity of contractions increase with walking

              e) Sedation does not stop contractions

          (ii) Bloody "show"—pink or blood-tinged mucous discharge from cervix may indicate loss of mucus plug

          (iii) Cervix dilates and effaces

          (iv) Presenting part has descended into pelvis

    (b) False labor

          (i) Contractions irregular in timing, duration and intensity

          (ii) Discomfort is felt mainly in abdomen

          (iii) Intensity of contractions not affected by walking

          (iv) No changes in cervix; no bloody show, dilatation or effacement

           (v)   Fetal head remains free in pelvis

           (vi) Sedation will stop contractions

   (c)   Rupture of membranes

           (i)   Occurs spontaneously at onset of labor in 50%

           (ii) Premature rupture of membranes associated with increased risk for:

                 a) PTL if occurs prior to 37 weeks gestation

                 b) Ascending intrauterine infection if not delivered within 24 hours

                 c) Prolapse of umbilical cord

2.   Interval visits

   a.   For low risk, routine monthly visits up to 28 weeks, every 2 to 3 weeks until 36 weeks, then weekly until delivery

   b.   Components of routine visits

      (1)   Measurement of maternal weight and blood pressure

      (2)   Screen urine for protein and glucose; ketones and nitrites if indicated

      (3)   Obtain interval history, evaluate client complaints and risk-related symptoms, answer questions and provide anticipatory guidance

      (4)   Assess fetal heart tones by fetoscope or doppler (normal rate is 120 to 160 beats per minute)

      (5)   Evaluate fetal growth

         (a)   Determine fundal height

         (b)   Leopold's maneuvers—abdominal palpation performed using four maneuvers to determine fetal presentation and position (used later in pregnancy—beginning approximately 26 weeks)

      (6)   Specific needs or screening tests as indicated by gestational age or patient history

         (a)   First trimester (LNMP through 13th week)

(i) Chorionic villus sampling (CVS)—refer when indicated for genetic reasons; optimal time 9 to 11 weeks

(ii) 1 hour postprandial 50 g glucose screen (initial visit or first trimester) for women with risk factors for gestational diabetes mellitus (GDM)—prior history of GDM; first degree relative with diabetes; prior delivery of macrosomic infant; previous unexplained stillbirth or spontaneous abortions; obesity; glucosuria; advanced maternal age ($\geq$ 35)

(iii) Assess physical and psychological impact of pregnancy, including support system

(iv) Discuss warning signs and early complications

(b) Second trimester (14th through 27th week)

(i) Maternal serum alpha-fetoprotein (MSAFP) and Multiple Marker Screening—screen at 15 to 19 weeks (16 to 18 weeks optimal)

a) Elevated levels of MSAFP associated with fetal congenital abnormalities—open neural tube defects, congenital nephrosis, abdominal wall defects; also elevated with multiple gestation

b) Low levels of MSAFP associated with Down Syndrome (Trisomy 21)

(ii) Amniocentesis—performed at 15 to 18 weeks if indicated

a) Genetic screening—mother of $\geq$ 35, history of previous child with chromosomal, congenital or metabolic abnormality

b) Rh sensitization—spectrophotometric examination of amniotic fluid predictive of severity of hemolytic disease

          c) Fetal lung maturity—lecithin/sphingo-myelin ration (L/S) ration $\geq$ 2:1 indicates lung maturity

    (iii) 1 hour postprandial 50 g glucose screen—screen all women between 24 to 28 weeks

          a) If 1 hr glucose screen is 140 to 199 mg/dL, order 3 hour 100 g glucose tolerance test (3 hr OGTT); if 2 or more values are abnormal, diagnosis of GDM is made

          b) If 1 hr glucose screen is > 200 mg/dL, order fasting blood sugar (FBS); if FBS is > 130 mg/dL, omit OGTT and refer for treatment

    (iv) Assess for fetal movements (quickening)—usually between 16 to 20 weeks

    (v) Evaluate for signs of PTL

  (c) Third trimester (28th week to term—usually 40 weeks)

    (i) Repeat VDRL and hemoglobin (Hgb)

    (ii) Re-evaluate antibody screen titer

    (iii) Rh (D) immune globulin (RhoGAM) to unsensitized Rh-negative mother—28 weeks

    (iv) Discuss importance of monitoring fetal movement as indicator of fetal well being

    (v) Review signs and symptoms of labor

    (vi) Perform cervical assessment for position, consistency, length and dilation

    (vii) Assess fetal lie and presentation (36 to 40 weeks)

3. Tests for assessment of fetal well-being

  a. Ultrasound (ultrasonography)

    (1) Definition: High-frequency sound waves reflected from tissues of varying densities and converted into images

(a) Level 1 (Basic Ultrasound)—establishes gestational age, location and grade of placenta; determines fetal presentation, number of fetuses, stage of fetal growth, cardiac activity; assesses amniotic fluid volume; detects gross fetal anomalies and maternal pelvic masses

(b) Level II (Targeted Ultrasound)—confirms information obtained in Level I and surveys fetal anatomy for malformations

(2) Indications—determination of gestational age; assess fetal growth pattern; size/date discrepancy; suspected ectopic pregnancy; determine fetal presentation/lie; suspected hydramnios/oligohydramnios; suspected fetal anomaly or fetal demise; determine placental location, integrity, maturity; identify number of fetuses; aid in diagnostic procedures, e.g., amniocentesis, CVS

b. Nonstress test (NST)

(1) Definition: Diagnostic test that monitors fetal heart rate acceleration in response to fetal movement (noninvasive); both NST and contraction stress test (CST) were developed to assess any indication of uteroplacental insufficiency and to predict ability of fetus to endure stress of labor

(2) Procedure—fetal heart rate (FHR), fetal movement and uterine contractions are assessed (using external monitoring) over a 20 minute period; may be extended to 40 minutes if no FHR accelerations occur

(3) Interpretation

(a) Reactive NST—appropriate heart rate accelerations; fetal well-being assured for one week (repeat weekly)

(b) Nonreactive NST—absence of appropriate heart rate accelerations over a 40 minute period; consider additional testing, e.g., contraction stress test (CST) or biophysical profile

c. Contraction stress test (CST)

(1) Definition: Diagnostic test performed to evaluate fetal response to uterine contractions; mimics labor

(2) Procedure—baseline tracing obtained prior to stimulating uterine contractions; if fewer than 3 contractions occur in 10 minutes, contractions stimulated by intravenous oxytocin infusion or nipple stimulation

(3) Interpretation

    (a) Positive CST—late decelerations following 50% or more of contractions; delivery recommended or further tests (test has 30% false-positive rate)

    (b) Negative CST—no late or variable decelerations; subsequent testing based on fetal and maternal conditions and institutional protocol

    (c) Equivocal CST—late decelerations in fewer than 50% of contractions, or significant variable decelerations; repeat in 24 hours or do biophysical profile

(4) Contraindications—premature rupture of membranes, history of PTL during current pregnancy, incompetent cervix or cerclage, previous vertical uterine incision, third trimester bleeding, polyhydramnios, placenta previa, multiple pregnancy

d. Biophysical profile (BPP)

(1) Definition: Use of real-time ultrasound combined with NST to assess four parameters of fetal well-being which include fetal tone, breathing, body movements and amniotic fluid volume

(2) Indications—high-risk pregnancy, e.g., post-date pregnancy, decreased fetal movement, maternal disease, suspected oligohydramnios, intrauterine growth retardation

(3) Interpretation—each of five components is scored as 2 (normal) or 0 (abnormal), with total possible score of 10

    (a) 8 to 10—normal

    (b) 6—equivocal (repeat according to agency protocol)

(c) ≤ 4—abnormal (consider delivery)

- Common Complaints in Pregnancy
    1. Nausea and vomiting
        a. Etiology—high levels of hCG in first trimester, changes in carbohydrate metabolism, delayed gastric emptying
        b. Management
            (1) Rule out hyperemesis gravidarum, pyelonephritis
            (2) Small, frequent high carbohydrate meals; avoid high-fat or spicy meals; avoid empty or overdistended stomach
    2. Backache
        a. Etiology—softening and relaxation of pelvic structures and joints; increased lordosis of spine caused by shift in center of gravity
        b. Management
            (1) Rule out pyelonephritis, labor, musculoskeletal disease
            (2) Teach pelvic tilt exercise; use proper body mechanics; avoid excessive twisting, bending and stretching
    3. Varicosities
        a. Etiology—pressure of enlarged uterus causing impaired venous circulation and increased venous pressure in lower extremities; relaxation of vein walls and valves; hereditary factors; weight gain
        b. Management
            (1) Rule out thrombophlebitis
            (2) Support pantyhose; frequent leg elevation; avoid standing for long periods, crossing legs, and knee high hose
    4. Hemorrhoids
        a. Etiology—pressure of enlarging uterus; constipation; predisposition to varicosities
        b. Management
            (1) Rule out abscessed or thrombosed hemorrhoids

        (2)   Topical anesthetics; prevent or treat constipation by increasing fluids and roughage in diet; warm or cool sitz baths; ice packs or cold compresses

5. Constipation

    a. Etiology—decreased intestinal motility caused by progesterone and compression of bowel by enlarging uterus; oral iron supplements

    b. Management—increase high-fiber foods and fluids; regular exercise; bulk-forming, nonnutritive laxative

6. Heartburn

    a. Etiology—decreased gastrointestinal peristalsis and relaxation of cardiac sphincter; reflux of gastric contents into lower esophagus; upward displacement and compression of the stomach by uterus

    b. Management

        (1)   Rule out cardiac, gallbladder, epigastric or pancreatic disease, PIH

        (2)   Small frequent meals; avoid fatty foods; fluids between but not with meals; do not lie down after eating for at least one hour; low sodium antacids

7. Pica and food cravings

    a. Etiology—unknown

    b. Management—evaluate diet to determine adequacy; explain need to maintain healthy diet; problems may occur if craved substance is substituting for nutritious food or is harmful to mother or fetus

8. Ptyalism (increased salivation)

    a. Etiology—unknown

    b. Management—reassurance of resolution following pregnancy; good oral hygiene; avoid excessive starch intake; adequate fluid intake

9. Fatigue—most common in first and third trimesters

    a. Etiology

      (1)   Early pregnancy—increased oxygen consumption, increased progesterone level, fetal demands

      (2)   Late pregnancy—sleep deprivation from physical discomforts

   b. Management

      (1)   Rule out iron deficiency anemia, depression

      (2)   Reassurance; encourage adequate sleep and rest periods

10. Headache

   a. Etiology—increased circulatory volume; vasodilation caused by high progesterone levels; vascular congestion; stress; fatigue; hypoglycemia

   b. Management

      (1)   Rule out PIH, migraine headache, sinus infection

      (2)   Teach symptoms of PIH; encourage adequate rest; stress reduction; massage; moist hot or cold compresses; avoid intake of foods that trigger headaches; acetaminophen

11. Vaginal discharge (leukorrhea)

   a. Etiology—estrogen-induced increase in vascularity and hypertrophy of cervical glands and vaginal cells

   b. Management

      (1)   Rule out ruptured membranes, vaginitis, cervicitis, sexually transmitted disease (STD)

      (2)   Reassurance; cotton underwear and loose clothing; avoid douching or tampon use; keep vulva clean and dry

12. Urinary frequency

   a. Etiology—enlargement of uterus compresses bladder; hyperplasia and hyperemia of pelvic organs and increased kidney output

   b. Management

      (1)   Rule out urinary tract infection (UTI)

      (2)   Void frequently; maintain adequate fluid intake; discontinue fluids 2 to 3 hours prior to bedtime; avoid caffeine

13. Leg cramps

    a. Etiology—pressure of uterus on pelvic nerves and blood vessels; imbalance in phosphorus/calcium ratio caused by inadequate or excessive calcium intake (postulated)

    b. Management

       (1) Rule out thromboembolic disease, varicosities

       (2) Avoid stretching legs, pointing toes, and lying on back; dorsiflexion of foot to relieve cramp in calf; diet evaluation to correct excessive or inadequate intake of calcium

14. Round ligament pain

    a. Etiology—growth of uterus causes round ligaments to stretch

    b. Management

       (1) Rule out PTL, ectopic pregnancy, ruptured ovarian cyst, appendicitis

       (2) Reassurance of resolution following pregnancy; avoid sudden, twisting movements; heating pad; avoid excessive exercise, standing or walking

15. Dyspnea (breathlessness)

    a. Etiology—increased sensitivity to lower levels of CO_2 (progesterone effect) in early pregnancy; later in pregnancy caused by displacement of diaphragm by enlarging uterus

    b. Management

       (1) Rule out upper respiratory infection, pulmonary or cardiac problem

       (2) Sleep with head elevated; reassure improvement will occur when fetus drops into pelvis; avoid exercise if a precipitating factor

16. Edema

    a. Etiology—increased capillary permeability (hormonal); pressure of uterus impedes venous return; increased fluid in intracellular spaces

    b. Management

       (1) Assess for PIH

      (2) Instruct about symptoms of PIH; rest in left lateral recumbent position for 1 to 2 hours during day and at night; elevate legs several times during day; avoid constrictive clothing; avoid long periods of sitting or standing

- Pregnancy Complications

  1. Bleeding disorders

     a. Spontaneous abortion (SAB)

        (1) Definition: Naturally occurring termination of pregnancy before 20 weeks gestation

        (2) Etiology—chromosomal abnormalities of fetus; maternal disease, infection, or endocrine imbalance; blighted ovum; faulty implantation; immune factors; advanced maternal age

        (3) Signs and symptoms/physical examination findings

            (a) Threatened abortion—occurs in 1 of 4 pregnancies

                (i) Vaginal bleeding with or without cramping; may be accompanied by low backache

                (ii) No cervical changes; cervix closed

            (b) Inevitable

                (i) Vaginal bleeding with contractions; possible gush of fluid from vagina

                (ii) Cervical dilatation and rupture of membranes

            (c) Missed abortion—prolonged retention of fetus after fetal death

                (i) Loss of symptoms of pregnancy; may have brownish vaginal discharge

                (ii) Gradual decrease in uterine size; cervix closed and firm

            (d) Incomplete abortion—incomplete expulsion of products of conception (POC), usually placenta retained

(i) Bleeding (may be profuse); cramping

(ii) May observe tissue in cervical canal

(e) Complete abortion—complete expulsion of all POC

(i) Bleeding; cramping

(ii) No retained POC; cervix dilated

(4) Differential diagnosis

(a) Vaginal infection

(b) Cervical polyp

(c) Ectopic pregnancy

(d) Molar pregnancy

(e) Incompetent cervix

(5) Diagnostic tests/findings

(a) Ultrasound for evidence of fetal heart action and uterine size

(b) Serial hCG levels

(c) Pelvic exam to evaluate cervical dilation, uterine size and bleeding

(6) Management/treatment

(a) Bedrest; pelvic rest; hydration; counsel regarding signs of infection and when to report symptoms

(b) May require hospitalization, dilatation and curettage (D & C), transfusion, IV fluids

b. Ectopic pregnancy

(1) Definition: Implantation of fertilized ovum outside the uterine cavity (usually in fallopian tube)

(2) Etiology—any condition that prevents or slows passage of fertilized ovum into uterus—e.g., tubal damage from previous pelvic infection, tubal surgery, previous ectopic; progestin-only contraceptive use

(3) Signs and symptoms/physical findings

        (a)   Before rupture—early pregnancy symptoms; amenorrhea followed by spotting/bleeding; lower abdominal pain, usually unilateral; uterus normal to slightly enlarged

        (b)   After rupture—sharp, unilateral abdominal pain, may radiate to shoulder; syncope/fainting/shock; spotting/bleeding; adnexal tenderness, possible fullness; cervical motion tenderness; bulging of posterior cul-de-sac

  (4)   Differential diagnosis

        (a)   Acute appendicitis

        (b)   Pelvic inflammatory disease (PID)

        (c)   Ruptured corpus luteum cyst

        (d)   SAB

  (5)   Diagnostic tests/findings

        (a)   Ultrasound—no evidence of intrauterine pregnancy

        (b)   CBC—may indicate anemia, slight leukocytosis

        (c)   Serum Beta hCG—positive, but hCG level lower than expected for gestational age

        (d)   Serial Beta hCG levels—level rises slowly or plateaus; with intrauterine pregnancy, doubles every 2 days

  (6)   Management/treatment—hospitalization; surgery for repair or removal of damaged tube; fluid replacement; transfusion if needed; RhoGAM administration for Rh-negative woman

c. Placenta previa

  (1)   Definition: Abnormal implantation of placenta in lower uterine segment

  (2)   Etiology—unknown; may be associated with multiparity, multiple gestation, previous cesarean, previous uterine surgery

  (3)   Signs and symptoms/physical findings

       (a)   Painless bleeding after 20 weeks gestation; usually in third trimester

       (b)   Uterus nontender; usually no evidence of fetal distress

   (4)   Differential diagnosis

       (a)   Abruptio placentae

       (b)   Cervical lesion or cervicitis

       (c)   Nonvaginal bleeding (rectal or urinary)

   (5)   Diagnostic tests/findings

       (a)   Ultrasound—indicates low-lying placenta

       (b)   *No* pelvic exam

   (6)   Management/treatment

       (a)   Gestation is less than 36 weeks—expectant management; hospitalization and bedrest; fetal surveillance; monitor mother for increased bleeding

       (b)   Gestation 36 weeks or more—anticipate delivery; may need amniocentesis to assess fetal lung maturity

 d.   Abruptio placentae

   (1)   Definition: Partial or complete detachment of normally implanted placenta anytime prior to delivery

   (2)   Etiology—unknown; contributing factors include PIH, cocaine use, decreased blood flow to placenta, advanced maternal age, multiparity, trauma, underlying vascular problems

   (3)   Signs and symptoms/physical findings

       (a)   Vaginal bleeding of varying amount with severe, unremitting abdominal pain

       (b)   Uterine tenderness, increased uterine tone, contractions, signs of fetal distress, signs of shock

   (4)   Differential diagnosis

       (a)   Placenta previa

(b) Appendicitis

(c) Ovarian cyst

(d) Hematoma of rectus muscle

(5) Diagnostic tests/findings—ultrasound for placental location

(6) Management/treatment

(a) Immediate transport for emergency care

(b) Immediate delivery if massive bleeding or fetal distress

(c) Expectant management in emergency facility if fetus immature, no evidence of fetal distress or maternal hypovolemia or anemia

2. Pregnancy induced hypertension (PIH)

a. Definition

(1) Hypertension (HTN)—blood pressure of at least 140/90 mm Hg, or systolic rise > 30 mm Hg or diastolic rise ≥ 15 mm Hg above baseline on at least 2 occasions, 6 hours or more apart

(2) Preeclampsia—HTN with proteinuria and/or generalized edema after 20 weeks gestation; may occur earlier with gestational trophoblastic disease

(3) HELLP Syndrome—variant of severe preeclampsia including **H**emolysis, **E**levated **L**iver enzymes, and **L**ow *P*latelets

(4) Eclampsia—when convulsions, not caused by neurological disease, occur in woman with clinical criteria for preeclampsia

b. Etiology

(1) Unknown

(2) Predisposing factors—primigravidas; maternal age < 20 or > 35; maternal family or personal history of preeclampsia; preexisting hypertensive, vascular, autoimmune or renal disease; multiple gestation; gestational trophoblastic disease

c. Signs and symptoms/physical findings

    (1) Preeclampsia—HTN, sudden weight gain; generalized edema; frontal or occipital headaches; visual disturbances, e.g., scotomata, blurred vision; hyper-reflexia; oliguria; decreased fetal movement; fetal size small for dates; proteinuria

    (2) HELLP Syndrome—preeclampsia signs and symptoms; fatigue; nausea with or without vomiting; jaundice; right upper quadrant tenderness; epigastric pain; enlarged, firm liver

    (3) Eclampsia—seizure; drowsiness following seizure; cyanosis and tachypnea; oliguria; decreased or absent FHT

d. Differential diagnosis

    (1) Brain tumor

    (2) Renal failure

    (3) Chronic HTN

e. Diagnostic tests/findings

    (1) Preeclampsia

        (a) Proteinuria—up to ≥ 5 g/24 hour urine collection with severe preeclampsia

        (b) CBC—hemoconcentration

        (c) AST, serum creatinine, uric acid—elevated

        (d) Ultrasound—may indicate intrauterine growth retardation

        (e) Coagulation studies—decreased clotting factors, platelets and increased fibrin

    (2) HELLP Syndrome—above plus

        (a) Extremely low platelets ($< 50,000$) and decreased clotting factors

        (b) Severe hemoconcentration (elevated hematocrit)

        (c) Serum glucose—may be significantly decreased

        (d) Elevated liver enzymes

      f. Management/treatment—delivery is only cure

        (1) Antepartum

          (a) Bedrest in left lateral recumbent position—indicated with mild to moderate preeclampsia

          (b) Adequate nutrition and hydration

          (c) Careful monitoring of mother and fetus—NST, CST, BPP, fetal movement counts

          (d) Hospitalization if condition worsens to decrease possibility of convulsions and increase chance for fetal survival

        (2) Intrapartum

          (a) Prevent convulsions and deliver

          (b) Medications used to control or prevent seizure activity

            (i) Magnesium sulfate

              a) Prevents convulsions without central nervous system depression

              b) Monitor for signs of toxicity—nausea, thirst, depression of reflexes, flushing

            (ii) Hydralazine—antihypertensive usually reserved for cases when diastolic BP is 110 mm Hg or higher

            (iii) Diazepam—reserved for most severe cases to arrest seizures

Contraception

- Oral Contraceptives

    1. Combined oral contraceptives (OC)

      a. Description

        (1) Pills containing both an estrogen and a progestin

          (a) Estrogenic compounds currently used in U.S.—ethinyl estradiol (EE) and mestranol

          (b) Currently available progestins

         (i)   First generation progestins—norethindrone; norethindrone acetate; ethynodiol diacetate; norgestrel; levonorgestrel

         (ii) New generation progestins—desogestrel; norgestimate; gestodene

  (2) Types of OC

     (a) Monophasic—constant dose of estrogen and progestin delivered throughout the cycle

     (b) Multiphasic—dosage of estrogen and progestin are varied during the cycle

b. Mechanism of action—suppression of ovulation through combined actions of estrogen and progestin

  (1) Estrogenic effects

     (a) Ovulation inhibited, partially by suppression of follicle stimulating hormone (FSH) and luteinizing hormone (LH)

     (b) Uterine secretions altered, inhibiting implantation

     (c) Acceleration of ovum transport

     (d) May cause degeneration of corpus luteum (luteolysis)

  (2) Progestin effects

     (a) Suppression of LH inhibits ovulation

     (b) Cervical mucus thickens, inhibiting sperm transport and sperm penetration of ovum

     (c) Ovum transport may be slowed

     (d) Alteration of endometrium hampers implantation

c. Effectiveness: First year failure rate

  (1) Perfect use—0.1%

  (2) Typical use—5%

d. Noncontraceptive benefits and advantages

  (1) Menstrual cycle effects

     (a) Regulation of menstrual cycle

        (b) Decreased menstrual cramps and pain

        (c) Decreased duration and amount of menstrual flow

    (2) Affords some protection against:

        (a) PID

        (b) Ovarian and endometrial cancer

        (c) Benign breast disease

        (d) Ectopic pregnancy

        (e) Functional ovarian cysts

        (f) Premenstrual symptoms

        (g) Iron deficiency anemia

    (3) Improvement of some medical conditions

        (a) Symptoms of estrogen deficiency—e.g., osteoporosis

        (b) Endometriosis

        (c) Acne

  e. Disadvantages

    (1) No protection against STD and HIV/AIDS

    (2) Must be taken every day

    (3) Potential side effects

        (a) Unwanted menstrual cycle changes—may include missed periods, scanty periods, spotting, breakthrough bleeding

        (b) Potential side effects caused by hormonal properties of OC—estrogenic, progestogenic and androgenic

            (i) Estrogenic effects—breast tenderness and possible increase in breast size; nausea; cyclic weight gain caused by fluid retention; cervical ectopia or erosion; growth of leiomyomata; spider angiomas; thromboembolism; pulmonary emboli; cerebrovascular accidents; hepatocellular adenomas and cancer

        (ii)   Progestogenic effects—breast tenderness; headaches; hypertension; myocardial infarction

        (iii) Androgenic effects—appetite increase and weight gain; depression, fatigue and tiredness; decreased libido; acne and oily skin; increased breast size due to alveolar tissue; increased LDL and decreased HDL cholesterol levels; diabetogenic effects including decreased carbohydrate tolerance; pruritus

  (4) Chlamydial cervicitis more common in women on OC

  (5) Potential but rare serious complications

    (a) Thrombophlebitis

    (b) Pulmonary emboli

    (c) Cardiovascular disease (CVD)

f. Precautions

  (1) Should not be provided to women who are pregnant or in whom pregnancy is strongly suspected

  (2) Should not be provided to women with current or previous diagnosis of:

    (a) Thrombophlebitis or thromboembolic disorder

    (b) Cerebrovascular accident

    (c) Coronary artery or ischemic heart disease

    (d) Known or strongly suspected breast cancer

    (e) Known or strongly suspected estrogen-dependent neoplasia

    (f) Benign hepatic adenoma or liver cancer

    (g) Markedly impaired liver function (currently)

    (h) Older than 35 and heavy smoker ($\geq$ 20 cigarettes per day)

  (3) Exercise caution in prescribing and monitor closely for development of adverse effects

    (a)   Older than 35 and light smoker (< 20 cigarettes per day)

    (b)   Migraine headaches that start after initiation of OC (without focal neurological symptoms)

    (c)   Hypertension with resting diastolic BP of ≥ 90 mm Hg or resting systolic BP of ≥ 140 mm Hg on 3 separate visits, or diastolic BP of ≥ 110 mm Hg on single visit

    (d)   Diabetes mellitus

    (e)   Impending major surgery requiring immobilization in next four weeks

    (f)   Undiagnosed abnormal vaginal bleeding

    (g)   Sickle cell disease or sickle C disease

    (h)   Lactation

    (i)   Gestational diabetes

    (j)   Active gallbladder disease

    (k)   Congenital hyperbilirubinemia

    (l)   Over age 50

    (m)   Completion of term pregnancy within past 21 days

    (n)   Current or past cardiac or renal disease

    (o)   Conditions likely to make it difficult for woman to take OC correctly and consistently

    (p)   Family history of dyslipidemia

    (q)   Family history of death of parent or sibling prior to age 50 due to myocardial infarction

g. Prescribing guidelines

    (1)   Most women started on OC containing ≤ 35 mcg estrogen (low-dose)

    (2)   Efficacy of low-dose OC may be lowered when used concurrently with medications that affect liver metabolism

      (a)   Anticonvulsants—phenobarbital, phenytoin, carba-mazepine, primidone, ethosuximide

      (b)   Antibiotics—particularly ampicillin and tetracy-cline

      (c)   Rifampin

      (d)   Griseofulvin

   (3)   OC may potentiate the effects of the following:

      (a)   Antidepressants—amitriptyline, desipramine, imipramine

      (b)   Benzodiazepines

      (c)   Beta-blockers—nadolol, propanolol, metoprolol, atenolol

      (d)   Theophylline

2. Progestin-only pills (minipills)

   a. Description—oral contraceptive containing fixed dose of a progestin only

   b. Mechanism of action

      (1)   Inhibition of ovulation—although does not consistently inhibit ovulation; regular, cyclic bleeding pattern indicates ovulation is not being suppressed

      (2)   Cervical mucus thickens and decreases in amount inhibiting sperm penetration

      (3)   Creation of thin, atrophic endometrium

      (4)   Premature luteolysis

   c. Effectiveness: First year failure rate

      (1)   Perfect use—0.5%

      (2)   Typical use—5%

   d. Noncontraceptive benefits and advantages

      (1)   No estrogen-related side effects or complications

      (2)   No adverse effects on lactation

(3) Scanty or no menses; decreased anemia; decreased dysmenorrhea

(4) Decreased risk of developing endometrial cancer, ovarian cancer, and PID

(5) Immediately reversible upon discontinuation

e. Disadvantages

(1) No protection against STD and HIV/AIDS

(2) Menstrual cycle disturbances—irregular bleeding

(3) Generally less effective than combined OC—must be taken consistently at the same time every day

(4) Functional ovarian cysts occur more often

(5) If pregnancy occurs, greater likelihood of ectopic

f. Precautions—exercise caution in prescribing and monitor closely for development of adverse effects

(1) Unexplained abnormal vaginal bleeding

(2) Liver conditions such as severe decompensated cirrhosis; adenoma or cancer; active viral hepatitis

(3) Breast cancer—effect of progestin not completely understood

(4) Use of rifampin and most antiseizure medications (phenytoin, carbamazepine, phenobarbital) which induce hepatic enzymes

- Implants and Injectables

  1. Norplant

     a. Description

        (1) Long-acting progestin-only contraceptive

        (2) Levonorgestrel administered through six slender, flexible silicone capsules that are 2.4 × 34 mm each

        (3) Silicone capsules are implanted under the skin of the upper, inner arm

        (4) Effective for five years

     b. Mechanism of action

     (1)   Ovulation inhibited

     (2)   Cervical mucus changes—thickens and decreases in amount making sperm penetration more difficult

     (3)   Creation of thin, atrophic endometrium

     (4)   Premature luteolysis

c. Effectiveness: First year failure rate

     (1)   Perfect use—0.05%

     (2)   Typical use—0.05%

d. Noncontraceptive benefits and advantages

     (1)   No estrogen-related side effects or complications

     (2)   Noncontraceptive benefits—scanty or no menses; decreased anemia; decreased dysmenorrhea; suppression of ovulation-related pain; decreased risk of endometrial cancer, ovarian cancer and PID

     (3)   Immediately reversible

     (4)   Extremely effective, long-term contraception

     (5)   Not related to intercourse

     (6)   Low risk of ectopic as compared with women not using a contraceptive method

e. Disadvantages

     (1)   No protection against STD and HIV/AIDS

     (2)   High initial cost

     (3)   Irregular bleeding patterns—most common reason for removal in first two years

     (4)   If pregnancy occurs, must consider ectopic

     (5)   Effectiveness significantly lowered with anticonvulsants and rifampin

     (6)   Implants may be visible or may cause scarring

     (7)   Side effects may include—bloating, weight gain, acne, hair loss, breast tenderness, local inflammation or infection at insertion site, depression

        (8)   Ovarian cysts—usually regress spontaneously

        (9)   Removal may be difficult—especially if insertion was too deep

  f.   Precautions

      (1)   Do not provide to women with following diagnoses

        (a)   Known or suspected pregnancy

        (b)   Unexplained abnormal vaginal bleeding

        (c)   Active thrombophlebitis or pulmonary emboli

        (d)   On antiseizure medications (except valproic acid) or rifampin

        (e)   Known or suspected current or past breast cancer

      (2)   Exercise caution in prescribing and monitor closely for development of adverse effects

        (a)   Intolerant of irregular bleeding

        (b)   Migraine or other headaches

        (c)   Heart lesions that predispose to subacute bacterial endocarditis

        (d)   History of heart attack, stroke, chest pain due to heart disease, thrombophlebitis, pulmonary embolism or blood clots in the eye, diabetes which predisposes to cardiovascular disease

        (e)   History of allergic reaction with use of pills containing levonorgestrel

        (f)   History of acne that worsened on combined OC

2. Depo-Provera (DMPA)

  a.   Description

      (1)   Injectable progestin (depo-medroxyprogesterone acetate)

      (2)   150 mg of DMPA administered by deep intramuscular injection every 12 weeks

  b.   Mechanism of action

      (1)   Inhibits ovulation by suppressing FSH and LH levels and eliminating LH surge

(2) Development of shallow, atrophic endometrium

(3) Thickens cervical mucus that decreases sperm penetration

c. Effectiveness: First year failure rate

(1) Perfect use—0.3%

(2) Typical use—0.3%

d. Noncontraceptive benefits and advantages

(1) Long-acting, highly effective, reversible contraceptive

(2) No estrogen-related side effects or complications

(3) No interference with intercourse

(4) Noncontraceptive benefits—scanty or no menses; decreased anemia; decreased dysmenorrhea; suppression of ovulation-associated pain; decreased risk of developing endometrial cancer, ovarian cancer, and PID

(5) Low risk of ectopic as compared with women not using any contraceptive method

(6) Decreases frequency of seizures

(7) No drug interactions

(8) No adverse effects on lactation

e. Disadvantages

(1) No protection against STD and HIV/AIDS

(2) Menstrual cycle changes—during first year of use, more spotting and breakthrough bleeding; the longer DMPA is used, the greater likelihood of amenorrhea

(3) Weight gain, depression, breast tenderness

(4) Return visits every 12 weeks for repeat injections

(5) No immediate discontinuation—side effects, including menstrual irregularities may continue for 6 to 8 months following discontinuation of method

(6) Lipid changes—decrease in HDL cholesterol levels

(7) Decrease in bone density; reversible when DMPA stopped

(8) Allergic reactions—anaphylactic reactions are rare, but may occur immediately following Depo-Provera injections

f. Precautions

(1) Should not be provided to women with following:

(a) Known or suspected pregnancy

(b) Unexplained vaginal bleeding past three months

(c) Breast cancer—current or past

(2) Exercise caution in prescribing and monitor closely for development of adverse effects

(a) Pregnancy planned in fairly near future

(b) Concern over weight gain

(c) Severe, acute liver disease, liver tumors, or gallbladder disease

(d) Diabetes with nephropathy, retinopathy, and neuropathy

g. Prescribing guidelines

(1) Administer

(a) During first five days after onset of menses

(b) Within first seven days postpartum if not breastfeeding

(c) At six weeks postpartum if breastfeeding

(2) Do not massage injection site—may lower effectiveness

- Intrauterine Device (IUD)

1. Description

a. Plastic contraceptive device inserted into uterus

b. Two types currently available in U.S.

(1) Progesterone T (Progestasert System)

(a) Must be removed and replaced every year

(b) Releases 65 mcg of progesterone per day

      (2)   Copper T 380A (Paragard)—most widely used in U.S.

          (a)   T-shaped polyethylene device with copper wound around vertical stem

          (b)   Approved for 10 years use

      (3)   Levonorgestrel-IUD (LNg IUD)—not currently approved in U.S., but approval is expected

          (a)   Releases 20 mcg levonorgestrel per day into uterus

          (b)   Effective for five years

2. Mechanism of action

   a.   Exact mechanism not completely understood

   b.   Immobilizes sperm

   c.   Interferes with migration of sperm from vagina to fallopian tubes

   d.   Speeds transport of ovum through the fallopian tubes

   e.   Local effects on endometrium

3. Effectiveness: First year failure rate

   a.   Copper T 380A

      (1)   Perfect use—0.6%

      (2)   Typical use—0.8%

   b.   Progesterone T

      (1)   Perfect use—1.5%

      (2)   Typical use—2.0%

   c.   LNg 20

      (1)   Perfect use—0.1%

      (2)   Typical use—0.1%

4. Noncontraceptive benefits and advantages

   a.   Less expensive per year and easier to use than some other methods

    b. Copper IUD can be used by women who have contraindications to hormonal methods

    c. IUD that release progesterone decrease menstrual blood loss and dysmenorrhea

5. Disadvantages

    a. No protection against STD and HIV/AIDS

    b. Increased risk of PID—greatest risk at time of insertion

    c. May have increased dysmenorrhea and minor increase in blood loss

    d. Spontaneous expulsion may occur—2 to 10% expelled within first year

    e. Pregnancy complications possible if pregnancy occurs with IUD in situ—if IUD left in place, 50% will end in spontaneous abortion; if IUD removed early in pregnancy, 25% will spontaneously abort

    f. Possible risks at time of insertion include—vasovagal reaction, uterine perforation, cramping and pain

    g. Potential side effects and complications

        (1) Spotting, bleeding, and hemorrhage—abnormal bleeding common in first 3 months; after first 3 months, may be a sign of infection or pregnancy

        (2) Anemia—remove IUD if Hgb < 9 g

        (3) Cramping and pain—except at time of insertion, may be sign of pregnancy, infection or expulsion

        (4) Expulsion—symptoms may include unusual vaginal discharge, cramping or pain, intermenstrual spotting, postcoital spotting, dyspareunia, absence or lengthening of IUD string, presence of hard plastic of IUD at cervical os or in vagina

        (5) Pregnancy—5% will be ectopic; higher risk of ectopic with Progesterone T

        (6) Uterine perforation, embedding and cervical perforation—most common sites are uterine fundus, body of the uterus, and cervical wall

   (7) PID—remove IUD and treat

6. Precautions

  a. Should not be provided to women with following:

   (1) Active, recent or recurrent pelvic infection—PID, post-partum endometritis, infection following abortion

   (2) Known or suspected pregnancy

   (3) Severely distorted uterine cavity caused by anatomical abnormalities of the uterus

  b. Exercise caution in prescribing, counsel thoroughly, and monitor closely for development of adverse effects

   (1) Risk factors for PID—purulent cervicitis; recent positive gonorrhea or chlamydia test; recurrent history of chlamydia or gonorrhea

   (2) High risk for STD—multiple partners or partner with multiple partners

   (3) Impaired response to infection—diabetes, steroid treatment, HIV disease

   (4) Risk factors for HIV infection and/or HIV disease

   (5) Undiagnosed, irregular, heavy or abnormal vaginal bleeding; known or suspected cervical or uterine cancer, including unresolved abnormal Pap smear

   (6) Previous problems with IUD use

   (7) History of vasovagal reactions or fainting

   (8) Lack of access to emergency medical care if complications occur

   (9) Valvular heart disease such as aortic stenosis; increased susceptibility to subacute bacterial endocarditis

   (10) Anatomical abnormalities that do not distort uterus—leiomyomata, endometrial polyps, cervical stenosis, bicornuate uterus, small uterus

   (11) Women who have never had a child tend not to tolerate the IUD as well as women who have carried to term

7. Prescribing guidelines

    a. Review IUD instructions with patient

       (1) Check strings

       (2) Be aware of infection signs or symptoms

       (3) Carefully monitor menstrual periods

    b. Teach patient IUD warning signs—PAINS

       (1) **P**eriod late (pregnancy), abnormal spotting or bleeding

       (2) **A**bdominal pain, pain with intercourse

       (3) **I**nfection exposure (any STD), abnormal discharge

       (4) **N**ot feeling well, fever, chills

       (5) **S**tring missing, shorter or longer

- Condoms

  1. Male condom

    a. Description

       (1) Sheath-like covering for the penis

       (2) Three types—Latex (rubber); polyurethane (plastic); lambskin (from intestinal membrane)

    b. Mechanism of action

       (1) Acts as a mechanical barrier, preventing sperm from entering vagina

       (2) Placed on erect penis before any contact with vagina

    c. Effectiveness: First year failure rate

       (1) Perfect use—3%

       (2) Typical use—14%

    d. Noncontraceptive benefits and advantages

       (1) Accessible and inexpensive—over 100 brands available, some with spermicide

       (2) Can effectively reduce transmission of STD and HIV/AIDS (latex and polyurethane)

       (3) Male involvement needed

        (4)   May help maintain erection and prevent premature ejaculation

        (5)   May prevent sperm allergy

  e. Disadvantages—interruption of foreplay; interference with erection; male involvement essential; reduced sensitivity; decreased pleasure; embarrassment; possibility of breakage; allergy to latex

  f. Precautions

        (1)   "Skin" condoms do not prevent STD and HIV transmission

        (2)   Petroleum-based lubricants and some vaginal medications break down latex

2.   Female condom

  a. Description—polyurethane sheath with flexible rings at each end

  b. Mechanism of Action—physical barrier that lines the vagina and partially covers the perineum

  c. Effectiveness: First year failure rate

        (1)   Perfect use—5%

        (2)   Typical use—21%

  d. Noncontraceptive benefits and advantages

        (1)   Polyurethane stronger than latex, may not tear as easily as male condom

        (2)   Theoretical protection against STD and HIV exposure—has been tested in laboratory

        (3)   Does not require prescription

        (4)   May be inserted up to eight hours prior to intercourse

  e. Disadvantages

        (1)   May be difficult for some women to insert

        (2)   May affect sexual sensation, cause irritation or discomfort

        (3)   May be used only once—expensive

       (4) May become displaced

   f. Precautions

       (1) Some may be allergic to polyurethane

       (2) May be difficult to use with some anatomic abnormalities

- Diaphragm

  1. Description

     a. Dome-shaped, latex rubber cup with flexible ring that is inserted into the vagina prior to intercourse, with anterior rim positioned behind the pubic bone and posterior rim in the posterior fornix; spermicidal jelly is placed within the dome and around rim prior to insertion

     b. Available in a variety of rim types (flat, coil, and arcing) and sizes (50 to 100 mm)

  2. Mechanism of action—barrier plus spermicide

  3. Effectiveness: First year failure rate

     a. Perfect use—6%

     b. Typical use—20%

  4. Noncontraceptive benefits and advantages

     a. No systemic side effects

     b. Some protection against STD, including gonorrhea and chlamydia; irritation related to spermicide may increase susceptibility to HIV transmission

     c. Protection against cervical neoplasia

  5. Disadvantages

     a. Requires fitting by clinician and instruction in use

     b. Slight increased risk for toxic shock syndrome

     c. Increases risk for vaginal and urinary tract infections

  6. Precautions—conditions that may preclude satisfactory use

     a. Allergy to spermicide, rubber, latex, or polyurethane

    b.   Abnormalities in vaginal anatomy that interfere with satisfactory fit or stable placement of diaphragm

    c.   Inability to learn correct insertion technique

    d.   History of toxic shock syndrome

    e.   Repeated urinary tract infections that persist despite refitting

    f.   Lack of trained personnel to fit or provide instruction

    g.   Full-term delivery within the past six weeks, recent spontaneous or induced abortion, vaginal bleeding

7. Prescribing guidelines

    a.   Review instructions for use

        (1)   Must be left in place six hours after last intercourse, with maximum time of 24 hours in vagina

        (2)   Avoid oil-based lubricants and medications

    b.   Teach warning signs for toxic shock syndrome—requires immediate treatment

- Cervical Cap (Prentif Cavity Rim Cervical Cap)

1. Description—deep, soft rubber cup with a firm round rim; covers the cervix and fits with suction around the base of the cervix; available in 4 sizes (22, 25, 28, 31 mm); small amount of spermicide placed in cap prior to insertion

2. Mechanism of action—barrier plus spermicide

3. Effectiveness: First year failure rate

    a.   Perfect use—parous women 20%; nulliparous women 9%

    b.   Typical use—parous women 40%; nulliparous women 20%

4. Advantages—continuous protection for up to 48 hours; STD and HIV protection has not been studied

5. Disadvantages

    a.   Requires trained clinician to fit

    b.   May be difficult for some women to insert or remove

    c.   May cause odor, especially with prolonged use

    d.   Slightly increased risk for toxic shock syndrome

6. Precautions—conditions that may preclude satisfactory use

   a. Allergy to latex or spermicide

   b. Anatomical abnormalities that interfere with satisfactory fit

   c. Inability to learn insertion or removal technique

   d. History of toxic shock syndrome

   e. Lack of trained personnel to fit and provide instruction

   f. Full-term vaginal delivery within past six weeks, recent spontaneous or induced abortion, vaginal bleeding

   g. Known or suspected cervical or uterine cancer, abnormal Pap smear, vaginal or cervical infection

- Spermicides

   1. Description—consists of two components

      a. Inert base or carrier—foam, jelly, cream, suppository, film

      b. Spermicidal chemical that kills sperm—Nonoxynol-9 or Octoxynol-9

   2. Mechanism of action—spermicides are surfactants that destroy sperm cell membrane

   3. Effectiveness: First year failure rate

      a. Perfect use—6%

      b. Typical use—26%

   4. Noncontraceptive benefits and advantages

      a. Relatively inexpensive; available without prescription or clinic visit

      b. Provide some protection against STD although protection greatest when used in conjunction with barrier method

      c. Can be used as back-up with other methods

   5. Disadvantages

      a. Possible allergic reaction to spermicide or base

      b. Increased colonization of *Candida albicans*

      c. Increased colonization of vagina with anaerobic bacteria and uropathogens (bacterial vaginosis)

    d. Relationship of spermicide use to HIV not completely established

6. Precautions—spermicide not the best choice in following circumstances

    a. Inability to learn correct insertion technique

    b. Allergy or sensitivity to spermicide or base ingredients

    c. Abnormal vaginal anatomy that interferes with appropriate placement or retention of spermicide

7. Guidelines for use

    a. Jellies, creams, foams—inserted into vagina prior to each act of intercourse; protection is immediate and remains effective for no more than one hour when used alone; jelly and cream when used with diaphragm remain effective for 6 to 8 hours

    b. Film and suppositories—inserted into vagina before each act of intercourse; contraceptive protection begins 10 to 15 minutes after insertion and lasts no more than one hour

- Emergency Contraception

  1. Description

    a. Postcoital contraception used after an act of unprotected intercourse

    b. Methods used include OC (Yuzpe method), danazol, synthetic estrogens and conjugated estrogens, antiprogestins and IUD insertion

    c. Yuzpe method is only emergency contraception currently approved by FDA as safe and effective for use

  2. Mechanism of action (Yuzpe method—emergency contraceptive pills)

    a. Are not effective if woman is already pregnant

    b. Act by delaying or inhibiting ovulation, and/or altering tubal transport of sperm and/or ova (inhibiting fertilization), and/or altering the endometrium (altering implantation)

  3. Effectiveness—depends on when unprotected intercourse occurs in cycle; effectiveness ranges from 55.3% to 94.2% (average effectiveness 74.0%)

4. Advantages

   a. Only option available after unprotected intercourse has occurred

   b. Simple, easy to use

   c. Side effects are of short duration

5. Disadvantages

   a. Nausea and vomiting are common side effects (nausea in 50% to 70%)

   b. May alter timing of next menstrual period—need to evaluate for pregnancy if no menstrual period within three weeks

6. Precautions—not appropriate for woman who has serious problems that would contraindicate OC

7. Guidelines for use

   a. Four regimens are currently approved by FDA—all require two doses, 12 hours apart, of an estrogen (ethinyl estradiol) and progestin (norgestrel or levonorgestrel)

   b. Must be initiated within 72 hours after unprotected intercourse

- Fertility Awareness Methods

  1. Description

     a. A variety of methods that help couples prevent or plan pregnancies by identifying fertile days of the menstrual cycle; natural family planning methods are based on fertility awareness

     b. Methods include calendar rhythm method, basal body temperature (BBT) method, cervical mucus charting (ovulation or Billings method), and sympto-thermal method

  2. Mechanism of action—calculation of fertile period based on four assumptions

     a. Sperm remain viable for two to seven days (average three days)

     b. Ovum remains fertile for 24 hours

     c. Ovulation occurs on day 14 ($\pm$ 2 days) before onset of next menses

      d.   Span of fertility may be from seven days before ovulation to three days after

3.   Effectiveness: First year failure rate

      a.   Perfect use—calendar 9%; ovulation method 3%; sympto-thermal 2%; BBT 1%

      b.   Typical use—25% for all

4.   Advantages

      a.   No serious side effects

      b.   Increases users' knowledge of reproductive physiology—can be used to plan conception, detect pregnancy, and prevent pregnancy

5.   Disadvantages

      a.   No protection against STD or HIV

      b.   Lack of cooperative male partner is an obstacle

      c.   Women must abstain (or use another method) when libido is at peak

6.   Precautions

      a.   Certain conditions may make fertility awareness more difficult to use—irregular menstrual cycles; irregular temperature charts; recent discontinuation of hormonal methods; recent menarche; approaching menopause; unable to keep careful records

      b.   Not recommended postpartum prior to resumption of normal menses

7.   Specific methods

      a.   Calendar charting—fertile days are predicted based on records of past menstrual cycles

          (1)   Earliest day of fertility is calculated by subtracting 18 days from length of shortest cycle

          (2)   Latest day of fertility is calculated by subtracting 11 days from length of longest cycle

      b.   Basal body temperature (BBT) charting—BBT is lowest body temperature of healthy person taken upon awakening

(1) Record BBT for 3 to 4 consecutive months to determine time of ovulation

(2) Drop in BBT sometimes precedes ovulation by 12 to 24 hours followed by sustained rise in BBT for several days

(3) Progesterone increases BBT by 0.4 to 0.8° F

(4) To avoid pregnancy, abstain until temperature elevation is sustained for three consecutive days

   c. Cervical mucus method (Ovulation, Billings)

(1) Mucus just before and at ovulation—clear, thin, watery, elastic, abundant

(2) Mucus following ovulation—thick, cloudy, whitish, tacky, scant

(3) To prevent pregnancy, avoid intercourse or use another method until day four after peak (ovulatory) mucus

   d. Sympto-thermal method

(1) Combines various charting techniques—mucus, cervix, BBT

(2) To prevent pregnancy, abstain or use another method until four days after peak mucus and three days after temperature rise

- Voluntary Sterilization

  1. Female sterilization

    a. Description—a surgical procedure in which the fallopian tubes are occluded to prevent the sperm and egg from uniting

    b. Mechanism of action

(1) Surgical interruption of fallopian tubes

(2) Methods for tubal interruption include—surgical ligation, excision, electrocoagulation, mechanical devices

    c. Effectiveness—first year failure rate 0.5% with perfect and typical use

    d. Advantages

(1) Safe operative procedure; no long-term side effects

(2) Permanent and highly effective

e. Disadvantages and precautions

    (1) Risks of surgery—anesthesia, infection, hemorrhage

    (2) Post-operative pain and discomfort

    (3) Expensive at time it is performed

    (4) No protection against STD and HIV

    (5) Considered permanent—reversibility difficult and expensive; success cannot be guaranteed

    (6) If pregnancy occurs, high probability of ectopic

2. Male sterilization—vasectomy

a. Description—male surgical procedure in which the vas deferens are blocked, preventing passage of sperm

b. Mechanism of action—surgical interruption of sperm

c. Effectiveness: First year failure rate

    (1) Perfect use:—0.1%

    (2) Typical use:—0.15%

d. Advantages

    (1) Extremely safe and effective

    (2) Permanent

    (3) Non-scalpel technique carries lower complication rate; simple procedure; very quickly performed

e. Disadvantages

    (1) Expensive in short term

    (2) Reversal is difficult, expensive, and results cannot be guaranteed

    (3) No protection against STD and HIV

    (4) Post-operative side effects—bruising, swelling, hematoma, infection at operative site

    (5) Vasectomy is not effective until sperm are ejaculated from reproductive system—usually 15 ejaculations

(6) One-half to two-thirds of men will develop sperm antibodies following vasectomy—no evidence that it causes pathology

f. Precautions—should not be provided to men with following diagnoses

(1) Local skin infection

(2) Varicocele, large hydrocele, inguinal hernia, scar tissue from previous surgery

(3) Special precautions with clotting disorders, diabetes and recent coronary artery disease

g. Counseling guidelines

(1) **B**enefits—permanent and highly effective

(2) **R**isks of surgery—small chance of future pregnancy

(3) **A**lternatives—other reversible contraceptive methods

(4) **I**nquiries—encourage and answer questions

(5) **D**ecision to change—without loss of medical or financial benefits

(6) **E**xplanation—of entire procedure and possible side effects

(7) **D**ocumentation—of method and timing of surgery, any complications

Menopause

- Definition: Ovarian failure marked by cessation of menses for 12 months or by a serum FSH level of over 40 mIU per mL on two occasions one week apart, outside of normal FSH surge; climacteric refers to transitional period of up to 15 years leading up to the last menstrual period marked by waning ovarian function; term "perimenopause" may be used interchangeably

- Etiology/Incidence

1. Results from changes in the ovary, with gradual atresia of ovarian follicles leading to decline in ovarian production of estrogen and progesterone; fewer available follicles to produce estradiol (most potent estrogen)

2. Estrogen deficiency increases woman's risk for cardiovascular disease and osteoporosis; also responsible for majority of symptoms associated with menopause

3. Cessation of menses usually occurs between 45 and 55 years—average age in U.S. is 50; ovarian failure prior to age 30 is premature; between 31 and 40 is considered early; after age 40 considered normal

- Signs and Symptoms of Menopause

    1. Menstrual changes—irregular menses with wide variations in cycle length and anovulatory cycles

    2. Hot flashes/hot flushes experienced during day or night

    3. Hormonal changes

        a. Immediately preceding menopause

            (1) Lower estradiol levels

            (2) Increased FSH levels

            (3) LH levels somewhat increased

        b. Following menopause

            (1) Primary estrogen is estrone—derived from conversion of androstenedione to estrone in extraglandular sites

            (2) FSH elevated 10 to 20 fold (> 40 mIU/mL)

            (3) LH elevated three fold

    4. Physical changes due to aging and estrogen loss

        a. Vulva—atrophy; pruritus; pubic hair thinning

        b. Vagina—decreased lubrication leading to dyspareunia; vaginitis; dryness; loss of rugae; becomes shorter and narrower; vaginal pH more alkaline (6.5 to 7.5)

        c. Pelvic floor—muscular tissue loss causing uterine prolapse, cystocele and rectocele

        d. Bladder/urethra—atrophy; frequency and urgency; stress incontinence

        e. Uterus—decreases in size and weight

  f. Breasts—decrease with gradual atrophy of glandular tissue; nipples smaller and flatter

  g. Skin—dryness; decreased sebaceous and sweat gland activity; less elasticity; hyperpigmentation/hypopigmentation; atrophy and thinning of epidermal and dermal skin layers; decrease in scalp, pubic and axillary hair

  h. Cardiovascular—changes in lipids (gradual increase in LDL and decrease in HDL) favor formation of atherosclerosis; coronary artery disease

  i. Lungs—lung expansion decreases; thorax more rigid and tissues less elastic

  j. Musculoskeletal—muscle tone related to exercise; if sedentary, tone and strength diminish; atrophy if muscles not used

    (1) Osteoporosis

      (a) Definition—imbalance between bone formation and bone resorption; associated with skeletal fractures

        (i) Type I—on average, occurs 15 to 20 years after menopause; trabecular bone loss; common fracture sites include vertebrae and distal radius

        (ii) Type II—occurs in men and women in 7th decade; common fracture site is hip

      (b) Risk factors—sedentary lifestyle, smoking, small-boned, Caucasian or Asian, low dietary intake of calcium throughout reproductive years, family history of osteoporosis

      (c) Management—estrogen replacement therapy to treat and prevent progression; adequate calcium intake to maintain calcium balance; weight-bearing exercise 30 minutes 3 times per week; eliminate smoking

  k. Neuroendocrine

    (1) Vasomotor instability (hot flashes and night sweats)

    (2) Sleep disturbances

     l. Psychological symptoms—anxiety; depression; irritability; libido changes; insomnia

- Diagnostic Tests/Findings

    1. Pregnancy test (if suspected)—negative

    2. Pap smear—low estrogen effect with predominantly parabasal cells

    3. Serum FSH—level > 40 mIU/mL is diagnostic of menopause

- Management/Treatment (see Osteoporosis in Musculoskeletal Disorders chapter)

    1. Discuss diet, exercise, stress management, calcium supplementation and hormone replacement therapy (HRT)

    2. Minimum daily calcium requirements—supplementation reduces bone loss and decreases fractures

        a. Women not on estrogen, 50 to 64 years of age 1500 mg

        b. Women on estrogen, 50 to 64 years of age 1000 mg

        c. All women over age 65 1500 mg

    3. Hormone replacement therapy (HRT)

        a. Indications

            (1) Relief of menopausal symptoms related to estrogen deficiency—hot flashes, urinary symptoms, vaginal dryness

            (2) Prevention and treatment of osteoporosis

            (3) Protection against cardiovascular disease

        b. Regimen options

            (1) Along with estrogen, progestin is indicated to decrease risk of endometrial hyperplasia or cancer if patient has a uterus

            (2) Sequential regimen—0.625 mg conjugated estrogen or 1.0 mg micronized estradiol daily or from day 1 to 25 each month; medroxyprogesterone acetate (Provera) 10 mg per day added for first 14 days of month or for last 10 days of estrogen administration

            (3) Continuous regimen—0.625 mg conjugated estrogen, or 0.625 estrone sulfate, or 1.0 mg micronized estradiol

daily with daily progestin administration of 2.5 or 5mg medroxyprogesterone acetate or 0.35 mg norethindrone

    (4)   Estradiol skin patch—0.05 to 0.1 mg estradiol; changed once or twice a week; add medroxyprogesterone acetate 10 mg for 12 days per month or 2.5 mg per day continuously for those women with intact uterus

  c. Contraindications to HRT

    (1)   Known or suspected breast cancer

    (2)   Known or suspected estrogen-dependent neoplasia

    (3)   Undiagnosed abnormal vaginal bleeding

    (4)   Past or present history of deep vein thrombosis

    (5)   Thrombophlebitis

    (6)   Liver dysfunction or disease

    (7)   Known or suspected pregnancy

    (8)   Active clotting disorders

  d. Guidelines for HRT provision

    (1)   If not contraindicated, decision for HRT should rest primarily with the woman

    (2)   Before initiating HRT—should have negative clinical breast examination and mammogram; endometrial biopsy indicated with abnormal vaginal bleeding

    (3)   For patients with abnormal vaginal bleeding beyond three to six months of initiating HRT, endometrial biopsy indicated

- General Guidelines

  1. Pharmacological and nonpharmacological options should be thoroughly discussed with patient

  2. Educate patient on nonpharmacological symptom relief strategies

  3. If HRT is prescribed, thoroughly discuss side effects

  4. Review/teach self breast examination

5. Annual mammogram

6. Annual breast examination by health professional

Note: This chapter was written by Susan Moskosky in her private capacity. No official support or endorsement by the Department of Health and Human Services or any component thereof is intended or should be inferred.

Questions
Select the best answer

1. Which of the following is a positive sign of pregnancy?

    a. Goodell's sign
    b. Urinary frequency/urgency
    c. Braxton-Hicks contractions
    d. Fetal movement felt by examiner

2. Which of the following statements is correct regarding maternal physiologic changes in pregnancy?

    a. Pulse rate decreases
    b. Insulin requirements decrease
    c. Increased sweat gland activity
    d. Increased intestinal peristalsis

3. Examination of the breasts in pregnancy may normally show:

    a. Increased nodularity
    b. Linea nigra
    c. Retractions in skin
    d. Loss of nipple pigmentation

4. Examination of a woman in the 30th week of pregnancy would normally reveal:

    a. Cervical dilation of 2 cm
    b. Complaint of nausea and vomiting
    c. Fundal height of 29 cm
    d. Increased platelet count

5. Examination of a woman in her 14th week of pregnancy would normally reveal:

    a. Fundal height of 14 cm
    b. Fetal heart tones audible with fetoscope
    c. Milk expressed from breasts
    d. Cyanosis of the cervix

6. Which of the following is considered to be a common complaint of pregnancy?

    a. Facial edema

b. Varicosities
c. Scotomata
d. Dysuria

7. Which of the following complications is most likely to occur in the first trimester?

a. Pregnancy induced hypertension
b. Bleeding
c. Placenta previa
d. Gestational diabetes

8. Recommended weight gain in pregnancy for a woman of normal weight for height is:

a. Less than 20 pounds
b. 20 pounds
c. 25 pounds
d. Over 30 pounds

9. How is the EDB determined using Nagele's rule?

a. Subtract 3 months from LNMP and add 7 days
b. Subtract 7 days and add 9 months from the start of the LNMP
c. Add 9 months from start of the LNMP
d. Subtract 7 from last day of LNMP and count back 3 months

10. During pregnancy, sexual relations are contraindicated when:

a. Increased whitish vaginal discharge is present
b. 36 weeks gestation has been reached
c. Rupture of membranes is suspected
d. Weight gain is inadequate

11. Which of the following statements is true regarding diagnostic testing during pregnancy?

a. Chorionic villus sampling is performed between weeks 14 and 24 when indicated for genetic reasons
b. Alpha-fetoprotein in maternal blood is assessed between weeks 16 and 18
c. Gestational diabetes screening is performed between weeks 15 and 18
d. Amniocentesis between weeks 22 and 26 when indicated for advanced maternal age

12. Which of the following should be avoided during pregnancy?

    a. Intercourse during the third trimester
    b. Swimming
    c. Daily caloric increase of 300 kcal
    d. Douching

13. True labor is characterized by:

    a. Contractions initially felt in back and radiate to lower abdomen
    b. Intensity of contractions decreases with walking
    c. Discomfort of contractions felt mainly in abdomen
    d. Contractions relieved with sedation

14. A predisposing factor for preterm labor is:

    a. Hypothyroidism
    b. Gestational diabetes
    c. Pyelonephritis
    d. Oligohydramnios

15. Which of the following is a risk factor for the development of gestational diabetes?

    a. Multiple gestation
    b. Prior macrosomic infant
    c. Oligohydramnios in prior pregnancy
    d. Maternal age under 19

16. A woman with a ruptured ectopic pregnancy is likely to have which of the following?

    a. Urinary frequency and urgency
    b. Hypertension
    c. Referred shoulder pain
    d. Fever with nausea and/or vomiting

17. Which of the following increase a woman's chances of having an ectopic pregnancy?

    a. Use of combined oral contraceptives
    b. Uterine myoma
    c. Endometriosis
    d. Previous ectopic pregnancy

18. Inevitable abortion refers to:

    a. Death of embryo or fetus without expulsion
    b. Gross rupture of membranes in the presence of cervical dilatation
    c. Expulsion of products of conception without medical intervention
    d. Presence of bleeding and uterine cramping without cervical dilation

19. Which of the following is a sign of increasingly severe preeclampsia?

    a. Hemoconcentration with decreased platelets
    b. Increased urinary output
    c. Patellar hyporeflexia
    d. Elevated serum glucose

20. Presentation with placenta previa is differentiated from abruptio placentae by:

    a. Abruptio placentae occurs earlier in gestation
    b. Amount of bleeding is more with placenta previa
    c. Severe abdominal pain with abruptio placentae
    d. PIH usually accompanies placenta previa

21. Typical failure rates for combined oral contraceptives approach:

    a. 0.5%
    b. 0.1%
    c. 1%
    d. 5%

22. Estrogen in combined oral contraceptives has which of the following effects?

    a. Decrease in HDL and increase in LDL
    b. Thickening of cervical mucus, inhibiting sperm transport
    c. Suppression of FSH and LH
    d. Ovum transport slowed

23. Noncontraceptive benefits of oral contraceptives include which of the following?

    a. Protection against ovarian and endometrial cancer
    b. Protection against breast cancer
    c. Increased libido
    d. Protection against cervical neoplasia

24. The efficacy of combined oral contraceptives may be lowered when used concurrently with which of the following?

    a. Antihypertensives
    b. Antiseizure medications
    c. Beta-blockers
    d. Antidepressants

25. Which of the following side effects is more characteristic of the minipill than the combined oral contraceptive?

    a. Nausea
    b. Increased breast size
    c. Cervical ectopia
    d. Irregular bleeding that persists after 3 months

26. A disadvantage of the minipill is:

    a. Incidence of functional ovarian cysts is increased
    b. Adversely affects lactation
    c. Delayed return to fertility after discontinuation
    d. Increased risk of PID

27. The Norplant system is effective for:

    a. 1 year
    b. 3 years
    c. 5 years
    d. 10 years

28. Which of the following statements about Norplant is true?

    a. Effectiveness not altered by medications
    b. Menstrual irregularities most common reason for removal
    c. Menstrual irregularities may continue for 6 to 8 months after removal
    d. Risk of decreasing bone density

29. A patient considering use of Depo-Provera should be counseled regarding:

    a. Failure rate of 3%
    b. Potential menstrual cycle changes
    c. Intensification of ovulatory pain
    d. Risk of developing hypertension

30. Which of the following is true with regard to administering Depo-Provera?

    a. Should be initiated within five days after onset of normal menses
    b. Injection site should be massaged to enhance absorption
    c. Should be initiated at six weeks postpartum if not breastfeeding
    d. Should not be used if breastfeeding

31. To be effective, emergency contraception must be initiated within:

    a. 24 hours
    b. 48 hours
    c. 72 hours
    d. 96 hours

32. A woman who had a ParaGard IUD inserted eight weeks ago is complaining of mild pelvic cramping and lengthening of the string. What is the most likely cause?

    a. Cervicitis
    b. Pregnancy
    c. Uterine perforation
    d. IUD expulsion

33. A woman with a ParaGard IUD is six weeks pregnant and wishes to continue the pregnancy. She should be told that:

    a. The IUD should be removed today and there is a risk of spontaneous abortion
    b. The IUD should be left in place to reduce the risk of spontaneous abortion
    c. There is an increased risk of fetal congenital anomalies from the copper in the IUD
    d. There is no increased risk of spontaneous abortion whether the IUD is left in or removed

34. Calculation of the fertile period rests on which of the following assumptions?

    a. Sperm remain viable for 24 hours
    b. Ovum survive an average of three days
    c. Ovulation occurs on day 14 ($\pm$ 2) before onset of next menses
    d. Progesterone decreases basal body temperature 0.4-0.8° F

35. Which of the following would not be considered a complication associated with IUD use?

    a. Infection
    b. Ectopic pregnancy
    c. Dysmenorrhea
    d. Ovarian cyst development

36. When counseling a patient who has a ParaGard IUD, emphasis should be placed on which of the following?

    a. Need to change IUD every five years
    b. Risk factors and signs of infection
    c. Risk of developing anemia
    d. Pain control for dysmenorrhea

37. Which of the following statements about the diaphragm is true?

    a. Has a 25% failure rate
    b. Association with increased incidence of urinary tract infections
    c. May be used with or without contraceptive jelly
    d. There are no contraindications for use other than latex allergy

38. What is the contraceptive ingredient in most vaginal spermicides?

    a. Sodium laurel sulfate
    b. Benzalkonium chloride
    c. Nonoxynol-9
    d. Surfactant

39. Which of the following statements about vaginal spermicides is incorrect?

    a. First year failure rates range from 6% to 26%
    b. Spermicides provide some protection against STD
    c. Use of spermicidal foam is most effective immediately following coitus
    d. Spermicides work by destroying sperm cell membranes

40. Which of the following statements about condoms is true?

    a. Petroleum based lubricants may deteriorate latex
    b. Skin condoms are equal to latex condoms in STD and HIV protection
    c. Condom use may exacerbate premature ejaculation
    d. Spermicide may weaken the latex in condoms

41. First year failure rates for male condom use range from:

    a. 1%-5%

b. 3%-14%
c. 5%-10%
d. 2%-15%

42. Which of the following is correct when calculating fertile days for a woman using calendar rhythm for contraception?

a. Subtract 15 days from the longest cycle, and 12 days from the shortest cycle
b. Subtract 15 days from the shortest cycle, and 12 days from the longest cycle
c. Subtract 11 days from the longest cycle, and 18 days from the shortest cycle
d. Subtract 11 days from the longest cycle, and add 7 days to the shortest cycle

43. A disadvantage of female sterilization is:

a. Less effective than Norplant
b. Long-term side effects
c. High incidence of ectopic pregnancy
d. Partner's consent is required

44. When compared to female sterilization procedures, male procedures:

a. Are more likely to result in complications
b. Have slightly lower failure rates
c. Are more expensive
d. Are more common

45. Which of the following is not a potential complication associated with a vasectomy?

a. Hematoma
b. Development of sperm antibodies
c. Prostatitis
d. Pregnancy

46. Which of the following is an indication for hormone replacement therapy?

a. Irregular vaginal bleeding
b. Bone pain
c. Uterine prolapse
d. Vasomotor instability

47. The average age a woman in the U.S. experiences menopause is:

    a. 40 years
    b. 45 years
    c. 50 years
    d. 55 years

48. With regard to menopause, which of the following statements is true?

    a. FSH and LH levels decrease
    b. Depo-Provera frequently used to treat symptoms
    c. Estradiol levels increase
    d. Estrone becomes primary type of estrogen in body

49. Which of the following is characteristic of estrogen deficiency?

    a. Atrophy of vaginal epithelium
    b. Increased sweat gland activity
    c. Thickening of skin epidermal and dermal layers
    d. Increased libido

50. Which of the following is a contraindication for hormone replacement therapy?

    a. Diabetes
    b. Hypertension
    c. Rheumatoid arthritis
    d. Liver disease

51. Which of the following may not be helpful in preventing or treating osteoporosis?

    a. Hormone replacement therapy
    b. Weight bearing exercise
    c. Vitamin E
    d. Calcium

Answers

1. d	18. b	35. d
2. c	19. a	36. b
3. a	20. c	37. b
4. c	21. d	38. c
5. d	22. c	39. c
6. b	23. a	40. a
7. b	24. b	41. b
8. c	25. d	42. c
9. a	26. a	43. a
10. c	27. c	44. b
11. b	28. b	45. c
12. d	29. b	46. d
13. a	30. a	47. c
14. c	31. c	48. d
15. b	32. d	49. a
16. c	33. a	50. d
17. d	34. c	51. c

$45/51$ 88%

Bibliography

Berek, J. S., Adashi, E. Y., & Hillard, P. A. (1996). *Novak's gynecology* (12th ed.). Baltimore, MD: Williams & Wilkins.

Centers for Disease Control and Prevention (CDC), National Center for Health Statistics (NCHS) (1995). Trends in pregnancies and pregnancy rates: Estimates for the United States, 1980-92. *Monthly vital statistics report,* 43 (11-S). Hyattsville, MD: U.S. Department of Health & Human Services, Publication No. 95-1120.

CDC, NCHS (1997). Births and deaths: United States, 1996. *Monthly vital statistics report,* 46(1-S2). Hyattsville, MD: U.S. Department of Health & Human Services, Publication No. 97-1120.

Cunningham, F. G., MacDonald, P. D., Gant, N. F., Leveno, K. J., Gilstrap, L. C., Hankins, G. D. V., & Clark, S. L. (1997). *Williams obstetrics* (20th ed.). Stanford, CT: Appleton & Lange.

Fogel, C. I., & Woods, N. F. (Eds.). (1995). *Women's health care: A comprehensive handbook.* Thousand Oaks, CA: Sage Publications.

Food and Drug Administration (1997). Prescription drug products: Certain combined oral contraceptives for use as postcoital emergency contraception; Notice. *Federal register, 62* (37). U.S. Department of Health & Human Services.

Hatcher, R. A., Trussell, J., Stewart, F., Cates Jr. W., Stewart, G. K., Guest, F., & Kowal, D. (1998). *Contraceptive technology* (18th ed.). New York: Ardent Media.

Lobo, R. (Ed.). (1994). *Treatment of the postmenopausal woman: Basic and clinical aspects.* New York: Raven Press.

Mishell, D., & Brenner, P. (1994). *Management of common problems in obstetrics and gynecology* (3rd ed.). Boston: Blackwell Scientific Publications.

Moore, K. L. (1998). *The developing human: Clinically oriented embryology* (6th ed.). Philadelphia: W.B. Saunders.

Olds, S.B., London, M.L., & Ladewig, P.W. (1996). *Maternal-newborn nursing: A family-centered approach* (5th ed.). Menlo Park, CA: Addison-Wesley.

Scott, J. R., Disaia, P. J., Hammond, C. B., & Spellacy, W. N. (1994). *Danforth's obstetrics and gynecology* (7th ed.). Philadelphia: J. B. Lippincott.

Speroff, L., & Darney, P. D. (1996). *A clinical guide for contraception* (2nd ed.). Baltimore, MD: Williams & Wilkins.

Speroff, L., Glass, R., & Kase, N. (1994). *Clinical gynecologic endocrinology and infertility* (5th ed.). Baltimore, MD: Williams & Wilkins.

Varney, H. (1997). *Varney's midwifery* (3rd ed.). Sudbury, MA: Jones & Barlett.

Youngkin, E. Q., & Davis, M. S. (Eds.). (1998). *Women's health: A primary care clinical guide* (2nd ed.). Norwalk, CT: Appleton & Lange.

Musculoskeletal Disorders

Madeline Turkeltaub

Osteoarthritis (OA)

- Definition: Degenerative disorder of movable joints which causes deterioration of articular and new bone formation at joint surfaces
- Etiology/Incidence
  1. Primary osteoarthritis—occurs without obvious cause
     a. Frequency
        (1) Ten times more frequent in females than males
        (2) 85% of cases are in people between 55 to 64 years of age
     b. Familial tendency
     c. Obesity
     d. Postural abnormalities
     e. Joint enlargement
     f. Gait changes
  2. Secondary osteoarthritis—results from underlying abnormality
     a. Trauma—old fracture
     b. Joint disorders—gout, congenital dysplastic hip
     c. Avascular necrosis—post trauma, post sepsis, use of steroids
- Signs and Symptoms
  1. Pain—aggravated by activity and relieved with rest; may become persistent as disease progresses
  2. Joints affected become edematous but not hot or red
  3. Limitation of movement in affected joint
  4. Joints most frequently involved
     a. Weight bearing
     b. Distal interphalangeal joints (DIP), proximal interphalangeal joints (PIP)
     c. Neck, low back, hip, knee, metatarsophalangeal (MTP)
- Differential Diagnosis
  1. Rheumatoid arthritis

2. Pseudogout

3. Reiter's syndrome

4. Arthritis of chronic ulcerative colitis

- Physical Findings

  1. Hands

     a. Heberden's nodes—enlargement of DIP joints

     b. Bouchard's nodes—enlargement of PIP joints

  2. Joints

     a. Localized tenderness

     b. Crepitus on movement

     c. Bony consistency to enlargement

  3. Neurologic—pain due to pressure on nerves by affected joints

  4. Hips—reduced internal rotation, pain may be referred to knee

- Diagnostic Tests/Findings

  1. Radiograph—four cardinal radiologic features

     a. Unequal loss of joint space

     b. Osteophytes

     c. Juxta-articular sclerosis

     d. Subchondral bone

  2. Synovial fluid aspirate is usually normal

- Management/Treatment

  1. Preserving function and decreasing pain are goals of treatment

  2. Treating biomechanical factors

     a. Weight loss

     b. Correct uneven leg length with heel wedge

     c. Use canes on opposite side or crutches to decrease weight bearing on affected joint

     d. Quadriceps setting for knee involvement

     e. Cervical collar for cervical spine pain

      f.   Isometric exercises for abdominal muscles decreases lumbosa-cral spine pain

      g.   Orthotic shoe modification

3. Local measures

      a.   Ice to improve range of motion (ROM) and exercise performance

      b.   Moist heat to decrease muscle spasm and relieve morning stiffness

      c.   Temporary rest such as removable splint to decrease motion

4. Medications

      a.   Acetaminophen 500 mg to 1 g t.i.d. or q.i.d.

      b.   Non-steroidal anti-inflammatory drugs (NSAID) e.g., ibuprofen 400 to 800 mg t.i.d.; indomethacin 50 to 200 mg/day up to 1 g q.i.d.

5. Consider H_2 blocker when using NSAID

6. Instruction on side effects of NSAID including:

      a.   Gastrointestinal intolerance

      b.   Fluid retention

      c.   Platelet abnormalities

      d.   Hepatic and renal dysfunction

7. Surgery—refer to physician for procedures, such as fusion or joint replacement

8. Educate regarding body mechanics, muscle strengthening, range of motion exercises and weight reduction strategies

Rheumatoid Arthritis (RA)

- Definition: Chronic multisystem disease resulting in symmetrical joint inflammation

- Etiology/Incidence

    1.   Cause unknown

    2.   Affects approximately 1% of the adult population

3. 30% of patients have mild disease with remissions and little deformity

4. 10% have a single period of active disease with only occasional exacerbations

5. About one-half of patients have progressive disease

6. Affects three times as many women as men

7. Onset most frequent in fourth and fifth decades; 80% develop disease between 35 and 50 years of age

8. Other diseases of joints, such as gout and OA may predispose to RA

- Signs and Symptoms

  1. Morning stiffness lasting several hours

  2. Pain—joint pain and/or stiffness develops insidiously over several weeks to months

  3. Fatigue, malaise, weakness, low-grade fever

  4. Proximal interphalangeal (PIP) and metacarpophalangeal (MCP) joints are the most commonly affected

  5. The first ROM loss is full extension

- Differential Diagnosis

  1. Ankylosing spondylitis

  2. Rheumatic fever

  3. Systemic lupus erythematosus

  4. Arthritis of inflammatory intestinal disease

  5. Psoriatic arthritis

  6. Reiter's syndrome

- Physical Findings

  1. Soft tissue swelling

     a. Most frequently in MCP joints, wrists and PIP joints

     b. Usually symmetrical

  2. Tenderness and pain on passive motion

3. Warmth at site of inflamed joint

4. Limited range of motion at joint

5. Permanent deformity in chronic disease

    a. Flexion contractures

    b. Subluxation

    c. Ulnar deviation of fingers at MCP joints or deformities of fingers (swan neck, boutonniere)

6. Synovial cysts can be visualized and palpated; Baker's cysts (synovial cysts of popliteal space) are common

- Diagnostic Tests/Findings

1. Erythrocyte sedimentation rate is elevated

2. Rheumatoid factor can be isolated in 70 to 80% of patients

3. Antinuclear antibodies are present in 20% of patients

4. Radiograph findings

    a. Early changes are often limited to periarticular osteoporosis

    b. In time, bony margins of joints show erosion

    c. In late stage, joint space will be narrowed

5. Joint fluid shows inflammatory changes

6. CBC—mild to moderate anemia

- Management/Treatment

1. The goals of treatment are

    a. To relieve pain

    b. To relieve inflammation

    c. To maintain optimal function

    d. To prevent deformity

    e. To educate the patient

2. Conservative management includes:

    a. Education

    b. Rest

    c. Physical therapy

    d. Nonsteroidal anti-inflammatory agents

3. If patient is unresponsive, additional medications from the following categories may be added

    a. Cytotoxic agents (methotrexate preferred)

    b. Antimalarials, e.g., hydroxychloroquine sulfate

    c. Gold salts—intramuscular or orally

    d. Corticosteroids (not more than 10 mg of prednisone or equivalent per day) on short term basis to relieve disabling symptoms

    e. Intra-articular corticosteroids if medications do not relieve symptoms

4. Education

    a. Explain what an autoimmune disease is

    b. Stress management and relaxation techniques

5. Multidisciplinary management

    a. Physical therapy

    b. Occupational therapy

6. Management plan for daily living

Gout

- Definition: Gout is a metabolic disease associated with abnormal accumulation of urates in the body and characterized by recurring acute arthritis; classic gouty attack is podagra, involving the big toe

- Etiology/Incidence

1. Due to deposition of crystals of monosodium urate (MSU)

2. Related to either excess production or decreased excretion of uric acid

3. Decreased uric acid excretion is present in 90% of patients

4. 90% of patients with primary gout are men over 30 years of age

5. The onset in women is usually at menopause plus 20 to 30 years

6. Rapid fluctuation of serum urate levels may be precipitated by alcohol and food excess; surgery, infection, diuretics or uricosuric drugs

- Signs and Symptoms

   1. Acute onset, frequently monarticular, affecting the first metatarsophalangeal joint, called Podagra

   2. Tophi due to accumulation of urate crystals may be found in ears, hands, feet

   3. Remissions and exacerbations

   4. Involved joint is swollen, tender, warm, red

   5. Temperature elevation to 39° C

   6. May become chronic with progressive loss and disability

- Differential Diagnosis

   1. Diagnosis may be confirmed based on dramatic response to NSAID or colchicine

   2. Acute stage may be confused with cellulitis

   3. Pseudogout presents with similar symptoms but normal serum uric acid

   4. Chronic gout may mimic rheumatoid arthritis

   5. Chronic lead intoxication may result in attacks of gout

   6. See rheumatoid arthritis

- Physical Findings

   1. Limited, painful range of motion in affected joint

   2. Elevated temperature during acute attack

   3. Palpation of tophi in areas indicated above

   4. Affected area hot to touch

- Diagnostic Tests/Findings

   1. Synovial fluid aspirate contains monosodium urate crystals

   2. In later stages of disease, radiograph may show punched-out areas in bone

   3. Erythrocyte sedimentation rate elevated

4. White cell count elevated

5. Uric acid elevated

6. Hyperuricemia—serum urate > 7.5 mg/dL

- Management/Treatment

   1. Acute attack should be treated first, hyperuricemia later

   2. NSAID—indomethacin, 50 mg every 8 hours, continued until symptoms resolve

   3. Colchicine

      a. Most effective during first 24 to 48 hours

      b. Dose—0.5 to 0.6 mg orally, every hour, until pain relieved or GI symptoms occur or maximum dose of 6 mg

   4. Corticosteroids—used for patients who cannot tolerate NSAID

   5. Analgesics—codeine or meperidine may be indicated; ASA is *contraindicated*

   6. Bed rest—for 24 hours after acute attack subsides

   7. Diet to maintain daily output of 2000 cc of urine; avoid obesity and prevent dehydration; low purine diet has little effect on blood levels

   8. Support is needed during remissions for patient to maintain medical regimen, including:

      a. Diet instruction

      b. Prophylactic medication

         (1) Uricosuric drugs—probenecid, 0.5 g/day, with gradual increase to 1 to 2 g/day; avoid use with salicylates

         (2) Allopurinol—100 mg/day for one week initially, then 200 to 300 mg/daily; observe for rash associated with hypersensitivity

   9. Comfort may be obtained with cold or hot compresses and elevation of affected area during acute attack

Osteoporosis

- Definition: Demineralization of bone, resulting in decrease in bone mass with an otherwise normal structural matrix

- Etiology/Incidence
    1. Most common metabolic bone disease in the U.S.
    2. Clinically evident in middle years and beyond
    3. Type I—affects women more frequently than men, especially post-menopausal women
    4. Type II—in men and women older than 75
    5. Caucasians have highest incidence, then Asians, then African-Americans
    6. Most frequently associated with
        a. Lack of estrogen (postmenopausal or postoophorectomy)
        b. Lack of activity (immobilization)
        c. Malabsorption (postgastrectomy, lactase deficiency)
        d. Vitamin D deficiency
        e. Low calcium intake
- Signs and Symptoms
    1. Loss of height
    2. Kyphosis
    3. Backache
    4. Spontaneous fracture or collapse of vertebrae
- Differential Diagnosis
    1. Adrenal cortical excess
    2. Hyperthyroidism
    3. Metabolic bone disease, such as hyperparathyroidism and osteomalacia
    4. Multiple myeloma
    5. Metastatic bone disease
- Physical Findings
    1. There may be no specific physical findings, unless a fracture is present
    2. Loss of height is most common

3. Kyphosis ("dowager's hump") is evident with vertebral compression fractures

- Diagnostic Tests/Findings

  1. Serum calcium, phosphorus and alkaline phosphatase are within normal limits.

  2. Standard radiography is not a reliable indicator since more than 25 to 30% of bone loss must occur for detection with this method

  3. Lateral radiograph of spine might show:

     a. Anterior wedging of thoracic vertebral bodies

     b. Widening intervertebral bodies

     c. New or old fractures of vertebrae

  4. Dual-energy x-ray absorptiometry (DEXA)—more sensitive to bone loss

  5. Additional laboratory tests may be ordered for older patients, including:

     a. Albumin (to allow interpretation of serum calcium)

     b. Serum and urine protein electrophoresis (differentiate multiple myeloma)

     c. BUN and creatinine (to rule out chronic renal disease)

- Management/Treatment: Treatment of established osteoporosis must take into consideration severity of disease, age and coexisting medical problems; prevention is key factor

  1. Prevention and treatment of osteoporosis includes:

     a. Balanced diet—protein not to exceed 20% of total calories; diet counseling to include dietary sources high in calcium and low in fat

     b. Exercise

        (1) Prevention

            (a) Weight-bearing, at least 30 minutes 3 to 4 times per week

            (b) Encourage life style changes related to importance of exercise

           (c)   Strength training, e.g., lifting weights, swimming

    (2)   Moderate walking for those with diagnosed osteoporosis, depending upon severity

    (3)   Active or passive range of motion for bedridden patients

c.   Hormone replacement therapy (HRT) in postmenopausal women or postoophorectomy—decreases rate of bone resorption

    (1)   Estrogen and progestin in women with intact uterus

    (2)   Estrogen may be used alone in women without uterus

    (3)   HRT should be initiated as soon as possible following menopause

    (4)   Major role is prevention; may be effective in mild to moderate disease

d.   Bisphosphonates

    (1)   Alendronate—inhibits osteoclast-mediated bone resporption, taken at least one half-hour prior to eating; used for both prevention and treatment

    (2)   Etidronate—not nearly as effective as alendronate

e.   Salmon calcitonin—decreases bone resorption

    (1)   Used primarily for treatment

    (2)   Alleviates bone pain

f.   Selective Estrogen Receptor Modules (SERMS)—raloxifene

    (1)   Antiestrogens

    (2)   Increase bone density

    (3)   Decrease lipid levels

    (4)   Negative effect on breast and uterus

g.   Adequate calcium intake

    (1)   Ages 11 to 24—1200 to 1500 mg/day

    (2)   Ages 25 to 49—1000 mg/day

    (3)   Ages 50 to 64—1500 mg/day (no HRT)

    (4)   Ages 50 to 64—1000 mg/day (on (HRT)

      (5)   All men and women over 65 years 1500 mg/day

   h. Calcium may be obtained through dietary sources or through calcium supplements; calcium carbonate—least expensive; calcium citrate—absorbed easily; calcium phosphate—decreased chance of constipation

   i. 400 to 600 IU vitamin D daily

2. Elderly patients must be protected from falls—educate family regarding safe environment

3. Alcohol and smoking should be avoided

4. Judicious use of glucocorticoids

5. Regular follow-up with mammogram and pelvic examination for women on HRT

6. Educate teens and young women regarding adequate calcium intake and dangers of excess exercise

7. Treatment for acute back pain includes:

   a. Rest

   b. Analgesia

   c. External support

   d. Heat

   e. Stool softeners

Low Back Pain (LBP)

- Definition: Acute, chronic or recurrent pain occurring in the lumbosacral spine region and associated musculoskeletal areas

- Etiology/Incidence

1. Most acute neck or back pain is caused by muscle strain and spasm of the paraspinal muscle groups

2. Low back pain from trauma or mechanical causes is most common from 30 to 40 years of age

3. 80% of the population will experience low back pain sometime during their lifetime

4. LBP is a self limited condition

       a. 40% remit in one week

       b. 60 to 80% in three weeks

       c. 90% in two months

- Signs and Symptoms
    1. Pain
    2. Numbness
    3. Weakness
    4. Bowel and bladder dysfunction
- Differential Diagnosis
    1. Congenital disorders, e.g., asymmetry
    2. Tumors involving nerve roots or meninges
    3. Trauma
        a. Lumbar strain
        b. Compression fracture
    4. Spondylosis and spondylolisthesis
    5. Metabolic disorders, e.g., osteoporosis
    6. Arthritis of the spine
    7. Degenerative diseases
    8. Herniated nucleus pulposus
    9. Infections
    10. Mechanical causes, e.g., weak abdominal muscles, pelvic tumors, prostate disease
    11. Psychogenic
- Physical Findings
    1. Postural deformity of the spine
    2. Gait and heel-and-toe walking will detect weakness of gastrocnemius and tibialis anterior muscles
    3. Straight leg raising—pain on early arc is associated with L_5-S_1 disc

4. Flexing thigh on pelvis (femoral stretch test)—associated with L_3 problems

5. Neurologic testing for motor weakness and sensory deficits

6. Local tenderness or spasm on palpation

7. Specific lesion-isolating findings

    a. L_{3-4} disc

        (1) Pain in lower back, hip, anterior leg to great toe

        (2) Numbness in anteromedial thigh and knee

        (3) Weakness in quadriceps leading to atrophy

        (4) Diminished patellar reflex

    b. L_{4-5} disc

        (1) Pain over sacroiliac joint, hip, lateral thigh

        (2) Numbness of lateral leg, web of great toe

        (3) Weakness on dorsiflexion, difficulty walking on heels

        (4) Reflexes usually unchanged

    c. L_5-S_1 disc

        (1) Pain over sacroiliac joint, hip, back of thigh and leg to heel

        (2) Numbness in back of calf and lateral foot to small toe

        (3) Difficulty walking on toes

        (4) Atrophy of gastrocnemius

        (5) Diminished or absent Achilles tendon reflex

8. Complete physical examination to rule out non-musculoskeletal etiology

- Diagnostic Tests/Findings

    1. If conservative management is not effective in 4 to 6 weeks then begin with standard radiography—AP, lateral and oblique to determine lumbar alignment, vertebral body size, bone density

    2. CT Scan—can detect lateral entrapment of spinal nerve roots

3. MRI—provides early detection of disc degeneration; can be used in pregnant women

- Management/Treatment: Key elements include:

1. Bedrest not indicated—limit select activities that increase pain
2. Analgesia
   a. Salicylates or acetaminophen
   b. Nonsteroidal anti-inflammatory drugs
   c. Occasionally, opiates may be required
3. Muscle relaxants
   a. Limit use to 1 to 2 weeks
   b. Avoid in older patients
4. Patient education
   a. Good body mechanics
   b. Diet—weight loss if indicated
   c. Appropriate exercise
   d. Sleeping posture
5. Traction
6. Back and abdominal exercises for prevention and recurrences; contraindicated during acute episode; walking better than jogging
7. Back massage
8. Many times there is a psychosocial overlay—a psychosocial assessment should be conducted for:
   a. Stress
   b. Depression
   c. Domestic violence
   d. Inadequate coping ability
   e. Marriage/family problems
9. Early return to work with limited activity
10. Stress management

Bursitis

- Definition: Inflammation of the synovial membrane lining of a bursal sac; more than 150 bursae throughout the body
- Etiology/Incidence
  1. Infection in a joint space
  2. Inflammation as part of a systemic process, such as rheumatoid arthritis or gout
  3. Occurs most commonly in middle and old age, following trauma or unaccustomed repetitive use of the part
  4. Most common locations
     a. Subdeltoid
     b. Olecranon
     c. Ischial
     d. Prepatellar
- Signs and Symptoms
  1. Abrupt onset of pain which increases on motion (superficial)
  2. Local tenderness, erythema, edema
  3. Regional tenderness and limited motion (deep bursitis)
- Differential Diagnosis
  1. Rheumatoid arthritis
  2. Gout or pseudogout
  3. Septic arthritis
- Physical Findings
  1. Restriction of movement
  2. Tenderness over rotator cuff
  3. Swelling and redness (prepatellar/olecranon)
- Diagnostic Tests/Findings: Aspirate fluid with 18 gauge needle and request laboratory analysis
  1. Culture
  2. WBC count—elevation is associated with bacterial infection

3. RBC count—associated with trauma

4. Glucose—decreased with bacterial infection

5. Crystals—associated with microcrystalline bursitis

6. Mucin clot—poor clot associated with bacterial infection

- Management/Treatment

    1. If bursitis is traumatic

        a. Splint part

        b. Apply heat 30 minutes t.i.d. or q.i.d.

        c. ASA or NSAID—Naproxen 250 mg b.i.d. or t.i.d.

    2. If symptoms recur and fluid reaccumulates inject long acting cortico-steroids into bursa

    3. If septic bursitis

        a. Incision and drainage

        b. Parenteral antibiotics

    4. Education regarding care of injured part

        a. Ice for first 24 hours

        b. After swelling is stabilized, warm, moist heat several times daily

Epicondylitis (Tennis Elbow)

- Definition: Inflammation in the region of the lateral epicondyle of the humerus at the origin of the common extensor muscles

- Etiology/Incidence

    1. Specific pathogenesis of tennis elbow is not known

    2. Occurs most frequently in the dominant extremity during mid-life (may be athletic or work related)

- Signs and Symptoms

    1. Pain exacerbated by constant motion of the forearm and twisting motions, aggravated by hand and wrist movements

    2. Gradual onset of dull pain along lateral aspect of elbow

    3. Point tenderness over the epicondyle

    4. Limited motion
- Differential Diagnosis
  1. Rheumatoid arthritis
  2. Localized intra-articular pathology
  3. Radial tunnel syndrome
- Physical Findings
  1. Burning or aching pain with grasping or lifting
  2. Point tenderness present at or just distal to lateral epicondyle
- Diagnostic Tests/Findings: Radiographs usually normal or show small calcium deposits
- Management/Treatment
  1. Pain relief
     a. Mild analgesics
     b. Rest
     c. Ice to tendon
  2. Counterforce brace; wrist splint
  3. Peri-tendon cortisone injection
  4. For continued pain
     a. Immobilize for 6 to 8 weeks in a long arm cast with 90° elbow flexion
     b. Physical therapy to restore strength and motion when cast is removed
  5. Reinforce an exercise program to condition muscle groups in the forearm and wrist
  6. If associated with a sport, evaluate whether improper technique was responsible for injury
  7. If nonoperative management fails surgical intervention recommended

Carpal Tunnel Syndrome

- Definition: Median nerve compression of wrist beneath transverse carpal ligament

- Etiology/Incidence
    1. Related to repeated forceful wrist flexion
    2. More common in women
    3. Frequently involves dominant hand
    4. May be associated with
        a. Pregnancy
        b. Endoneural edema in diabetes mellitus
        c. Thyroid disease
        d. Occupational activities
- Signs and Symptoms
    1. Burning, tingling, numbness sensation along distribution of median nerve
    2. Pain exacerbated with dorsiflexion of wrist
    3. Night pain that interferes with sleep
    4. Clumsiness in performing fine hand movements
    5. May be unilateral or bilateral
- Differential Diagnosis
    1. Compression syndromes of median nerve
    2. Mononeuritis multiplex
- Physical Findings
    1. Decreased two point discrimination on affected side
    2. Positive Tinel's sign—sensation of electric shock on percussion of volar aspect of wrist
    3. Positive Phalen's sign—pain and/or paresthesia when hands are held in forced flexion for 30 to 60 seconds
    4. Decreased sensation and muscle atrophy of thenar eminence
- Diagnostic Tests/Findings
    1. Electromyography—assists in documenting motor involvement
    2. Segmental sensory and motor conduction testing

- Management/Treatment
    1. Elevate extremity
    2. Splint hand and forearm
    3. Injection of corticosteroids into carpal tunnel, if bursitis is involved
    4. Refer to M.D. for surgical intervention
    5. Notification of health care provider if symptoms increase
        a. Numbness and tingling persists
        b. Sensation in fingers decreases
    6. Take NSAID with food and report any gastric distress
    7. Consideration of occupational changes if appropriate

Knee Pain

- Definition: Knee pain is due to mechanical, inflammatory and/or degenerative problems
- Etiology/Incidence
    1. Trauma
    2. Most frequently exercise related condition
    3. Tears of medial meniscus 10 times more common than lateral meniscus
- Signs and Symptoms
    1. Locking—most frequently indicative of meniscal tear or loose bodies
    2. "Giving way" or "buckling"—related to patella dislocation or ligamentous instability or anterior cruciate tear
    3. Effusions around knee—associated with hemarthrosis and anterior cruciate ligament; fluid under patella noted on ballottement
    4. Crepitus
- Differential Diagnosis
    1. Single painful knee with minimal edema
        a. Dislocated patella
        b. Degenerative joint disease (DJD)

      c. Prepatellar bursitis

  2. Single edematous knee

      a. Baker's cyst

      b. Torn ligaments

      c. Loose bodies

      d. Meniscal tears

- Physical Findings—the physical examination is confirmatory, following a careful history

  1. McMurray's test—a palpable or audible click when knee is raised slowly with foot externally rotated; examiner's hand rests on joint line; positive = medial meniscal injuries

  2. Anterior drawer test—positive = anterior cruciate ligament (ACL) tear
     Posterior drawer test—positive = posterior cruciate ligament (PCL) tear

  3. Lachman test—(anterior drawer test for ACL tear) most sensitive and easy to perform test on a swollen, painful knee; place knee in 20° to 30° flexion, grasp leg with one hand with anterior force to proximal tibia (to stress ACL) while opposite hand stabilizes thigh; graded 1+ to 3+ grade of displacement

  4. Pain on resisted knee extension

  5. Appley's grind test—flex knee to 90° with patient prone; put pressure on heel with one hand while rotating the lower leg internally and externally; pain or click = positive = medial or lateral collateral ligament damage

- Diagnostic Tests/Findings

  1. Radiographs of knees—AP and lateral

  2. Laboratory examination indicated if arthritis suspected

- Management/Treatment

  1. Rest, cold pack, immobilization

  2. NSAID

  3. ROM of knee, if possible, to prevent stiffness

  4. Quadriceps setting

5. Aspirate effusion

6. Review range of motion and muscle strengthening exercises

7. ACL/PCL tears not responsive to conservative management should be referred to orthopedic surgeon

Ankle Sprain

- Definition: Stretched, partially torn or completely ruptured ligaments

- Etiology/Incidence

  1. Lateral ankle sprains most frequent sports-related injury

  2. Most commonly involved structures include the anterior talofibular and fibulocalcaneal ligaments

  3. 10% of ankle sprains are injuries to the medial ligament, as a result of pronation and eversion of the ankle

- Signs and Symptoms

  1. Sprains are classified on a grading system of 1 through 3; signs and symptoms are associated with each grade as follows:

     a. Grade 1—related to a stretched ligament; mild or minimal sprain

        (1) Mild localized tenderness

        (2) Normal range of motion

        (3) No functional disability

     b. Grade 2—characterized by incomplete or partial rupture of ligament fibers

        (1) Moderate to severe pain with weight bearing; difficulty walking

        (2) Abnormal range of motion

        (3) Swelling and local ecchymosis

        (4) Pain immediately after injury

     c. Grade 3—complete disruption of ligament

        (1) Ambulation is impossible

        (2) Resists any motion of the foot

        (3)   Marked pain, edema, hemorrhage

        (4)   Egg-shaped swelling within 2 hours of injury

- Differential Diagnosis

    1.   Avulsion fractures of the malleoli or tarsal bones

    2.   Epiphyseal fractures in young patients

    3.   Fracture of the calcaneus

    4.   Fracture of the fifth metatarsal base

    5.   Injury to the bifurcate ligament

- Physical Findings: Drawer sign determines anterior talofibulor rupture—tibia is stabilized with one hand with foot in neutral and plantar flexed position, force applied to heel with other hand, if positive anterior displacement of talus occurs

- Diagnostic Tests/Findings

    1.   Radiograph to detect fractures

    2.   Arthrography—determines site and extent of ligamentous injury

    3.   MRI

- Management/Treatment: Treatment depends upon the degree of injury

    1.   General treatment

        a.   Rest

        b.   Ice—15 to 20 minutes every 1 to 2 hours for 72 hours, then begin contrast baths

        c.   Compression

        d.   Elevation

        e.   Non-weight bearing

        f.   NSAID for 10 to 14 days

        g.   Begin ROM when asymptomatic

        h.   Refer grade 3 sprains for casting

    2.   Rehabilitation may begin on the first day after injury and is individualized

        a.   ROM

    b.   Achilles tendon stretching

    c.   Isometrics

    d.   Manual resistance exercises

    e.   Build up ankle strength after healing to prevent subsequent injury

Muscle Strain

- Definition: Overuse of muscle tendons, resulting in inflammation, often associated with repetitive motion; does not include disruption of tissue

- Etiology/Incidence: Strains occur during mild stress by overusing muscle groups not usually used

- Signs and Symptoms: Pain after overuse or injury

- Differential Diagnosis

  1. Sprain

  2. Fracture

- Physical Findings

  1. Pain on range of motion

  2. Edema

  3. Ecchymosis

  4. Pain of muscle strain resolves after 1 to 2 days.

- Diagnostic Tests/Findings: Usually none indicated unless symptoms persist or to rule out suspected fracture

- Management/Treatment

  1. Rest of affected part with assistive devices, if needed

  2. Ice t.i.d. for 20 minutes

  3. Compression

  4. Elevation

  5. Analgesics

  6. NSAID

  7. Education efforts focus on prevention

8. Increase awareness of repetitive motion

9. Identify possible changes which will decrease stress on the extremity

10. Emphasize warm up and stretching before any activity—occupational or sports related

Questions
Select the best answer

1. Mr. Johnson, age 55, has developed a slight limp and pain in his right leg which is worse with weight bearing. These complaints are most frequently associated with:

   a. Rheumatoid arthritis
   b. Osteoarthritis
   c. Gout
   d. Osteoporosis

2. On history, Mr. Johnson indicated that he had suffered a fracture of his right leg in a car accident 10 years ago. Based on this history, it is likely that his present symptoms are:

   a. Unrelated
   b. Related to infection
   c. Secondary to the trauma
   d. Associated with obesity

3. On physical examination, enlargement of an 83-year-old patient's distal interphalangeal joints is noted. Enlargement of these joints is known as:

   a. Heberden's nodes
   b. Bouchard's nodes
   c. Tinel's sign
   d. Tenosynovitis

4. Most frequently, synovial fluid aspirate to diagnose osteoarthritis:

   a. Is high in protein
   b. Has a poor mucin clot
   c. Is normal
   d. Has WBC

5. Osteoarthritis is often associated with:

   a. Systemic symptoms of disease
   b. Restricted joint motion
   c. Elevated temperature
   d. Inflammation of the proximal interphalangeal joints

6. Which of the following is not a radiological feature of osteoarthritis?

    a. Unequal loss of joint space
    b. Subchondral bone
    c. Osteophytes
    d. Osteoporosis

7. Applications of ice to arthritic joints is more frequently done to:

    a. Decrease muscle spasm
    b. Improve range of motion
    c. Numb the affected extremity
    d. Reposition the joint

8. Rheumatoid arthritis is often associated with:

    a. Systemic symptoms
    b. Weight bearing joints
    c. Obesity
    d. High purine diet

9. Nonsteroidal anti-inflammatory medications are frequently used in the treatment of musculoskeletal conditions. It is important to remind a patient to:

    a. Take antacids one hour after taking NSAID
    b. Exercise at least one-half hour after taking medication
    c. Take the medication at least one time per day
    d. Take NSAID with food

10. The onset of rheumatoid arthritis is most frequent:

    a. During 20s and 30s
    b. During 60s and 70s
    c. During 30s and 40s
    d. During 40s and 50s

11. Mrs. Franklin has been complaining of fatigue and painful, hot, swollen PIP joints. Mrs. Franklin's symptoms occurred six months ago, and recurred one week ago. It would not be unusual for a CBC to show:

    a. Positive antinuclear antibodies
    b. Mild to moderate anemia
    c. Elevated hematocrit
    d. Elevated WBC

12. The joints most commonly affected by rheumatoid arthritis are the:

    a. Proximal interphalangeal and metacarpophalangeal joints
    b. Distal interphalangeal joints
    c. Spinous processes
    d. Elbow and shoulder

13. When diagnosing rheumatoid arthritis, which of the following would not be considered as a potential differential diagnoses?

    a. Reiter's syndrome
    b. Multiple sclerosis
    c. Rheumatic fever
    d. Ankylosing spondylitis

14. Which of the following would not be considered a goal of treatment for rheumatoid arthritis?

    a. Pain relief
    b. Independence
    c. Prevention of deformity
    d. Reversal of deformity

15. Which category of medication is not currently used for the treatment of rheumatoid arthritis?

    a. Antimalarials
    b. Gold salts
    c. Antibiotics
    d. Cytotoxic agents

16. Podagra is an example of:

    a. Pseudogout
    b. Gout
    c. Osteosarcoma
    d. Septic arthritis

17. Tophi associated with gout are often found in:

    a. Ear lobes
    b. Kidneys
    c. Fingernails
    d. Ankle and knee joints

18. Mr. Adams, age 55, has a history of chronic exposure to lead. He presents with pain and swelling of his left foot. These facts are both associated with:

    a. Rheumatoid arthritis
    b. Gout
    c. Fracture
    d. Osteoarthritis

19. The most common metabolic bone disease in the U.S. is:

    a. Rickets
    b. Scurvy
    c. Osteomyelitis
    d. Osteoporosis

20. When providing dietary counseling for a patient at risk for osteoporosis, it would be best to recommend:

    a. Baked potato and one ounce of sour cream
    b. A dish of ice cream with whipped cream
    c. A glass of skim milk and an apple
    d. Spinach salad with oil and vinegar

21. When a patient with gout experiences mild pain, the medication indicated is:

    a. ASA
    b. NSAID
    c. Allopurinol
    d. Probenecid

22. Mr. Jones, age 27, is complaining of acute onset lower back pain after helping to move a refrigerator. His pain is on the right and shoots down the back of his thigh. The intervertebral space most likely affected is:

    a. L_4-L_5
    b. L_5-S_1
    c. L_3-L_4
    d. T_{10}-L_1

23. Mr. Jone's pain persists for one week. He has been treated with activity limitation and NSAID with minimal relief. The first diagnostic test to be ordered is:

    a. Anteroposterior and lateral radiograph of the spine
    b. MRI

c. CT scan
d. Spinal tap

24. A scan for a patient with back pain would be indicated if:

a. Spinal nerve entrapment is suspected
b. The history and physical exam do not suggest a cause
c. The pain radiates to one or both legs
d. The patient is pregnant

25. Aspirate from a joint space affected by bursitis may be indicative of a bacterial infection, when:

a. WBC are decreased
b. Glucose is decreased
c. RBC are increased
d. Glucose is increased

26. Tennis elbow is a type of:

a. Tenosynovitis
b. Rheumatic disease
c. Epicondylitis
d. Osteoarthritis

27. Mrs. Thomas was seen, complaining of pain and point tenderness in the area of her elbow which has increased since one week ago, following a day of gardening. A physical finding which differentiates the diagnosis of ''tennis elbow'' is:

a. Burning or aching pain with extension
b. Burning or aching pain with lifting
c. Inability to pronate arm
d. Inability to push down against resistance

28. Positive Tinel's and Phalen's signs are associated with:

a. Carpal tunnel syndrome
b. Torn medial meniscus
c. Baker's cyst
d. Epicondylitis

29. ''Loose bodies'' in the knee would result in the following symptom

a. Inflammation

b. "Click" on extension
c. "Locking"
d. Instability

30. Mrs. Abbott, age 32, "turned" her ankle when stepping off a curb. She immediately experienced pain on weight bearing and had limited range of motion on examination. The most likely diagnosis is:

a. Muscle strain
b. Grade 2 ankle sprain
c. Fractured calcaneus
d. Grade 3 ankle sprain

Answers

1. b	11. b	21. b
2. c	12. a	22. b
3. a	13. b	23. a
4. c	14. d	24. a
5. b	15. c	25. b
6. d	16. b	26. c
7. b	17. a	27. b
8. a	18. b	28. a
9. d	19. d	29. c
10. d	20. c	30. b

29/30 97%

Bibliography

Downs, D. (1997). Non-specific work-related upper extremity disorders. *American Family Physician, 55*(4), 1296-1302.

Fan, P. (1997). An approach to rheumatoid arthritis, evaluation, early management and patient involvement. *Family Practice, 19*(2), 37-51.

Fenstermacher, K., & Hudson, B. (1997). *Practice guidelines for family nurse practitioners.* Philadelphia: W. B. Saunders.

Ham, R., & Sloane, P. (1997). *Primary care geriatrics, a case based approach.* St. Louis: Mosby.

Masear, V. (1996). *Primary care orthopedics.* Philadelphia: W. B. Saunders.

Millonig, V. L. (1996). *Today and tomorrow's woman—menopause: Before and after.* Potomac, MD: Health Leadership Associates, Inc.

Morgan, R., & Linder, M. (1997). Common wrist injuries. *American Family Physician, 55*(3), 857-868.

Noble, J. (Ed.). (1996). *Textbook of primary care medicine.* St. Louis: Mosby.

Ross, C. (1997). A comparison of osteoarthritis and rheumatoid arthritis: Diagnosis and treatment. *The Nurse Practitioner, 22*(9), 20-39.

Schnare, S. (1995). Evaluating and managing acute low back pain. *Contemporary Nurse Practitioner, 1*(6), 10-16.

Smith, B., & Green, G. (1995). Acute knee injuries: Part I. *American Family Physician, 51*(3), 615-621.

Tierney, L., McPhee, S., & Papadakis, M. (Eds.). (1998). *Current medical diagnosis and treatment.* Stamford, CT: Appleton & Lange.

Neurological Disorders

Sally K. Miller

Headache

- Definition: Very common complaint in primary care; may be actual product of a disease or syndrome (tension or migraine), or symptom of an underlying disorder (giant cell arteritis, structural lesion); since there are many types of headaches, all with varying degrees of severity, proper assessment of headache and associated symptoms is critical

- Etiology/Incidence

    1. Tension (accounts for 90% of all headaches)

    2. Migraine

        a. Classic (occurs with aura)

        b. Common (no aura)

    3. Cluster headaches

    4. Toxic

        a. Viral infection

        b. Medication induced

    5. Subdural hematoma

    6. Subarachnoid hemorrhage—medical emergency requiring immediate hospitalization

    7. Meningeal irritation

    8. Giant cell arteritis

    9. Structural lesion—infrequently presents as headache but must be considered

    10. Referred pain from eyes, ears, sinuses, teeth

    11. Visual strain

    12. Narrow angle glaucoma

    13. Hypertensive headache

- Components of Headache Evaluation

    1. Chronology is most important item—headache of recent onset that becomes progressively more frequent and/or severe is more ominous than extremely intense headache that has presented in same fashion over a period of time

2. Location, duration and quality—should be evaluated as they will provide clues to the underlying cause

3. Associated activity—exertion, sleep, tension, relaxation

4. Timing of menstrual cycle in women

5. Presence of associated symptoms such as neurological symptoms, systemic symptoms of illness (rhinitis, pharyngitis), symptoms of anxiety or depression (sleep disturbance, inability to concentrate)

6. Presence of triggers—things that seem to be associated with headache onset such as certain foods, stress, alcohol, weather changes

7. Age of onset

Tension Headaches

- Definition: Single most common type of headache evaluated in primary care
- Etiology/Incidence
  1. Physical or emotional stress
  2. Tension producing circumstances
  3. Most common headache in adults
- Signs and Symptoms
  1. Associated complaints of poor concentration and other vague, non-specific symptoms
  2. Usually lasts for several hours
  3. Usually described as generalized about the head—may be most intense about the neck or back of head
  4. Described as vise-like or tight in quality
  5. Occur frequently during or following stressful circumstances
  6. No associated focal neurological symptoms
  7. No aura
- Differential Diagnosis
  1. Evaluation of social history very important in differentiating tension headache
     a. Work history

          b.   Family circumstances

          c.   Recent life changes—birth, death, marriage, divorce

    2.   Other syndromes producing similar headache patterns

          a.   Common migraine

          b.   Toxic headache

          c.   Hypertensive headache

          d.   Referred pain from other structures in the head

          e.   Meningeal irritation

- Physical Findings

    1.   Often no physical findings

    2.   May find cervical muscle pain/tenderness

    3.   Other findings depending upon severity

          a.   Tremor

          b.   Disinterest in appearance

- Diagnostic Tests/Findings

    1.   None specific to tension headache

    2.   Radiographic imaging of head as appropriate to rule out organic disorder

- Management/Treatment

    1.   Over the counter analgesics

          a.   Acetaminophen 650 to 1000 mg q.i.d.

          b.   Aspirin 650 to 1000 mg q.i.d.

          c.   Ibuprofen 400 mg q.i.d.

    2.   Relaxation or stress reducing techniques

          a.   Biofeedback

          b.   Massage

          c.   Hot baths

    3.   Explore underlying cause of stress

4. When initial measures fail, a trial of anti-migraine agents is appropriate

Migraine Headache

- Definition: An extremely painful headache syndrome that is disabling during acute attack; commonly divided into two categories:
    1. Classic migraine occurring after an aura—aura precedes pain and may include visual disturbances, auditory, visual or olfactory hallucinations, or other neurological symptoms
    2. Common migraine—not associated with an aura
- Etiology/Incidence
    1. Etiology unknown, but theories include:
        a. Dilation and excessive pulsation of the external carotid artery
        b. Excess release of the neurotransmitter serotonin, leading to an inflammatory process involving the trigeminal nerve
    2. Variety of triggers
        a. Emotional or physical stress
        b. Lack of/or excess sleep
        c. Missed meals
        d. Specific foods
        e. Alcoholic beverages
        f. Menstruation
        g. Changes in weather
        h. Nitrate containing foods
    3. Onset usually in adolescence or early adult years
    4. Often family history of migraine
    5. Females more often affected than males
- Signs and Symptoms
    1. Episodic unilateral, lateralized, throbbing headache
    2. Builds up gradually and lasts several hours or longer
    3. Focal neurologic disturbances may precede or accompany migraines

    4. Visual disturbances frequently occur

        a. Visual field defects

        b. Luminous visual hallucinations (stars, sparks, zigzag of lights)

    5. Aphasia, numbness, tingling, clumsiness or weakness

    6. Nausea and vomiting

    7. Photophobia

    8. Phonophobia

- Differential Diagnosis

    1. Subarachnoid hemorrhage

    2. Cluster headaches

    3. Hypertensive headache

    4. Cerebrovascular accident

    5. Space occupying lesion

- Physical Findings

    1. Many times physical examination normal

    2. Patient appears acutely ill during migraine

    3. Thorough neurological examination

        a. Focal deficits may accompany migraine

        b. Focal deficits may indicate tumor

- Diagnostic Tests/Findings

    1. None available specific to migraine

    2. Patients with new onset migraine require baseline studies to rule out organic cause; abnormalities may indicate organic cause of pain

        a. Blood chemistries

        b. Complete blood count

        c. Syphilis screen

        d. Erythrocyte sedimentation rate

        e. Radiographic imaging of the head

        f. Other studies indicated by history and physical examination

- Management/Treatment: Prophylactic

  1. Avoidance of trigger factors very important

  2. Relaxation and stress management techniques described in management of tension headache

  3. Pharmacologic therapy if attacks occur more than 2 to 3 times per month

     a. Aspirin 650 to 1950 mg daily

     b. Propranolol 10 to 20 mg b.i.d. starting dose, gradually increase to effective dose of 80 to 120 mg daily—contraindicated in congestive heart failure, obstructive pulmonary disease, diabetes and severe depression

     c. Amitriptyline 10 to 150 mg daily

        (1) Other tricyclic antidepressants helpful

        (2) Must be taken for 2 to 4 weeks before improvement seen

        (3) Contraindicated in cardiac dysrhythmia, narrow angle glaucoma, and urinary difficulties

     d. Selective serotonin reuptake inhibitors (SSRI)

        (1) Newest category, fewer side effects than tricyclic antidepressants

        (2) Better choice for geriatric patients and those with cardiac disoders

        (3) Fluoxetine, sertraline, paroxetine and venlafaxine are common choices

            (a) Start 10 mg every day at 7 a.m., build to 20 mg in 7 to 10 days

            (b) Contraindicated in severe depression

     e. Calcium channel blockers widely used but not as effective

        (1) Verapamil 40 mg t.i.d., increased to 80 mg t.i.d. over 2 to 3 weeks; maximum dose 160 mg t.i.d.

        (2) Contraindicated in congestive heart failure, heart block, hypotension

- Management/Treatment: Acute Attack

1. Rest in dark, quiet room

2. Simple analgesics (aspirin) taken immediately upon onset may provide some relief

3. Nonsteroidal agents

   a. Naproxen 250 mg repeat in 1 to 4 hours as needed

   b. Ketorolac 10 mg repeat in 1 to 4 hours as needed

4. Butalbital-containing medications

   a. Aspirin, caffeine, butalbital combination

   b. Acetaminophen, caffeine, butalbital combination

5. Opiates—may be effective but should be used with caution

   a. Butorphanol 1 mg every 4 hr

   b. Meperidine 75 to 100 mg with hydroxyzine 50 mg IM every 4 hr

6. Sumatriptan

   a. 6 mg SQ, may repeat in one hour but no more than three times per day

   b. Also available in 25 and 50 mg oral dose and as nasal spray

   c. Contraindicated in coronary artery disease, Prinzmetal's angina, basilar and hemiplegic migraine, uncontrolled hypertension, history of anaphylaxis, and recent ergotamine use

7. Ergot alkaloids orally or as suppository—contraindicated in pregnancy, uncontrolled hypertension, peripheral vascular disease, coronary artery disease, liver and kidney disease, and concomitant use of sumatriptan

8. Migranal 2 mg intranasal spray

9. Medicate for nausea as indicated

10. Acetaminophen, aspirin, and caffeine preparation (oral)

Cluster Headaches

- Definition: Among the most painful of all pain inducing conditions
- Etiology/Incidence

1. Intrinsic histamine-mediated dilation of external carotid artery

2. Decreased oxygen saturation due to intrinsic hypothalamic abnormality stimulates brainstem causing pain

3. Episodic (90%); chronic (10%)

4. Cycles occur the same time each year—most often during fall and spring

5. Males more often affected than females at 5:1 ratio

- Signs and Symptoms

    1. Severe unilateral orbital, supraorbital and/or temporal pain occuring in clusters of days or weeks with pain free period in between

    2. Pain lasts 15 minutes to 3 hours

    3. Attacks occur 1 to 8 times daily

    4. May rock, pace, or put fist against the painful eye

- Differential Diagnosis

    1. Migraine headache

    2. Narrow angle glaucoma

    3. Structural lesions

- Physical Findings

    1. May be none

    2. Conjunctival injection

    3. Ipsilateral nasal congestion

    4. Rhinorrhea

    5. Forehead or facial sweating

    6. Miosis

    7. Ptosis

    8. Eyelid edema

- Diagnostic Tests/Findings

    1. None diagnostic of cluster headache

    2. As indicated to rule out organic disorders

    a.   Computerized axial tomography (CT) scan of the head

    b.   Magnetic resonance imaging (MRI) of the head

    c.   Complete blood count

    d.   Serum chemistries

    e.   Erythrocyte sedimentation rate

    f.   Electroencephelogram (EEG)

- Management/Treatment: Prophylaxis

  1. Ergotamine tartrate 2 mg every day, 0.5 to 1.0 mg per rectum, or 0.25 mg SQ t.i.d. 5 days weekly

  2. Prednisone 20 to 40 mg daily or q.o.d. for 2 weeks, then taper

  3. Verapamil 240 to 480 mg every day

  4. Methysergide 4 to 6 mg every day

- Management/Treatment: Acute Attack

  1. Oral drugs usually not successful

  2. Sumatriptan 6 mg SQ

  3. Ergotamine tartrate aerosol inhalation may be effective

  4. Inhalation of 100% oxygen—typically only effective in case of cluster headache

Transient Ischemic Attack (T.I.A.)

- Definition: Interruption in the cerebral vascular flow, causing ischemia and resultant temporary focal neurologic deficits; two types of T.I.A—carotid and vertebrobasilar; treatments are same for either type but presenting signs and symptoms differ

- Etiology/Incidence

  1. Embolization is an important cause

     a. Cardiac dysrhythmia

     b. Rheumatic heart disease

     c. Mitral valve disease

     d. Ulcerated plaque on a major artery

     e. Infective endocarditis

      f. Mural thrombus following myocardial infarction

  2. Fibromuscular dysplasia

  3. Inflammatory disorders

      a. Giant cell arteritis

      b. Systemic lupus erythematosus

  4. Hypotension in clients with extracranial artery stenosis

  5. Hematologic disorders

      a. Polycythemia

      b. Sickle cell disease

      c. Severe anemia

  6. Risk factors for vascular disease are often present

      a. Diabetes mellitus

      b. Tobacco use

      c. Hypertension

      d. Elevated serum cholesterol

  7. Patients with acquired immune deficiency syndrome (AIDS) at increased risk

  8. 30,000 to 150,000 occur annually (may be under reported)

- Signs and Symptoms (Carotid T.I.A.)

  1. Weakness of the contralateral arm, leg, or face, singly or in combination

  2. Numbness or paresthesia of the contralateral side may occur alone or in combination with motor deficits

  3. Homonymous hemianopsia

  4. Ipsilateral monocular vision loss

  5. Symptoms usually disappear within one hour and must resolve completely within 24 hours for a diagnosis of T.I.A.

  6. Any of the above symptoms may occur singly or in combination with other symptoms

- Signs and Symptoms (Vertebrobasilar T.I.A.)

1. Unilateral or bilateral weakness

2. Vertigo

3. Ataxia

4. Diplopia

5. Dysarthria

6. Perioral numbness

7. Drop attacks may occur due to bilateral leg weakness

8. Dysphasia

9. Hearing loss

10. Symptoms may occur singly or in any combination

11. Symptoms usually resolve in < 1 hour, must resolve in < 24 hours to be diagnostic of T.I.A.

- Differential Diagnosis

  1. Focal seizures

  2. Classic migraine

  3. Hypoglycemia

- Physical Findings

  1. Physical findings present only during event

  2. Hyperactive deep tendon reflexes

  3. Slowness of movement

  4. Flaccid weakness with pyramidal distribution

  5. May identify sensory impairment

  6. May see atherosclerotic changes on funduscopic exam

  7. Carotid artery bruit

  8. Cardiac examination may suggest source

     a. Murmur

     b. Dysrhythmia

  9. Physical findings absent if patient examined after resolution of symptoms

- Diagnostic Tests/Findings

  1. Clinical and laboratory evaluation must include assessment of risk factors for vascular disease

     a. Complete blood count

     b. Serum glucose

     c. Serum cholesterol

     d. Syphilis screening

     e. Electrocardiogram

     f. Chest radiograph

  2. Echocardiography if cardiac emboli suspected

  3. Evaluate for hypertension

  4. Holter monitor if transient disturbance in cardiac rhythm suspected

  5. CT scan of the head to rule out small hemorrhage, infarct or tumor

  6. Ultrasound to evaluate cerebral circulation and major vessels to head

  7. Arteriography is definitive study of vasculature—should be considered if patient is good operative risk, CT scan is normal, and no apparent source of cardiac emboli present

- Management/Treatment

  1. Medical management aimed toward preventing further attacks as 30% of patients with cerebrovascular accident have history of T.I.A.

     a. Cessation of tobacco use

     b. Control of underlying medical conditions

        (1) Hyperlipidemia

        (2) Diabetes mellitus

        (3) Hypertension

        (4) Arteritis

        (5) Hematologic disorders

     c. Immediate anticoagulation when cardiac emboli is strong possibility—intravenous heparin followed by oral warfarin sodium

    d. Aspirin 325 mg daily when cardiac emboli not strong possibility

    e. Platelet inhibitors in those intolerant of aspirin

        (1) Clopidogrel bisulfate 75 mg daily—caution with severe liver disease

        (2) Ticlopidine 250 mg b.i.d.—monitor for neutropenia or agranulocytosis

  2. Carotid thromboendarterectomy considered when:

    a. Arteriography reveals a surgically accessible stenosis > 70%

    b. Relatively little atherosclerosis elsewhere

    c. Patient is a good surgical candidate

Seizure Disorder

- Definition

  1. A disorder characterized by transient disturbance of cerebral function due to an abnormal paroxysmal neuronal discharge in the brain

  2. Two main classifications of seizure

    a. Partial seizures

        (1) Simple partial seizure

        (2) Complex partial seizure

    b. Generalized seizures

        (1) Absence (petit mal) seizure

        (2) Myoclonic seizure

        (3) Tonic-clonic (grand mal) seizure

  2. Partial seizures result from an activation of part of one hemisphere (unilaterally)

  3. Generalized seizures result from a generalized activation of the brain (bilateral)

- Etiology/Incidence

  1. Congenital abnormalities and perinatal injuries may result in seizures presenting in infancy and early childhood

2. Metabolic disorders

    a. Hypocalcemia

    b. Hypoglycemia

    c. Hyponatremia

    d. Pyridoxine deficiency

    e. Renal failure

    f. Acidosis

    g. Alcohol withdrawal

3. Infectious diseases

    a. Bacterial meningitis

    b. Herpes encephalitis

    c. Neurosyphilis

4. Trauma an important cause in young adults

5. Tumors and other space occupying lesions

6. Vascular disease, an increasingly frequent cause in the older population—most common cause when seizure onset is after age 60

7. May be due to unknown cause

8. Overall affects approximately 0.5% of the population in the U.S.

- Signs and Symptoms: Simple Partial Seizure

    1. No loss of consciousness

    2. Lasts approximately one minute

    3. Focal motor symptoms (convulsive jerking)

    4. Speech arrest or vocalizations

    5. Jacksonian march

    6. Special sensory symptoms

        a. Light flashes

        b. Buzzing

    7. Paresthesias

    8. Autonomic symptoms

      a. Flushing

      b. Diaphoresis

      c. Pupillary dilation

    9. Dysmnesic symptoms (déjà vu)

- Signs and Symptoms: Complex Partial Seizures—any symptoms of simple partial seizure accompanied by a period of impaired consciousness before, during or after episode

- Signs and Symptoms: Absence (Petit Mal) Seizures

    1. Impairment of consciousness

    2. Mild tonic, clonic, or atonic components

    3. Occasional autonomic components

      a. Flushing

      b. Diaphoresis

      c. Enuresis

    4. Onset and termination very brief, lasting seconds—individual may break off in midsentence for a few seconds

    5. Almost always begin in childhood

    6. Frequently cease by age 20, occasionally replaced by other forms of generalized seizure

- Signs and Symptoms: Myoclonic Seizures

    1. Single or multiple myoclonic jerks

    2. No loss of consciousness

- Signs and Symptoms: Tonic Clonic (Grand Mal) Seizure

    1. Sudden loss of consciousness

    2. Patient becomes rigid, falls to the ground

    3. Respiration is arrested

    4. Clonic phase follows tonic phase—jerking of body musculature lasting 2 to 3 minutes followed by stage of flaccid coma

    5. Urinary and/or fecal incontinence may occur

    6. Lips or tongue may be bitten

7. After one tonic-clonic cycle, patient may:

   a. Recover consciousness

   b. Fall into deep sleep (postictal state)—headache, disorientation, soreness, nausea and drowsiness common upon awakening

   c. More attacks after recovering consciousness (serial seizures)

   d. More attacks without recovering consciousness (status epilepticus)

   e. Display postepileptic automatism

      (1) Behave in an abnormal fashion in immediate postictal period

      (2) No subsequent memory of events

** *AN EYEWITNESSES ACCOUNT OF SEIZURE ACTIVITY IS EXTREMELY VALUABLE AND SHOULD BE OBTAINED IF AT ALL POSSIBLE* **

- Differential Diagnosis: Partial Seizures

  1. Transient ischemic attacks

  2. Rage attacks

  3. Panic attacks

- Differential Diagnosis: Generalized Seizures

  1. Syncope

  2. Cardiac dysrhythmia

  3. Brain stem ischemia

  4. Pseudoseizures

- Physical Findings

  1. May be none

  2. May show evidence of underlying disorder

     a. Trauma

     b. Focal neurological deficits (brain lesion)

     c. Hyperactive reflexes

3. Muscle soreness following grand mal seizure

4. Tongue trauma

- Diagnostic Tests/Findings

    1. As indicated to investigate underlying cause as indicated by history and age of patient

    2. Initial evaluation in patients over 10 years of age should include the following tests in order to investigate cause and provide a baseline for subsequent monitoring of long term treatment

        a. Complete blood count

        b. Serum glucose

        c. Liver function tests

        d. Renal function tests

        e. Serologic test for syphilis

    3. Electroencephelogram (EEG) for paroxysmal abnormalities containing spikes or sharp waves

        a. May help classify disorder

        b. Support clinical diagnosis of seizure

        c. Evaluate candidates for surgical treatment by localizing epileptogenic source

    4. CT scan or MRI to rule out lesion or neoplasm when:

        a. Focal neurological signs and symptoms present

        b. EEG findings suggestive of focal disturbance

        c. Onset after age 30

        d. Seizure disorder is progressive

    5. Chest radiograph to rule out primary or secondary neoplasms

    6. Lumbar puncture (LP)—rule out infectious process

- Management/Treatment: Acute Seizure

    1. Diazepam 5 to 10 mg slow IV

    2. Lorazepam 4 mg slow IV

    3. Treatment not indicated for alcohol withdrawal seizures

- Management/Treatment: Preventive
    1. May need to be reported to Department of Motor Vehicles
    2. Treat underlying problem as appropriate
        a. Infectious process
        b. Metabolic disturbance
    3. Pharmacologic choice depends upon type of seizure
    4. Pharmacologic options for generalized tonic-clonic or partial seizures
        a. Phenytoin 200 to 400 mg daily or in divided doses
            (1) Maintain serum level 10 to 20 μg/mL
            (2) Contraindicated in patients with sinoatrial or atrioventricular block
        b. Carbamazepine 600 to 1200 mg in two divided doses daily
            (1) Maintain serum level 4 to 8 μg/mL
            (2) Contraindicated in patients with known hypersensitivity to tricyclic antidepressants, patients with past or present bone marrow depression, and patients on monoamine oxidase inhibitors
        c. Valproic acid 1500 to 2000 mg in three divided doses daily
            (1) Maintain serum level 50 to 100 μg/mL
            (2) Contraindicated in patients with known hepatic disease
    5. Pharmacologic choices for petit mal seizures
        a. Ethosuximide 100 to 1500 mg in two divided doses daily
            (1) Maintain serum level 40 to 100 μg/mL
            (2) Use with extreme caution in patients with hepatic or renal disease
        b. Valproic acid at doses indicated for tonic-clonic seizure
        c. Clonazepam 0.05 to 0.2 mg/kg in two divided doses daily
            (1) Maintain serum level 20 to 80 ng/mL
            (2) Contraindicated in patients with known hypersensitivity

to benzodiazepines, hepatic disease, chronic respiratory disorders, and untreated glaucoma

6. Pharmacologic choice for myoclonic seizure

    a. Valproic acid at doses indicated for tonic-clonic seizure

    b. Clonazepam at doses indicated for petit mal seizure

7. Patients should be advised to avoid dangerous situations

8. When first drug choice does not provide control, add second drug until therapeutic levels obtained, then first drug gradually withdrawn

9. Prophylactic medication not generally indicated based on one seizure unless further attacks occur or investigation identifies untreatable pathology

10. Withdrawal of medication should only be considered when patient has been free of seizure activity for at least four years

    a. Dose reduction over a period of weeks/months

    b. Reinstitution of same drug(s) if seizure recurs

Parkinson's Disease

- Definition: Degenerative central nervous system disorder characterized by any combination of tremor, rigidity, bradykinesia or progressive postural instability

- Etiology/Incidence

    1. Degeneration of the dopaminergic nigrostriatal system leads to dopamine depletion and consequently a dopamine/acetylcholine imbalance

    2. Most commonly idiopathic, but causes may include:

        a. Exposure to toxins

            (1) Manganese dust

            (2) Carbon disulfide

            (3) Carbon monoxide

        b. Postencephalitic parkinsonism

    3. Onset usually between 45 and 65 years of age

4. Approximately equal gender distribution

5. Occurs in all ethnic groups

- Signs and Symptoms
    1. Any combination of:
        a. Tremor
        b. Rigidity
        c. Bradykinesia
        d. Progressive postural instability
    2. Wooden facies
    3. Impaired swallowing
    4. Decreased automatic movement
    5. Seborrhea of scalp and face

- Differential Diagnosis
    1. Side effects of high potency neuroleptics
    2. Brain tumor
    3. Depression
    4. Benign essential tremor
    5. Dementia
    6. Huntington's disease
    7. Creutzfeldt-Jakob Disease

- Physical Findings
    1. Relatively immobile face with wide palpebral fissures
    2. Infrequent blinking
    3. Seborrhea
    4. Myerson's response—repetitive tapping over bridge of nose produces sustained blinking response
    5. Drooling
    6. Bradykinesia
    7. Slow cycle tremor

8. No muscle weakness

9. No alteration in deep tendon reflexes or plantar response

10. Slow shuffling steps; loss of automatic arm swing

- Diagnostic Tests/Findings

    1. None specific to Parkinson's disease

    2. As indicated to rule out toxins

    3. As indicated to rule out differential diagnoses

- Management/Treatment

    1. Levodopa/carbidopa 25/100 or sustained release form 50/200 t.i.d.

        a. Improves all clinical features but does not halt progression

        b. Contraindicated in:

            (1) Narrow angle glaucoma

            (2) Psychotic illness

            (3) Patients taking monoamine oxidase A inhibitors

        c. Use caution with malignant melanoma or active ulcer disease

    2. Dopamine agonists—stimulate dopamine receptors in brain; may be used as monotherapy or in combination with levodopa/carbidopa

        a. Ropinirole 0.25 mg to 3 mg t.i.d.—adverse effects include orthostatic hypotension, syncope, hallucinations

        b. Pramipexole 1.5 mg to 6 mg daily—adverse effects include orthostatic hypotension, hallucinations, somnolence, nausea, vomiting

        c. Bromocriptine 1.25 mg b.i.d. titrate to symptom improvement—contraindicated in:

            (1) History of mental illnes

            (2) Recent myocardial infarction

            (3) Peripheral vascular disease

            (4) Bleeding ulcers

    3. Catechol-o-methyl transferase (COMT) inhibitors

        a. Tolcapone 100 to 200 mg t.i.d.

    b. Inhibits enzyme that breaks down levodopa

    c. Should be used with levodopa

    d. Use cautiously in patients with liver desease, particularly women

4. Selegiline 5 mg b.i.d with breakfast and lunch with Levodopa

    a. Clinical responses not consistent

    b. Evidence that it arrests the progression of disease requires it be considered for patients with early disease or mild forms

5. Anticholinergics to alleviate tremor and rigidity

    a. Benztropine mesylate 1 to 6 mg daily

    b. Trihexyphenidyl 6 to 20 mg daily

    c. Biperiden 2 to 12 mg daily

    d. Poorly tolerated by elderly; side effects include:

        (1) Urinary retention

        (2) Increased intraocular pressure

        (3) Dysrhythmia

        (4) Constiption

    e. Contraindicated in:

        (1) Narrow angle glaucoma

        (2) Prostatic hypertrophy

        (3) Obstructive gastrointestinal disease

6. Amantadine 100 mg b.i.d.

    a. Mode of action unclear

    b. Improves clinical features in mild disease

    c. Side effects include confusion, depression, restlessness, hypotension and cardiac abnormalities

7. Physical therapy and speech therapy may be helpful

8. Surgical thalamotomy or pallidotomy a consideration for those with severe disease and medication intolerance

Multiple Sclerosis

- Definition
    1. Pathological focal areas of demyelination with reactive gliosis scattered in white matter of brain and in optic nerve; single lesions cannot explain clinical findings
    2. Months or years may pass between initial symptom appearance and recurrence or exacerbation, but eventually progressive disability usually results
    3. Less commonly, symptoms worsen steadily from onset and disability occurs early
- Etiology/Incidence
    1. Cause unknown
    2. May be familial incidence
    3. Association with HLA-DR2 antigen suggests genetic predisposition
    4. Immunological basis suspected
    5. Greatest incidence in young adults—onset usually < 55 years of age
    6. More common in persons of Western European descent
    7. Certain factors may trigger exacerbation
        a. Pregnancy and postpartum period
        b. Infection
        c. Trauma
- Signs and Symptoms
    1. Weakness, numbness, tingling or unsteadiness in a limb
    2. Spastic paraparesis
    3. Diplopia
    4. Disequilibrium
    5. Urinary urgency or hesitancy
    6. Vertigo
    7. Sphincter disturbance

- Differential Diagnosis

    1. Anxiety

    2. Brain tumor

    3. Spinal cord lesion

    4. Neurosyphilis

    5. Systemic lupus erythematosus

    6. Metastatic carcinoma

- Physical Findings

    1. Optic atrophy

    2. Nystagmus

    3. Ataxia

    4. Dysarthria

    5. Muscle weakness

    6. Decreased vibratory sense

    7. Hyperactive deep tendon reflexes

    8. Positive Babinski with clonus

    9. Sensory deficits in some or all limbs

- Diagnostic Tests/Findings

    1. Definitive diagnosis cannot be based on laboratory findings alone

    2. Diagnostic tests as indicated to rule out other causes of symptoms

    3. Mild lymphocytosis

    4. Cerebrospinal fluid abnormalities

        a. Slightly elevated protein

        b. Elevated IgG

        c. Discrete bands of IgG called oligoclonal bands—presence of oligoclonal bands not specific but supportive

    5. Magnetic resonance imaging (MRI) preferred to computerized axial tomography (CT) scan

        a. Demonstrates multiplicity of lesions

    b. Rule out surgically treatable lesions

    c. Visualize foramen magnum to rule out Arnold-Chiari malformation

    d. Neurophysiological assessment of electrocerebral responses to evaluate subclinical involvement of cerebral pathways

- Management/Treatment

  1. No definitive method of arresting disease process, but areas of investigation include:

    a. Immunosuppressive therapy

    b. Plasmaphoresis

    c. Beta interferon used in relapsing-remitting form of disease

    d. Cop 1 (a random polymer-stimulating myelin basic protein) may be helpful to patients with relapsing-remitting form

  2. Methylprednisolone 1 g intravenously for three days followed by prednisone 80 mg daily for one week then tapered for 2 to 3 weeks

    a. May hasten recovery from acute exacerbation

    b. Does not improve the extent of recovery

    c. Does not slow progression of disease

  3. Treatment of urinary retention

    a. Various pharmacologic options to stimulate urination

    b. Intermittent self-catheterization

    c. In-dwelling foley catheter last option

  4. Diazepam and carbamazepine may relieve paresthesias

  5. Antidepressant medications may relieve fatigue

  6. Rest/activity balance

  7. Treatment of constipation

    a. High fiber diet

    b. Stool softeners/laxatives as indicated

  8. Emotional support/patient teaching

    a. Sexual dysfunction may be a problem

b. Other social/intimacy issues

    (1) Questions regarding marriage

    (2) Questions regarding having children

9. Avoidance of triggers

Questions
Select the best answer

1. The most commonly diagnosed headache is:

   a. Tension
   b. Toxic
   c. Common migraine
   d. Classic migraine

2. Which of the following causes of headache is a medical emergency?

   a. Toxic headache
   b. Classic migraine
   c. Subarachnoid hemorrhage
   d. Subdural hematoma

3. Headache can be a symptom of any variety of medical conditions, as in the case of a structural lesion, or it can be the primary manifestation of a condition as in tension headache. A systematic and thorough assessment of the headache is important in making the appropriate diagnosis. Which of the following components of headache assessment is the most important?

   a. Presence of associated symptoms
   b. Chronology of headache
   c. Presence of triggers
   d. Age of onset

4. Your patient describes a headache that is quite painful and vise-like in quality. The pain is generalized about the head, and lasts for several hours at a time. There does not appear to be an aura, and the patient does not report any symptoms suggestive of focal neurological deficits. Based upon your knowledge of headache evaluation, you know that the most likely diagnosis is:

   a. Cluster headache
   b. Common migraine
   c. Tension headache
   d. Hypertensive headache

5. Migraine and cluster headache are both extremely painful headache syndromes that may be difficult to differentiate. Based on known epidemiological patterns, who is most likely to suffer from migraines?

   a. A 45-year-old male with history of excess alcohol use

b. A 35-year-old female with history of excess alcohol use
c. A 19-year-old female with family history of migraine
d. A 24-year-old male with family history of migraine

6. Excess release of serotonin is proposed as possible etiological factor in:

   a. Migraine headache
   b. Seizure disorder
   c. Parkinson's disease
   d. Multiple sclerosis

7. Which of the following is not typically a trigger of migraine headache?

   a. Menstruation
   b. Excess sleep
   c. Changes in weather
   d. Loud noise

8. Space occupying lesions, subarachnoid hemorrhage, and cerebrovascular accident are all differential diagnoses of migraine headache. If there is any question as to the etiology of the pain, the most appropriate diagnostic intervention would be:

   a. Cerebral arteriogram
   b. Doppler ultrasound of the carotid artery
   c. Complete bloodcount
   d. Computerized axial tomography (CT)

9. When a new diagnosis of migraine is being considered a variety of baseline studies must be performed to rule out an organic cause of the pain. Which of the following would suggest an organic cause of the pain?

   a. Cortical atrophy by CT scan
   b. Elevated erythrocyte sedimentation rate
   c. WBCs $6,000 \times 10^6$/L, Hgb 14.2 g/dL, Hct 43%, Platelets 300,000/μL
   d. Na+ 140 mEq/L, K+ 3.2 mEq/L, Cl 104 mEq/L, CO_2 mEq/L, BUN 11 mg/dL, Cr 0.9 mg/dL

10. Propranolol is a pharmacologic agent used in the prophylactic management of migraine, but there are several contraindications to its use. In which of the following patients is propranolol not contraindicated?

    a. A 40-year-old man with emphysema
    b. A 39-year-old man with angina

c. A 32-year-old woman with type 1 DM

d. A 24-year-old man with severe depression

11. Amitriptyline is an antidepressant medication that can be useful in the prophylactic management of migraine headache. Which of the following statements is true regarding amitriptyline therapy for migraine prophylaxis?

    a. It is the only antidepressant that is useful in migraine prophylaxis
    b. Improvement is usually seen in 2-4 weeks
    c. It is contraindicated in severe depression
    d. It has less side effects than paroxetine

12. Cluster headache is among the most painful of all pain inducing conditions. Acute attacks are difficult to manage. Which of the following therapies is known to be effective only in the case of cluster headache?

    a. Oxygen
    b. Butalbital
    c. Naproxen
    d. Verapamil

13. Many headache inducing conditions are difficult to diagnose because there are no associated physical exam findings. Ptosis, eyelid edema, conjunctival injection and ipsilateral nasal congestion are findings associated with:

    a. Classic migraine
    b. Toxic headache
    c. Narrow angle glaucoma
    d. Cluster headache

14. Tapered corticosteroids are a recommended prophylactic regimen in the treatment of:

    a. Cluster headache
    b. Tension headache
    c. Migraine headache
    d. Subdural hematoma

15. Which of the following is diagnostic criteria for transient ischemic attack?

    a. Numbness or parasthesia with motor deficits
    b. Symptoms resolve in < 24 hours
    c. Symptoms include homonymous hemianopsia
    d. Lacunar infarct on CT scan

16. Medical management of transient ischemic attack (T.I.A.) is aimed toward preventing further attacks and subsequent cerebrovascular accident (CVA). When atrial fibrillation is discovered during the clinical examination, therapy of T.I.A. should include:

    a. Aspririn 325 mg daily
    b. Heparin infusion at 1000 u/hr
    c. Ticlopidine 250 mg b.i.d.
    d. Verapamil 80 mg b.i.d.

17. When is ticlopidine preferred in the management of T.I.A.?

    a. When the patient is intolerant of aspirin
    b. When cardiac emboli is suspected
    c. When heparin has been administered for 5 to 7 days
    d. When the patient is dysrhythmic

18. The most common cause of seizure disorder in the elderly population is?

    a. Congenital abnormalities
    b. Renal failure
    c. Neurosyphilis
    d. Vascular disease

19. A seizure that consists of focal motor symptoms, autonomic symptoms, no loss of consciousness and lasts approximately one minute is most likely a:

    a. Petit mal seizure
    b. Myoclonic seizure
    c. Simple partial seizure
    d. Complex partial seizure

20. Which type of seizure is almost exclusively found in children and young adults?

    a. Myoclonic
    b. Simple partial
    c. Absence
    d. Tonic-clonic

21. Postepileptic automatism is characterized by:

    a. More tonic clonic attacks with periods of consciousness in between
    b. Headache, disorientation and nausea

    c. More tonic clonic attacks without periods of consciousness in between

    d. Abnormal behavior in the immediate postictal period

22. The most important information in seizure assessment is usually provided by

    a. An eyewitness

    b. An electroencephelogram (EEG)

    c. A CT scan

    d. Magnetic resonance imaging (MRI)

23. Initial evaluation of all patients over 10 years of age who present with seizure disorder should not include which of the following?

    a. Serum glucose

    b. Syphilis serology

    c. Renal function tests

    d. Sleep study

24. An EEG is helpful in the evaluation of seizure disorder for several reasons. Which of the following is not accomplished with an EEG?

    a. Classification of the disorder

    b. Etiology of the disorder

    c. Localization of the epileptogenic source

    d. Support of clinical diagnosis

25. The drug of choice for acute seizure management includes:

    a. Phenytoin

    b. Clonazepam

    c. Lorazepam

    d. Valproic acid

26. Phenytoin is not indicated for which type of seizure?

    a. Tonic-clonic

    b. Absence

    c. Simple partial

    d. Complex partial

27. When is it appropriate to withdraw seizure medication?

    a. When the patient is pregnant

    b. When the patient has been seizure free for four years

c. When the patient is an alcoholic

d. When the patient has untreatable pathology

28. The most common cause of Parkinsonism is:

    a. Postencephalitic
    b. Manganese dust
    c. Exposure to toxins
    d. Idiopathic

29. Immobile face with wide palpebral fissures is a common physical finding in the patient with:

    a. Absence seizure
    b. Depression
    c. Multiple sclerosis
    d. Parkinson's disease

30. Amantadine improves clinical features of mild parkinsonism but has several side effects. Which of the following is not a side effect of amantadine?

    a. Urinary retention
    b. Restlessness
    c. Hypotension
    d. Cardiac abnormalities

31. Which of the following is true regarding the use of corticosteroids in treating multiple sclerosis?

    a. It hastens recovery from exacerbation
    b. It improves the extent of recovery
    c. It slows progression of the disease
    d. It relieves paresthesias

Answers

1. a	11. b	21. d
2. c	12. a	22. a
3. b	13. d	23. d
4. c	14. a	24. b
5. c	15. b	25. c
6. a	16. b	26. b
7. d	17. a	27. b
8. d	18. d	28. d
9. b	19. c	29. d
10. b	20. c	30. a
		31. a

Bibliography

Allen, T. G. (1997). Seizure disorders: A primary care guide. *Advance for Nurse Practitioners, 5*(10), 32-34, 40, 66.

Aminoff, M. J. (1998). Nervous system. In L.M. Tierney, Jr., S.J. McPhee, & M.A. Papadakis (Eds.). *Current medical diagnosis and treatment* (37th ed., pp. 916-972). Stamford, CT: Appleton & Lange.

Bergman, G. D., Saper, J. R., & Solomon, G. D. (1996). Chronic headache: Management strategies that make sense. *Patient Care, 30*(2), 54-66.

Brodie, M. J., & Dichter, M. A. (1996). Drug therapy: Antiepileptic drugs. *New England Journal of Medicine, 334*(3), 168-175.

Cusack, T. (1996). Multiple sclerosis: Clues to diagnosis and recommended management recertification series. *Physician Assistant, 20*(10), 24, 27-28, 37-39.

Fenstermacher, K., & Hudson, B. (1997). *Practice guidelines for family nurse practitioners.* Philadelphia: W. B. Saunders Company.

Fischer, J. H., French, J., & Leppik, I. E. (1996). Making the most of new seizure treatments. *Patient Care, 30*(1), 53-54, 56, 61-63.

Haider, A., Tuchek, J. M., & Haider, S. (1996). Seizure control: How to use the new antiepileptic drugs in older patients. *Geriatrics, 51*(9), 42-45.

Hely, M. A., & Morris, J. G. L. (1996). Controversies in the treatment of parkinson's disease. *Current Opinions in Neurology, 9*(4), 308-313.

Jones, J. M. (1996). Treating acute pain in the desperate headacher. *Journal of the American Academy of Physician Assistants, 9*(3), 26-28, 33-36, 44.

Psychosocial Disorders

Sister Maria Salerno

Depression (Major)

- Definition: A clinical syndrome consisting of physical, affective, and cognitive symptoms that range from mild to severe, commonly categorized as:
    1. Adjustment Disorder with Depressed Mood
        a. Occurring within three months of an identifiable stressor
        b. Depressed mood and impairment of function or symptoms in excess of those normally expected
        c. Symptoms ease as stressor passes
        d. Often self limiting but can lead to major depression
    2. Major Depression (MD)
        a. Five of nine symptoms are present continuously during the same two week period
            (1) Presence of depressed mood, OR
            (2) Anhedonia (loss of interest or pleasure in most all activities most of the day) with:
                (a) Increased or decreased appetite or significant weight loss or gain—more than 5% of body weight in a month
                (b) Sleep disturbance—hypersomnia or insomnia
                (c) Psychomotor agitation or retardation
                (d) Fatigue or loss of energy
                (e) Feelings of worthlessness or inappropriate guilt or low-self-esteem
                (f) Decreased ability to think, concentrate or make decisions
                (g) Recurrent thoughts of death, suicidal ideation without an attempt or specific plan (American Psychiatric Association, 1994)
        b. The symptoms represent a change from previous functioning and are severe and disabling
        c. The onset is variable and may be superimposed on Dysthymia

3. Dysthymia (chronic depression)

   a. Milder than MD

      (1) Depressed mood

      (2) At least two other symptoms

      (3) Loss of self esteem prominent

   b. Poor coping skills

   c. Often associated with chronic drug use

   d. More chronic—symptoms present for two years or more

   e. No clear onset

4. Depressive Disorder Not Otherwise Specified (NOS)

   a. Depressed mood and 2 to 4 moderate to severe symptoms

   b. Does not meet criteria for MD or Dysthymia

   c. Includes several sub-categories

      (1) Atypical Depression—characterized by:

         (a) Hypersomnia

         (b) Hyperphagia

         (c) Lethargy

         (d) Rejection sensitivity

      (2) Seasonal Affective Disorder

         (a) Disturbance of circadian rhythm

         (b) Related to light spectrum exposure

         (c) Carbohydrate craving, lethargy, hyperphagia, and hypersomnia are characteristic

      (3) Premenstrual Dysphoric Disorder—symptoms occur year round during the late luteal phase of the cycle

      (4) Prenatal and Post-Partum Depressions

         (a) 10 to 15% accompanied by obsessive concerns about ability to care for infant or fear of doing harm to the infant

         (b) Usually occurs 2 weeks to 6 months postpartum

5. Bipolar Disorder—recurrent episodes of depression interspersed with bouts of mania

   a. Heredity a strong factor

   b. Tricyclic antidepressants (TCA) often precipitate a manic response called "hypomania"

   c. Early onset, usually before age 30

   d. Incidence in African-Americans and Whites similar

   e. Incidence is similar in males and females

6. Organic Mood Syndrome—major depressive episode associated with a general medical condition or medications (see Table 1); examples include:

   a. Substance abuse (alcoholism is a common cause)

   b. Endocrinopathy, e.g., hypothyroidism, Cushing's disease, Addison's disease

   c. Neurological disorders—left sided stroke, Parkinsonism

   d. Pancreatic cancer

   e. Antihypertensives

- Etiology/Incidence

   1. Psychosocial and/or biochemical causes for depression have been theorized

      a. Psychosocial

         (1) Psychoanalytical

            (a) Anger turned inward

            (b) Regression to a less mature stage of functioning

         (2) Environmental

            (a) Stressful life events

            (b) Changes or inadequacies in social support

         (3) Psychodynamic

            (a) Personality development

               (i) Passive/dependent

Table 1

Some Medications and Medical Conditions Which Cause Depressive Symptoms

Anemias
Cardiovascular
    Congestive heart failure
    Hypertension
    Myocardial infarction
    Stroke
Neurological
    Brain tumors
    Dementia
    Parkinsonism
    Multiple sclerosis
    Seizure disorders
Endocrinopathies
    Addison's disease
    Cushing's syndrome
    Diabetes mellitus
    Thyroid disorders
Electrolyte imbalances
Malignancies
    Pancreatic cancer
    Lymphomas
Other
    Chronic fatigue syndrome
    Chronic obstructive pulmonary disease
    Chronic pain
    Hepatitis
    Substance abuse/stimulant withdrawal
    Rheumatoid arthritis
    Renal disease
Medications
    Anabolic steroid withdrawal
    Analgesics
    Antihypertensives (methyldopa, reserpine, clonidine)
    Antitubercular
    Benzodiazepines
    Barbiturates
    Chemotherapeutic agents
    Corticosteroids
    Levo-dopa
    Withdrawal of psychostimulants (amphetamines, cocaine)
    Analgesics

        (ii)   Obsessive/compulsive

    (b)   Effects of past relationships and developmental task on coping styles, particularly use of defense mechanisms

        (i)   Denial

                       (ii)   Suppression

                       (iii) Sublimation

        (4)   Cognitive

            (a)   Self-reinforcing habit of unrealistic negative ideas

            (b)   Recent or past style of thinking and relating

            (c)   Learned "helplessness"

   b.   Biochemical

      (1)   Catecholamine

         (a)   Poorly functioning neurotransmitter

         (b)   Primarily dopamine, norepinephrine, epinephrine, and serotonin

      (2)   Endocrine

         (a)   Cortisol

         (b)   Thyroid releasing hormone

2.   Incidence

   a.   Depressive illness most common mental health problem seen in general practice

   b.   Estimated 9 to 16 million Americans suffer from depressive illness, yet fewer than a third will receive treatment

   c.   Twice as many women as men with major depression worldwide

   d.   Lifetime risk for developing depressive illness

      (1)   20% for females

      (2)   10% for males

   e.   Major depression can occur in any age group

      (1)   Adolescents and the elderly at higher risk

      (2)   Other risk factors

         (a)   Family history of depressive illness, alcoholism, or major medical illness

         (b)   Prior depressive episode

         (c)   Being post partum

         (d)   Unanticipated or prolonged stress

   f.   Major depression has a 50% to 85% recurrence rate within three to nine years

- Signs and Symptoms

   1.   None specific

       a.   Aggravation of any physical pathology

       b.   Pains of undetermined etiology in a variety of anatomical sites

   2.   Mnemonic device to recall major symptoms—IN SAD CAGES

       a.   *I*nterest—loss of interest or pleasure in just about any activity

       b.   *S*leep disturbances

          (1)   Hypersomnia or insomnia

          (2)   Early morning awakenings with painful ruminations

       c.   *A*ppetite change/weight change

       d.   *D*epressed mood

          (1)   Tends to be most pervasive symptom

          (2)   May manifest as crying spells

       e.   *C*oncentration poor; indecisiveness, inability to act, procrastination

       f.   *A*ctivity—agitation or retardation

       g.   *G*uilt/low self-esteem

       h.   *E*nergy loss/fatigue

       i.   *S*uicidal ideation, thoughts of death, suicide attempts

- Differential Diagnosis

   1.   Since depression may be a manifestation of many illnesses the differential diagnosis must include a thorough search for factors or organic diseases which may be responsible for symptom manifestation including:

       a.   Infections, inflammation

       b.   Neurological neoplasms, stroke, trauma

      c.   Endocrine disorders

      d.   Nutritional deficiencies

      e.   Electrolyte disturbances

  2.   Differentiate major depression from other mental disorders, e.g., schizophrenia, dementia, adjustment disorder with depressed mood

  3.   Currently the trend is to address the signs and symptoms of major depression; if criteria presented previously are met the diagnosis is made regardless of co-morbidity

- Physical Findings

  1.   General—may show lack of personal grooming and hygiene, inattention to dress, slouched posture, slowed speech and movements, long pauses in response to questions, tearfulness; weight may be less than or more than ideal for body size, may appear dehydrated

  2.   Mental status—poor concentration, decreased memory, indecision, pessimism

- Diagnostic Tests/Findings

  1.   Initial tests

      a.   CBC—normal

      b.   Chemical profile including liver function—normal

      c.   Urinalysis and urine toxicology screen—normal

      d.   Thyroid function—normal

      e.   VDRL—normal

      f. B_{12} level—normal

      g.   EKG—normal

      h.   Chest radiograph—normal

      i.   In first or second episode

          (1)   Computer tomography (CT) scan or magnetic resonance image (MRI) of the brain—normal

          (2)   HIV screen—normal

  2.   Depression screening instruments—scores indicative of depression

      a.   Beck Depression Inventory

    b.   Yesavage Geriatric Depression Scale

    c.   Zung Self-Rating Depression Scale

3.   Special tests (primarily used in psychiatric and research settings)

    a.   Thyroid stimulating hormone (TSH) response to thyroid releasing hormone (TRH) may be decreased

    b.   Dexamethasone suppression test (DST) used to distinguish between major and minor depression

    c.   EEG sleep profile—may show reduction in REM sleep

    d.   Platelet monoamine oxidase (MAO) activity—increased

    e.   Biogenic amines (norepinephrine, serotonin)—increased levels

- Management/Treatment

1.   General considerations

    a.   Assess degree of problem related to daily functioning

    b.   Refer those with evidence of:

        (1)   Hallucinations, delusions

        (2)   Loss of contact with reality

        (3)   Suicidal thoughts, wishes, tendencies (see section on suicide)

2.   Mild depression (no clear criteria but general functional status tends to be high)

    a.   Structured monitoring with weekly appointments with phone contact for backup

    b.   Use therapeutic communication skills to:

        (1)   Encourage verbalization, clarification of feelings and fears, as well as relationship of feelings to specific events if known

        (2)   Assess and discuss losses that have occurred and their meaning

        (3)   Help correct cognitive errors in thinking

    c.   Use crisis or social skills models to teach and promote more effective coping strategies

      (1)   Help client recognize need for and identify alternative coping methods

      (2)   Encourage interaction with other people

      (3)   Encourage planned, regular physical activity

      (4)   Teach relaxation techniques

      (5)   Provide client with anticipatory guidance regarding feelings and usual course of the problem, e.g., gradual improvement and abatement of symptoms

  d.   Provide consistency and caring, avoiding a judgmental or blaming attitude

  e.   Reinforce positive behaviors

  f.   Avoid actions or response that could be interpreted as punishment

  g.   Consult with physician or psychiatrist regarding psychotherapy and use of antidepressants; both have been shown to be of help in mild depression; see Tables 2 and 3

3.   Moderate to severe depression

  a.   Hospitalization of those thought to:

      (1)   Be a potential danger to self or others; unable to meet basic needs; suicidal ideation or behavior

      (2)   Have impaired cognition or judgment

      (3)   Need skilled observation for diagnosis, assessment, or monitoring of therapy

      (4)   Have inadequate social supports for outpatient treatment

  b.   Antidepressant and/or antianxiety medications; most appropriate initial therapy for reasonably healthy individual; see Tables 2 and 3

      (1)   Those with delusions, hallucinations, profound psychomotor retardation less responsive

      (2)   Only 65% have complete remission with any one drug

      (3)   No concrete evidence that any one is more efficacious than another

Table 2

Antidepressants

Drug Name	Anticholinergic Effect	Sedative Effect	Orthostatic Hypotension	Cardiac Conduction	Adult dose range per day (mg)[a]
Tertiary tricyclics					
Amitriptyline	+4	+4	+4	+4	25–300
Clomipramine	+3	+2	+3	+3	25–250
Doxepine	+3	+4	+4	+2	25–300
Imipramine	+3	+2	+4	+4	25–300
Trimipramine	+3	+4	+3	+4	25–300
Secondary Tricyclics					
Amoxapine	+3	+2	+1	+2	50–600
Desipramine	+2	+2	+2	+3	25–300
Nortriptyline	+2	+3	+1	+3	25–250
Protriptyline	+2	+1	+4	+4	15–60
Tetracyclics					
Maprotiline	+2	+4	+2	+3	50–225
Mirtazapine	+3	+2	+2	+2	15–45
Others					
Alprazolam[b]	0	0	0	0	5–6
Buproprion	0	0	0	+1	100–450
Nefazodone	0	+3	+2	0/+1	200–600
Trazadone	0	+4	+4	+1	50–600
Venlafaxine	+1	0	0	+1	75–375
Selective Serotonin Reuptake Inhibitors (SSRI)					
Fluoxetine	0	0	0	0	20–80
Fluvoxamine	0	0	0	0	50–300
Sertraline	0/+1	0	0	0	50–200
Paroxetine	+1	0	0	0	20–50
Monoamine Oxidase Inhibitors (MAO)					
Phenelzine	+1	+1	+1	+3	45–90
Tranylcypromine	0	+1	+1	+2	30–60

Note: Data derived from Bhatia & Bhatia, 1997; Eisendrath, 1997; Pinkowish, 1997; Sussman & Stahl, 1997.
[a]Generally lower doses are recommended for adolescents and the elderly
[b]Only benzodiazepine approved for depression

(4) Choice based on predominant symptoms, side effects, cost, and complexity of dosing—affect compliance

(5) Most will respond within three weeks of reaching therapeutic levels

(6) Continue medication full 6 to 12 months after complete remission of symptoms

(7) When drugs are discontinued taper over 6 to 8 weeks

(8) Long term prophylaxis—full treatment dosage for those with recurrent episodes (at least three)

(9) Some controversy regarding efficacy in Minor Depression, Dysthymia, and Adjustment Disorder

(10) Heterocyclics (tricyclics, tetracyclics, and others)

   (a) Major advantage over newer agents is cost

   (b) Start with low dose and build to therapeutic level

   (c) Plasma levels provide crude indication of compliance with regimen

   (d) May require up to three weeks at therapeutic levels before effects are noticed

   (e) Side effects—anticholinergic, antihistaminic, antiadrenergic, and quinidine-like (except trazadone) effects

   (f) Among tricyclics, desipramine and nortriptyline are least anticholinergic, sedating, and least likely to cause postural hypotension

   (g) Among heterocyclics, trazodone lacks conduction problems and anticholinergic effects, but very sedating; also very low lethality in overdose

   (h) Dispense in small amounts; 10 day supply in many cases can be lethal

(11) Newer agents include the serotonin reuptake inhibitors (SSRI) and the phenylaminoketones

   (a) Relatively safe for use in elderly

   (b) Do not cause postural hypotension

    (c)   Little if any effect on cardiac conduction

    (d)   Do not have antihistaminic effects

    (e)   With the exception of paroxetine do not have anti-cholinergic effects

    (f)   Starting dose may be effective treatment dose

    (g)   SSRI all inhibit cytochrome P-450 system in the liver; must monitor for potential toxicity of other drugs such as anticonvulsants, digitalis, and coumadin

    (h)   Buproprion has no effect on liver enzymes, and does not cause sexual side effects common to other antidepressants

    (i)   Side effects of anxiety, insomnia, agitation with newer agents may require concomittant use of sedating antihistamine, antidepressant, or anxiolytic

    (j)   Pharmacokinetic differences in the elderly can lead to toxicity or efficacy at lower than expected doses

  c. Psychotherapy

  d. Electroconvulsive therapy (ECT)

    (1)   More rapid improvement than with pharmacologic agents

    (2)   Indicated for severely depressed or suicidal persons for whom pharmacologic agents are contraindicated or ineffective

    (3)   Barbiturates and muscle relaxants used prior to the procedure

    (4)   Confusion, headache, temporary amnesia lasting one to two weeks are common side effects in about 40%; may be clinically apparent up to one month

    (5)   Avoided in persons with brain tumor, recent (three months) MI, CVA, or perforated viscus repair

  e. Other options include exercise and light therapy

Table 3

Antidepressants and Anti-Anxiety Medications: Contraindications and Precautions

Drug Group	Contraindications	Precautions
Antidepressants		
Tricyclics	Acute M.I., hypersensitivity; concurrent administration of MAO inhibitors	In patients with urinary retention; prostatic hypertrophy; narrow angle glaucoma, convulsive disorders; cardiovascular disease; thyroid disease; pregnant patients
MAO inhibitors	Hypertension, cardiovascular disease, headaches, liver disease or advanced renal disease, concurrent use of a tricyclic; schizophrenia	Safety during pregnancy not established; avoid fermented foods, pickles, cheeses, red wine, beer, fava beans, raisins, chocolate; cold remedies, weight reduction meds, e.g., anything with tyramine
Lithium Carbonate	Significant renal disease, dietary salt restriction; cardiovascular disease; brain damage	Use caution with pregnant patients; elderly; patient who is breast feeding; persons with thyroid disease; mild renal and cardiovascular disease; epilepsy
Anti-anxiety Drugs		
Benzodiazepines	Glaucoma, hypersensitivity	Use caution if hx of allergies; psychological addiction to these drugs; hepatic or renal impairment; lower dose for elderly or breast feeding mothers
Carbamazepine	Severe renal, cardiovascular, or liver disease	Use with caution if liver, renal disease, or blood dyscrasias
SSRI[a]	Do not administer with MAO inhibitors or with tryptophan supplements	Caution in persons with history of seizures; impaired renal or hepatic function; mania or hypomania; in pregnant or nursing women; in the elderly

[a]Selective Serotinin Uptake Inhibitors

4. Client education

   a. Disease course, expected outcomes, and usual treatment modalities

   b. Purpose, dosage, side effects of medication

      (1) Improvement in symptoms not evident for 3 to 4 weeks

      (2) Importance of adhering to prescribed pharmacologic regimen; avoid abrupt discontinuation of medications

      (3) Caution against concomitant use of over-the-counter preparations

      (4) Interactions with food or other medications; see Table 3

5. Persons with major depression should be followed at least weekly for first 6 to 8 weeks, preferably by a mental health professional for medication adjustment and brief psychotherapeutic support

6. Persons known to be on antidepressants or receiving care for depression, who are being seen for other reasons should be routinely checked for:

   a. Suicidal feelings, plans, intentions, risks

   b. Tremor, blurred vision, dry mouth, tachycardia, postural hypotension

Suicide

- Definition

  1. The intentional taking of one's own life

  2. Usually described as:

     a. Attempted—unsuccessful conscious attempt to take one's own life

     b. Threatened—verbal or physical indication of intent for self-destruction

     c. Ideation—thoughts or behaviors indicating conscious intent for self-destruction

- Etiology/Incidence

  1. Often a manifestation or complication of depressive illness or anxiety states

  2. About 15% of depressed patients commit suicide

  3. Risk factors include:

     a. Sudden crisis or loss

     b. Destructive coping mechanisms

     c. Few or no significant others

     d. Poor social or personal resources

     e. Past suicide attempts or family history of suicide

     f. Previous psychotic problems

     g. Unstable life style

     h. Specific plan

     i. Substance abuse

4. Eight of 10 persons who state an intent to commit suicide do so; risk for depressed patients is greatest during the first month of treatment when the individual begins to feel better and has more energy

5. In the U.S. women attempt suicide more often, but men are three times as likely to succeed; in elderly, suicide among males outnumber those among women

    a. Female rates peak at age 55

    b. Male rates peak at age 75

6. Adolescents and white males over the age of 45 have a higher incidence rate; second leading cause of death in adolescent

7. In adolescents increased risk has been associated with:

    a. Extreme parental control or permissiveness

    b. Loss of communication with parents and teachers

    c. Hostility and difficulty in school or with the law

    d. Lack of social supports (peers, social, work, and school)

- Signs and Symptoms

    1. Feelings of worthlessness and/or helplessness

    2. Preoccupation with a dead relative or friend

    3. Excessive denial, indignation, or anger in response to being questioned about suicide

    4. Verbalization of a plan or rehearsal of a plan

    5. Sudden mood elevation in a depressed patient often accompanied by more energy and calmer, more placid manner

    6. Giving possessions away

    7. Setting affairs in order

    8. Making a will

    9. Presence of hallucinations or delusions

    10. Intuition on the part of the health professional

    11. In adolescents these may be more prominent

        a. Taking excessive risks

        b. Self-destructive behaviors, e.g., drug abuse, accident proneness

    c.   Negative self-concept

    d.   Expression of wish to die

    e.   Withdrawal from family and persons

    f.   Increased interest and companionship with animal/pets

12.   All depressed clients need to be asked about suicide. If client does not volunteer information, ask directly about thoughts of taking their own life. Also ask direct questions to elicit information about a plan, its lethality, and any mental or actual rehearsals of the plan. Risk is highest if planned in 24 hours; low or moderate if planned for a later time

    a.   Presence of five or more risk factors constitutes high risk

    b.   Mnemonic device to recall risk factors—SAD PERSONS

        (1)   *S*ex

        (2)   *A*ge

        (3)   *D*epression

        (4)   *P*revious attempt

        (5)   *E*thanol abuse

        (6)   *R*ational thinking diminished

        (7)   *S*ocial support loss or absence

        (8)   *O*rganized plan

        (9)   *N*o spouse

      (10)   *S*ick

- Differential Diagnosis

   1.   Depression with melancholic features

   2.   Depression with seasonal pattern (seasonal affective disorder)

   3.   Organic disease

- Physical Findings

   1.   No specific physical findings, however those of depression may be evident

    a.   General appearance—unkempt, slumped or stooped posture, slow speech pattern, lack of expression or dejected look or agitation, hostility, tremulousness

   b. Mental status—disorientation, poor concentration, agitation, hallucinations or delusions

  2. Old scars or evidence of injury from past attempts or high risk behaviors

- Diagnostic Tests/Findings: There are no specific laboratory tests. See Diagnostic Tests/Findings in section on Depression

- Management/Treatment

  1. Treatment usually includes hospitalization with psychotherapy, antidepressant medications, and/or ECT; see previous section on Management and Treatment of Depression

  2. If a client is deemed suicidal or if there is concern about the client's potential for suicide, do not leave the client alone but obtain immediate psychiatric consultation

Anxiety

- Definition

  1. An unpleasant feeling of dread, apprehension, foreboding, or tension resulting from an unexpected threat to one's feelings of self-esteem or well-being

  2. Major categories

   a. Generalized Anxiety Disorder—unrealistic or excessive anxiety and worry about life circumstance

   b. Panic Disorders—unfounded morbid dread of seemingly harmless object or situation often leads to agoraphobia

   c. Obsessive Compulsive Disorder (OCD)—repetitive thoughts (obsession) that a person is unable to control and/or urge to perform an act that cannot be resisted without great difficulty (compulsion), and which interferes with functional abilities

   d. Post-traumatic Stress Disorder (PTSD)—delayed (at least six months) anxiety after a severe trauma often perceived as a threat to physical integrity or self-concept; intrusive thoughts, flashbacks, and nightmares form the symptomatic triad

   e. Other categories include adjustment disorder with anxious mood, simple and social phobias; refer to psychiatric or major primary care text for detailed discussion

- Etiology/Incidence

    1. Various theories related to etiology include:

        a. Psychodynamic

            (1) Freudian—conflict between id and superego; ego not strong enough to resolve the conflict

            (2) Sullivanian—fear of disapproval from mother figure; conditional love leads to fragile ego, lack of self-confidence, lack of self-esteem, fear of failure

            (3) Dollar and Miller—learned response to innate drive to avoid pain; anxiety the result of two competing drives or goals

        b. Biologic

            (1) Genetic influence with high family incidence

            (2) Autonomic nervous system response—fight or flight mechanism

            (3) Biologic abnormalities of neurotransmitter receptors in the central nervous system, particularly gamma aminobutyric acid (GABA) receptors

        c. Family dynamics

            (1) Individual with dysfunctional behavior is representative of family system problems

            (2) Carrier of problems resulting from disrupted interrelationships

    2. Incidence

        a. Anxiety disorders occur in 10% to 15% of clients seen in health care settings

            (1) Only 1 in 4 diagnosed and treated

            (2) 3% of Americans will experience an anxiety disorder in their lifetime

            (3) Slight preponderance in woman

        b. Panic disorders

(1) Occur more frequently in women than in men

(2) Onset usually in late teens or early adulthood

(3) More common in those who have had an early traumatic event, e.g., the death of a parent

c. Obsessive compulsive disorder

(1) Most often seen in adolescence and early adulthood

(2) Males and females affected equally

(3) More frequent in upper middle class and in persons with higher levels of intellectual functioning

- Signs and Symptoms

   1. Generalized anxiety and panic attacks

      a. A feeling of tightness in the throat

      b. Difficulty breathing; feelings of suffocation

      c. Palpitations

      d. Chest tightness or pain

      e. Tachypnea, tachycardia

      f. Gastric distress or discomfort

      g. Nausea

      h. Diarrhea

      i. Feeling of weakness in lower limbs

      j. Tingling, numbness of extremities

      k. Feeling of light-headedness

      l. Dryness of the mouth

      m. Feeling of something caught in the throat

      n. Cold sweaty hands

      o. Feelings of loss of control; irritability; impatience

      p. Motor tension—shakiness, jitteriness, trembling, restlessness

      q. Anxiety insomnia, difficulty falling asleep

      r.   Symptoms of panic generally develop suddenly and have been related to mitral valve prolapse

  2. OCD

      a.   Recurrent, persistent thoughts, ideas or images experienced as intrusive

      b.   Repetitious, purposeful, intentional behaviors which are distressing, time consuming, or interfere with functioning

  3. PTSD

      a.   Intrusive thoughts, flashbacks, nightmares related to the traumatic event

      b.   Poor impulse control, unpredictability, and/or aggressiveness

      c.   Avoidance symptoms

          (1)   Avoids reminders of event

          (2)   Memory difficulty

          (3)   Detachment and restricted affect

      d.   Hyperarousal symptoms

          (1)   Hypervigilance

          (2)   Insomnia

          (3)   Irritability, poor concentration

- Differential Diagnosis

  1. Drug abuse, withdrawal, or intoxication

  2. Thyrotoxicosis

  3. Hypoglycemia

  4. Acute hypoxia

  5. Myocardial infarction

  6. Pheochromocytoma

  7. Seizure disorder

  8. Side effects of chemical agents or medications, e.g., caffeine, nicotine, antihistamines, tricyclics

- Physical Findings
  1. Between attacks may all be within normal limits
  2. During an attack
     a. General appearance—looks worried, frightened, restless
     b. Vital signs—tachycardia, increased respirations, elevated BP
     c. Integumentary—pallor, flushed face, cold clammy hands
     d. Gastrointestinal—possible loss of bowel or bladder control
     e. Mental status—hypervigilence; easy distractibility; poor concentration
     f. Motor tension—shakiness, jitteriness
- Diagnostic Tests/Findings.
  1. Serum drug analysis—negative
  2. Thyroid function tests—normal
  3. Serum glucose—normal
  4. ECG—normal
- Management/Treatment
  1. Depends on careful workup and identified anxiety subtype
  2. Obtain consult regarding testing for other emotional or physical disorders
  3. Cognitive behavioral therapy more effective for generalized anxiety than for panic attacks
     a. Assess usual coping mechanisms, life style, social supports
     b. Establish a trusting, warm, empathetic, respectful relationship
     c. Assist client to identify and describe emotional and physical feelings and to identify the relationship between them
     d. Identify patient behaviors that cause anxiety in the health care provider
     e. Use supportive confrontation as needed
     f. Keep focus of responsibility on the client

g. Encourage use of and teach or refer for relaxation techniques, biofeedback, and meditation

4. Anti-anxiety medications (see Tables 3 and 4)

   a. Most have behavioral profile similar to alcohol

   b. All have hypnotic properties

   c. All have varying potential for tolerance and physiologic dependence

   d. Benzodiazepines most widely used

      (1) Therapeutic doses usually do not result in physiologic dependence

      (2) May be misused to ''boost'' effects of methadone

   e. Antihistamines for those with COPD or potential for abuse of benzodiazepines

   f. Beta adrenergic blockers, e.g., propranolol more effective in reducing marked autonomic symptoms (tachycardia, palpations, breathlessness)

   g. Tricyclics and MAO inhibitors good for panic attacks but not for generalized anxiety

   h. Buspirone only anxiolytic not classified as a tranquilizer

      (1) Not linked to dependence or depressant effects

      (2) Does not impair motor skills

      (3) Does not potentiate alcohol effects

   i. Optimal duration of treatment not well established

5. Refer to psychiatric mental health professional for counseling and more specific therapy

6. Obtain consult regarding testing for other physical or emotional disorders

7. Patient education

   a. Disease course, expected outcome

      (1) Reassurance that anxiety rarely evolves into a more serious disorder

Table 4

Anti-anxiety Medication

Generic	Average daily dose*
Benzodiazepines (Longer acting)	
Chlordiazepoxide	15–40 mg
Clorazepate dipotassium	15–60 mg
Diazepam	4–40 mg
Halazepam	60–160 mg
Benzodiazepines (Shorter acting)	
Alprazolam	0.75–1.5 mg
Lorazepam	2–6 mg
Oxazepam	30–60 mg
Nonbenzodiazepines	
Buspirone	20–30 mg
Hydroxyzine	30–300 mg
Meprobamate	400–2000 mg
Paroxetine	40 mg
For control of aggression/and mania	
Carbamazepine	100–200 mg initially
	Increase to 400–1500 mg until serum level is
	8–12 μg/ml

*Most divided in 2 to 4 portions per day. Elderly would have lower averages and treatment resistent patients might have much higher averages than those shown.

        (2)   Reassurance that symptoms can be alleviated with appropriate therapy

        (3)   Condition is temporary and with appropriate therapy and time, anxiety may be alleviated

        (4)   Dosage, side effects, expected action of pharmacologic agents

    b.   Chart attacks—date, time, situation, level of anxiety or symptoms on a scale of 0 to 10

Alcoholism

- Definition

    1.   Recurrent use of alcohol to the extent it significantly interferes with the individual's physical, social, and/or emotional life

    2.   Characterized by preoccupation with the drug, loss of control over its use, physical dependence, and tolerance

- Etiology/Incidence

  1. Multifactorial and poorly understood; several etiologic theories have been developed

     a. Psychological

        (1) Retarded ego, weak super ego

        (2) Fixed in lower level of psychosocial development

            (a) Dependent personality with poor impulse control

            (b) Low frustration tolerance

            (c) Low self-esteem

        (3) No evidence to support distinct personality predisposition

     b. Biologic

        (1) Physiologic changes in enzymes, genes, brain chemistry, hormones cause the disorder

        (2) May be familial, inherited or acquired

  2. About 1 in 12 persons have serious problems related to alcohol use

     a. Children of alcoholics are four times as likely to develop alcoholism as children of non-alcoholics

     b. Three times as many men as women are alcoholics and they are more likely to develop the problem early in life

     c. Highest prevalence of drinking problems in 18 to 29 year olds

  3. Risk factors include:

     a. Use of alcohol or other psychoactive substance

     b. Family history of alcohol abuse

     c. Being a young single male

     d. Heavy drinking—five or more drinks in one sitting or getting drunk once a week

     e. Family or social background that accepts or promotes intoxication

     f. Ready accessibility

- Signs and Symptoms
  1. Definite (Level I)
     a. Blackouts
     b. Alcoholic hepatitis
     c. Withdrawal symptoms—hallucinations; fine tremors of face, tongue and hands; disorientation; seizures
     d. Memory loss, confabulation
     e. Nystagmus
     f. Prior exhibition of signs and symptoms of levels II and III
  2. Probable (Level II)
     a. Previous diagnosis of:
        (1) Cirrhosis
        (2) Pancreatitis without cholelithiasis
     b. Loss of control over alcohol intake/increased alcohol tolerance
     c. Numbness of hands and feet
     d. Increased incidence of infection
     e. Weight loss
     f. Forgetfulness
     g. Trauma from accidents or altercations—cigarette burns, healed fractures
     h. Hypothermic injuries
     i. Attempted suicide
     j. Symptoms of associated diseases; see Table 5
  3. Possible (Level III)
     a. Blurred or dim vision
     b. Nocturnal diuresis
     c. Anxiety or depression
     d. Impotence
     e. Symptoms of associated diseases; see Table 6

    f. History of chronic gastritis, anemia, clotting disorders, marital discord or loss of significant relationships (job, family, friends)

- Differential Diagnosis

    1. Distinguish from a wide variety of medical and psychiatric problems that may account for signs and symptoms, e.g., depression, anxiety, endocrinopathies, viral hepatitis

    2. Determine level of alcoholism and look for concurrent abuse of other substances

        a. Use history and physical evidence to determine stage and further testing

        b. Use of CAGE screening test (Buck, Shaw, Cleary, Delbanco & Aronson, 1987)

            (1) Four questions related to drinking patterns

            (2) Scores > 2 indicate alcoholism

        c. Use of an addiction severity tool such as the Michigan Alcohol Screening Test (MAST)

            (1) 25 item questionnaire with 90% sensitivity and 74% specificity

            (2) Scores > 5 indicative of alcoholism

        d. Short MAST (SMAST) (Pokorny, Miller & Kaplan, 1972)

            (1) 13 questions

            (2) Score > 3 indicative of alcoholism

            (3) Sensitivity 70%, specificity 74%

Table 5

Conditions Commonly Associated With Substance Abuse

1.	Frequent upper respiratory infection
2.	Slowly healing skin ulcers
3.	Recurrent vaginal infections
4.	Hepatitis
5.	Sexually transmitted disease
6.	Mononucleosis
7.	Malnutrition
8.	HIV infection
9.	Pancreatitis
10.	Tuberculosis

- Physical Findings

    1. Definite (Level I)

        a. General appearance—fearful, anxious, stuporous, hyperactive, or incoherent

        b. Vital signs—mild fever, tachycardia, increased or labile B.P.

        c. Integumentary—flushed face and/or palms, spider nevi, angiomas on face, numerous scars, ecchymotic areas; generalized tissue edema, and dry, dull hair

        d. HEENT—pupil constriction, nystagmus, parotid adenopathy, inflamed buccal cavity, alcoholic odor to breath, fissures at corners of mouth

        e. Cardiovascular—tachycardia; dysrhythmias; weak, irregular peripheral pulses

        f. Abdomen—gastric distention, ascites, enlarged liver, tenderness

        g. Musculoskeletal—muscle wasting, healed or new fractures

        h. Neurological—memory loss, confabulation, hallucinations, disorientation, fine motor tremors, unsteady ataxic gait

    2. Probable (Level II) and Possible (Level III)

        a. General appearance—no major abnormalities

        b. Vital signs—normal or possible tachycardia, hypertension, and cardiac dysrhythmias

        c. Integumentary—unexplained ecchymosis

        d. HEENT—parotid adenopathy, angiomas

        e. Abdomen—hepatomegaly, tenderness

        f. Neurological—hyperreflexia; unsteady walk, ataxia (Wernicke-Korsakoff Syndrome)

- Diagnostic Tests/Findings

    1. Blood alcohol/drug levels—may or may not be severely elevated depending on amount and time of consumption

        a. 300 mg/100 mL at anytime = definite diagnosis

        b. 100 mg/mL on routine exam = definite diagnosis

    c. 150 mg/mL without evidence of intoxication = alcohol tolerance

2. CBC—increased or depressed white count; microcytic, hypochromic or macrocytic, megaloblastic anemia; decreased platelets

3. Blood glucose—hyper or hypoglycemia

4. Electrolytes—hypokalemia and hypomagnesemia

5. Liver function—all may be increased

    a. Gamma glutamyl transferase (GGT)— > 30 units/L suggests heavy drinking

    b. Alanine aminotransferase (ALT)

    c. Aspartate aminotransferase (AST)

    d. Lactate dehydrogenase (LDH)

6. Total bilirubin, triglycerides, cholesterol, amylase—increased

7. Prothrombin time—prolonged

8. Urinalysis—infection, ketones

9. Nutritional—albumin and total protein decreased, folic acid low

10. Chest radiograph—enlarged heart, right lower lobe pneumonia

11. ECG—dysrhythmias, cardiac myopathies, ischemic heart disease

- Management/Treatment

1. Consult with physician regarding treatment and possible need for detoxification

2. Confront client with diagnosis "Alcoholism"

3. Do not use nebulous statements, e.g., "We think you might have a drinking problem" or "You need to cut down on your drinking"

4. Tell the client it is a disease and treatable

5. Tell the client it is not his/her fault but he/she IS responsible for accepting treatment and the goal of therapy is abstinence

6. Describe treatment options; many treatment programs will not accept pregnant women

7. Make appropriate referral for treatment and follow-up

    a. Alcoholics Anonymous (most successful)

      b. Behavioral approaches

      c. Rational emotive psychotherapy

      d. Psychodrama

  8. Provide family members with information on alcoholism and encourage involvement in Al-Anon (for families of alcoholics) and/or Ala-Teen and Ala-Tots (for teenagers and young children of alcoholics)

  9. General considerations

      a. Alcoholic women have a higher incidence of suicide attempts than both alcoholic men and the female population as a whole; see section on suicide

      b. Females, even with less alcohol consumption are more likely to develop liver disease than males

      c. Alcohol use by pregnant women is the leading cause of mental retardation

      d. Women's drinking and drug problems are often viewed as less serious than men's and are more frequently misdiagnosed

      e. If seeing a patient who was referred for treatment of alcoholism, reinforce participation in treatment and use of any agreed upon treatment aids

      f. Avoid compounding the problems or hindering recovery by prescribing sedatives or other depressants (cross tolerance)

Psychoactive Substance Abuse

- Definition

  1. Misuse of any substance capable of producing altered state of consciousness and/or euphoria

  2. Addiction or compulsive use includes:

      a. Psychologic craving

      b. Physiologic dependence (withdrawal symptoms with discontinuance)

      c. Tolerance (need for larger and larger doses to produce desired effect)

- Etiology/Incidence

1. As with alcohol abuse, several theories have been developed to explain the cause of substance abuse which include:

   a. Psychologic

      (1) Failure to complete developmental tasks

      (2) Underdeveloped ego

      (3) Dependent personality

      (4) Poor impulse control

      (5) Ego breakdown with subsequent drug use as a coping mechanism

   b. Biologic hereditary/genetic factors

      (1) Neurotransmitter deficiency

      (2) Enzyme deficiency

   c. Family dynamics

      (1) Dysfunctional family system

      (2) Absent parent

      (3) Tyrannical or weak ineffective parent

      (4) Negative role models

      (5) Drugs used for stress relief

      (6) Cultural perceptions of drug abuse

2. Incidence

   a. Drug use is the leading cause of death among teens

   b. 26% of female and 24% of males between the age of 12 to 17 years have used an illicit drug

   c. More than 1 million women on legal psychoactive drugs

   d. 66% of psychoactive drugs are prescribed for women

   e. Most commonly used substances alone or in combination (see Table 6)

      (1) Depressants—benzodiazepines, barbiturates, opiates, morphine, heroin, alcohol, sedatives, hypnotics, and minor tranquilizers

(a) Most widely used and abused drugs

(b) Often prescribed for anxiety, depression, or sleep disorders

(2) Stimulants (amphetamines, cocaine, caffeine, tobacco)

(a) Most commonly abused stimulants other than caffeine and nicotine are amphetamine and cocaine

(b) Twice as many males as females use stimulants primarily in the 21 to 44 year age range

(3) Hallucinogens (lysergic acid diethylamide, L.S.D.; myristicene, nutmeg; dimethyltryptamine, DMT; psilocybin, magic mushroom; phencyclidine, PCP or angel dust; mescaline, peyote; cannabis, hashish and marijuana; and chemically related substances)

f. Solvents/gases

(1) Used to reproduce effects of depressants, stimulants, hallucinogenics

(2) Produce inebriation similar to volatile anesthetics.

(3) Examples include gasoline, paint thinners, correction fluid

- Signs and Symptoms

  1. Depressants

      a. Nausea/vomiting

      b. Myalgia, deep bone or muscle pain (methadone abusers)

      c. Rhinorrhea, sneezing, excessive lacrimation

      d. Headache

      e. Miosis

      f. Euphoria

      g. Apathy, dysphoria, depression

      h. Drowsiness, psychomotor retardation, slurred speech

Table 6

Commonly Abused Drugs

Generic or Trade Name	Street/Slang name
Depressants	
Codeine	School boy
Meperidine HCL (Demerol)	Demies
Hydromorphone HCL (Dilaudid)	Little D
Heroin	H; horse; junk; downtown; hard stuff; scag; white stuff
Methadone HCL	Meth; dollies
Morphine	M; Miss Emma; morph
Opium	Black stuff; blue velvet
Methaqualone (Qualude)	Ludes; 714s; Qs; soapers
Pentobarbital	Downers; yellow jackets
Amobarbital/secobarbital (comb.), Phenobarbital	Blues; red hearts; purple hearts; reds; F40s; rainbows
Benzodiazepines (Librium, Valium)	Tanks, downs
Stimulants	
Cocaine	Coke; snow; flake; toot; uptown; crack; blow
Dextoamphetamines;	Bennies; black beauties; copilots
Methamphetamines (Benzedrine)	Dexies; speed; meth; crank
Biphetamine (Desoxyn; Dexedrine)	Crystal; uppers
Hallucinogens	
Lysergic acid diethylamide	LSD; acid
Mescaline (peyote)	Buttons; cactus; mesc.
Myristicin	Nutmeg
Dimethyltryptamine	DMT, STP
Psilocybin	Magic mushroom
Phencyclidine HCL	PCP; angel dust; DOA; peace pill, hog
Marijuana	Pot; maryjane, chronic

    i.   Impaired attention, memory, social judgment (disinhibition)

    j.   Ataxia, tremors, lack of coordination

    k.   Mood swings, aggression, combativeness; loss of impulse control

    l.   Auditory hallucinations, paranoia

    m.   Fever, perspiration (with withdrawal)

2. Stimulants

    a.   Restlessness, irritability, anxiety, confusion, aggression

    b.   Tachycardia, cardiac dysrhythmia, chest pain (cocaine), increased blood pressure

    c.   Elation, grandiosity

    d.   Perspiration or chills

      e.   Hyper or hypothermia

      f.   Abdominal pain, nausea/vomiting, diarrhea, frequent urination

      g.   Insomnia

      h.   Paranoia, hallucinations (visual and tactile with cocaine)

      i.   Dilated pupils

3. Hallucinogenics

      a.   Dilated pupils, vertical and horizontal nystagmus

      b.   Flushed skin

      c.   Increased pulse and B.P.

      d.   Marked anxiety; panic paranoia

      e.   Hallucinations, visual and sensory distortions

      f.   Rapid, severe mood changes, hostility, aggression, violence

      g.   Depression, suicidal thoughts

      h.   Grandiosity, euphoria

      i.   Tremors

      j.   Flashbacks

      k.   Insensitivity to pain

4. Solvents/gases (inhaled)

      a.   Euphoria

      b.   Slurred speech

      c.   Hallucinations/confusion

      d.   Unconsciousness

      e.   Cardiopulmonary depression or failure

- Differential Diagnosis

1. Poly abuse is common and may present with intoxication, overdose, and/or in various stages of withdrawal

2. Rule out other disorders that may account for presenting signs and symptoms, e.g.

      a.   Seizure disorders

    b. Hypo or hyperthyroidism, thyroid storm

    c. Hyper or hypoglycemia

    d. Schizophrenia, mania

    e. Head injury

- Physical Findings: In addition to drug specific signs, some general physical findings might include:

  1. General appearance—unkempt, poor hygiene

  2. Vital signs—temperature elevation, increased or decreased BP, tachycardia, tachypnea

  3. Integumentary—bruises, burns, needle marks, infections, cellulitis, ulcerations, abscesses

  4. HEENT—changes in pupil size, reaction to light, and extraocular movements; poor oral hygiene, puncture wounds under the tongue, pharyngitis, inflammation and or erosion of the nasal mucosa

  5. Abdomen—tenderness, organomegaly

  6. Cardiovascular—dysrhythmia

  7. Neuromuscular—incoordination; decreased pain perception (PCP); alterations and distortions in consciousness, attention, sensory perceptions

- Diagnostic Tests/Findings

  1. CBC—leukocytosis; anemia

  2. Urine and drug screens—positive for abused substance(s)

  3. If associated diseases are present other alterations will be noted, e.g., abnormal liver enzymes, thyroid function tests, or glucose levels; positive HIV test

- Management/Treatment

  1. Depressant abuse

      a. Identify drugs taken, when taken, and route of administration if possible

      b. Assess level of consciousness

      c. Evaluate for evidence of head trauma

     d.   Refer to physician, emergency room, or drug detoxification unit if acute overdose or intoxication is noted

     e.   In the meantime provide quiet, lighted room and do not leave patient alone

     f.   Monitor vital signs

     g.   In consultation with physician determine need for starting an IV

2.   Stimulant abuse

     a.   In cases of intoxication, overdose, or withdrawal refer to physician or emergency room

     b.   In the meantime provide quiet area with reduced stimuli and high staff profile; aggressive behavior is associated with amphetamine use

     c.   Monitor cardiac rate and rhythm; ventricular arrhythmia/cardiac arrest may occur with toxic levels of cocaine

     d.   Persons experiencing stimulant withdrawal may be suicidal as a result of profound CNS rebound depression; use suicide precautions until patient is transferred to emergency room or detoxification unit

     e.   For non-emergency cases refer to drug rehabilitation unit

3.   Hallucinogenic abuse

     a.   Hallucinogenics do not have a withdrawal syndrome and do not require detoxification as such

     b.   Refer patients with psychotic symptoms to the psychiatric unit

     c.   Protect client and others from injury

         (1)   Darkened, quiet, non-threatening environment to decrease the likelihood of confusion, fear, and violent behavior

         (2)   Speak in a soft, non-threatening voice

            (a)   If LSD has been taken provide reassurance verbally and by touch and orient the individual ("talking down")

            (b)   If PCP intoxication is present do not attempt

"talking down" it will increase the patient's agitation and tendency for violent behavior

(3) Suspiciousness and paranoia, visual and auditory hallucinations, and agitation make suicide or accidental injury a likely possibility; take precautions early

(4) If frightened and hallucinating avoid the use of physical restraints, however, use of restraints with PCP users may be necessary for the safety of self and others; PCP is an anesthetic and alters thinking; persons on PCP are a danger to themselves as well as to others

4. General considerations

   a. Primary role is diagnosis and referral

   b. Consult with physician on medication use

      (1) Period of drug free observation usually recommended

      (2) Haloperidol may be given to control psychotic and assaultive behaviors

      (3) Diazepam is used to reduce muscle spasm and restlessness

      (4) Phenothiazine neuroleptics should be avoided in patients on PCP because of the possibility of potentiating the anticholinergic effects of PCP

      (5) Vitamin C tablets (ascorbic acid) or cranberry juice may be used to acidify the urine and promote excretion of PCP

   c. Many treatment programs will not accept pregnant women

   d. Many treatment programs do not provide child care or other alternatives for woman and can be a significant barrier to help

   e. Alcoholics Anonymous, Al-Anon will also accept other substance abusers; family members should be given information on Al-Anon and Ala-Teen even if patient refuses treatment

   f. Narcotics Anonymous (substance abusers) and Nar-Anon (families of substance abusers) groups are available in some areas

Delirium (Acute Confusion)

- Definition: A transient global disorder of attention, with clouding of consciousness and cognitive impairment
- Etiology/Incidence
  1. Usually the result of systemic problems e.g. medications, hypoxia, dehydration, or electrolyte imbalance—examples include:
     a. Intoxication—alcohol, analgesics, bromides, sedatives, psychedelics
     b. Withdrawal from alcohol, sedatives, hypnotics, or corticosteroids
     c. Infections—urinary, respiratory, meningitis, encephalitis, septicemia, syphilis
     d. Endocrine disorders—diabetes, hyper or hypothyroidism, Addison's disease, Cushing's syndrome
     e. Nutritional deficiencies especially of B_1, B_6, B_{12}
     f. Medications—anticholinergics, antidepressants, digoxin, H_2 blockers
     g. May be related to sensory deprivation or overload
     h. Sleep deprivation
     i. Psychological stress
  2. Can occur in any age group but the elderly are particularly vulnerable
  3. Estimated that 40% to 80% of elderly patients hospitalized for acute physical illness exhibit delirium at time of admission or soon after
- Signs and Symptoms
  1. Cognitive impairment
     a. Inability to focus attention/short attention span
     b. Impaired recent memory and recall
     c. Problems in perceptual processing
     d. Disorientation
     e. Impaired judgement

2. Emotional lability

3. Impaired impulse control

4. Anxiety/irritability

5. Mild to moderate depression

6. Visual and auditory hallucinations

7. Confabulation

8. Fluctuating mental status; worse in the evening "sundowning," more common in those with pre-existing dementia

9. Psychomotor restlessness with insomnia

10. Tachycardia, dilated pupils, sweating

- Differential Diagnosis

   1. Dementia

   2. Pseudodementia

   3. Amnestic syndrome

   4. Substance induced hallucinosis

   5. Schizophrenia

   6. Other psychoses

- Physical Findings: Varies according to the underlying cause

   1. General appearance—may be restless, hyper or hypovigilant; dazed expression

   2. Tachycardia, elevated blood pressure, increased temperature, tachypnea

   3. Focal neurological symptoms may be present

- Diagnostic Tests/Findings

   1. Thorough history and physical examination with mental status and neurological examination—may reveal clues to etiology

   2. Basic laboratory workup may include:

      a. CBC with differential, chemical screen, blood gas analysis

      b. Electrocardiogram

      c. Chest radiograph

      d.   Urinalysis and urine toxicology screen

   3.   Special tests as needed

      a.   EEG—tends to show general slowing in delirium

      b.   Computer tomography (CT) scan or magnetic resonance imaging (MRI) of the brain—expect to be normal

      c.   Blood levels for medications

- Management/Treatment

   1.   Diagnostic consult with physician

   2.   Identify suspected cause

   3.   Remove or modify etiology when possible, e.g., treat infections with antimicrobials, discontinue or simplify medication regimens

   4.   Nonpharmacologic interventions

      a.   Provide adequate nutrition, hydration, oxygenation

      b.   Institute environmental controls to control stimuli levels

      c.   Provide reassurance and institute safety measures

      d.   Institute reorientation measures; provide patient and family with sensitive reassurance

   5.   Pharmacologic intervention

      a.   Judicious use of sedation to promote rest, reduce anxiety, decrease agitation and restlessness

      b.   No ideal drug

      c.   Short acting anxiolytics without active metabolites

         (1)   Oxazepam 10 to 50 mg/day

         (2)   Lorazepam 0.5 to 2 mg/day

         (3)   Alprazolam 0.5 to 4 mg/day

      d.   For immediate calming of acute agitation—haloperidol 0.5 mg IV combined with 0.5 to 1 mg lorazepam, repeated in 30 minutes

         (1)   Repeat every hour till calming achieved

         (2)   Once delirium cycle is broken sedation may be continued particularly in evening and night hours

6. General considerations

    a. Anticipate delirium when risk factors are present

        (1) Being >80 years of age

        (2) Having visual or hearing impairments

        (3) Pain

        (4) Multiple medications

        (5) Urine elimination problems

        (6) Fracture injury

        (7) Multiple chronic diseases

        (8) Pervious history of acute confusion

        (9) Immobilized

        (10) Low scores on mental status examinations

    b. Prevention strategies

        (1) Avoid polypharmacy

        (2) Monitor medication intake and monitor for side effects, interactions, toxicity

        (3) Maintain adequate hydration and oxygenation

        (4) Maintain adequate nutrition

        (5) Assess for adequate pain control

        (6) Control environmental stimuli to avoid sensory deprivation or overload

        (7) Provide assistive devices to supplement sensory alterations, e.g., glasses, hearing aids, controlled lighting

Questions
Select the best answer.

1. Which of the following is associated with higher risk for Major Depression?

   a. Being male
   b. Having had a traumatic experience in the last six months
   c. Being middle aged
   d. Having a family history of alcoholism

2. Which is true of Major Depression?

   a. Majority of patients will have a reoccurrence
   b. It may be a normal grief reaction
   c. It is often self-limiting
   d. Strongly associated with chronic drug use

3. Dysthymic Disorder is distinguished from Major Depression by which of the following?

   a. It usually first manifests itself in old age
   b. It is rarely associated with drug use
   c. It has milder more chronic symptoms
   d. It is rarely chronic

4. Post-traumatic Stress Disorder is marked by which triad of findings?

   a. Intrusive thoughts, nightmares, flashbacks
   b. Tendency to globalize, psychomotor retardation, hypersomnia
   c. Weight loss, feelings of helplessness, irritability
   d. Indifference, decreased concentration, hyperphagia

5. Mrs. S. is a 65-year-old who comes in complaining of feeling depressed. She would like a prescription to make her feel better. Her husband died three weeks ago.

   The data you have at this point indicates:

   a. Her problem is a normal grief reaction, but will require surveillance
   b. Diagnostic tests will not be needed
   c. Pharmacologic intervention would not be warranted
   d. Major depression is a possibility

6. Your next step would be to:

   a. Refer her for psychologic evaluation
   b. Prescribe antidepressants
   c. Obtain additional information
   d. Reassure her that the problem is self-limiting

7. In a patient of this age it would be important to remember that:

   a. Somatic signs may be overlooked as normal changes
   b. Elderly may require higher doses of antidepressants for therapeutic effect
   c. Previously undiagnosed bipolar disorder is probable
   d. Tricyclics may cause "hypomania"

8. With further exploration you determine that Mrs. S. has had intermittent episodes of anorexia, difficulty sleeping, has been feeling tired and listless. She has had to force herself to go out with her friends, although she did enjoy her grandson's birthday party a week ago. She denies any thoughts of harming herself. Routine physical and lab work are unremarkable.

   The most likely diagnosis for this patient is:

   a. Adjustment disorder with depressed mood
   b. Primary major depression
   c. Dysthymic disorder
   d. Bipolar disorder

9. Mrs. S. tells you that she can't help thinking that her husband might not have died if she had done things differently.

   Which response would be most appropriate?

   a. Telling her that these thoughts will decrease in a few weeks
   b. Encourage her to elaborate on these thoughts
   c. Tell her a psychologist or psychiatrist will best help her with her guilt
   d. Suggest an antidepressant will correct this kind of thinking

10. A 17-year-old male student comes into the student health service complaining of weight loss, fatigue, anorexia. He states that the symptoms began about a month ago after he broke up with his girl-friend. He has difficulty sleeping and says he wakes up thinking about her. He says that since she left him he just doesn't enjoy going out anymore and has been spending most of his free time

in his room. His affect is flat and he shows little expression as he relates his problem. The physical examination is within normal limits.

You suspect depression to be his problem. Your next step would be to:

a. Prescribe an anti-anxiety medication
b. Find out how he has coped with losses in the past
c. Explain that this is a temporary situation and will probably clear up in another couple of weeks
d. Ask him directly about feelings or thoughts of harming himself

11. Which factors in the available data might lead you to suspect that he might be suicidal?

a. Weight loss, fatigue, anorexia
b. Insomnia, loss of pleasure, social withdrawal
c. Age, gender, emotional loss, signs of depression
d. Intrusive thoughts, flat affect, with normal physical exam

12. Upon further questioning he admits to suicidal ideation. Knowing which of the following would be most helpful in assessing his suicide risk?

a. Whether there have been any suicides in his family
b. If he rooms alone or has a roommate
c. If his family lives nearby
d. If he has a plan for suicide in the next 24 hours

13. This patient has a roommate, but his family lives in another state. He denies substance abuse, or definite plan or time for suicide. What would be the best action at this point?

a. Consult with a physician regarding psychotherapy and antidepressants
b. Consult with a physician and arrange for hospitalization
c. Give him a prescription for antidepressants and arrange to have him stay with his family for a week
d. Give him a prescription for antidepressants, call his roommate, and have them both check with you in 24 hours

14. A 38-year-old married male comes to the clinic asking for an AIDS test. He has been awakening at night with sweating and his heart pounding. He has read in *Time* magazine that night sweats were a sign of AIDS and a few years ago he had to have a transfusion after a car accident. He would also like to have a radiograph of his throat as he feels like there's something stuck in it

and wonders if it might be cancer. At times he feels like he's losing control. He denies IV drug use or high risk sexual activities. He denies marital or work problems. In fact, he just got a promotion two weeks ago and he and his wife have bought a new home.

What other information would be most helpful to you in your diagnosis?

a. How long has he had these symptoms
b. Whether he has nightmares
c. If anyone in his family has had a major mental health problem
d. If he has a prolapsed heart valve

15. If he denies nightmares and has had the symptoms for about two weeks and the physical findings are normal, you should:

a. Order a barium swallow
b. Refer to a gastroenterologist
c. Consider a post traumatic stress syndrome as the probable diagnosis
d. Consider situational anxiety as the probable diagnosis

16. Benzodiazepines are used in anxiety disorders. They are:

a. Contraindicated in glaucoma
b. Not helpful for short term use in situational anxiety
c. Usually physiologically addicting
d. As effective as beta blockers for control of palpitations

17. The most common mental health problem seen in general practice is:

a. Anxiety
b. Depression
c. Alcoholism
d. Schizophrenia

18. Which of these symptoms is least characteristic of anxiety?

a. Sleep disorder
b. Decreased concentration
c. Irritability
d. Indifference

19. Which of the following would least likely be a cause of anxiety symptoms?

a. Thyrotoxicosis

b. Hyperglycemia
c. Hormone-releasing tumor
d. Prolapsed mitral valve

20. Tricyclics are not used for bipolar disorders because:

a. They may precipitate mania
b. They cause liver dysfunction
c. They may lead to physiologic dependance
d. They may cause a hypertensive crisis

21. Mrs. J. is a 65-year-old widow who completed a series of E.C.T. treatments a week ago with positive results. Both she and her daughter are concerned that she continues to experience a significant memory loss.

You could be most helpful by:

a. Reporting the problem to her psychiatrist
b. Allow her to ventilate her feelings without any comment regarding the memory loss
c. Explain that the loss is temporary and full memory will return
d. Inform her that many individuals of her age begin to experience memory loss

22. Mr. P. is a 45-year-old divorced male who comes in for a physical exam required for a new job. During the interview he reveals previous hospitalization for pancreatitis and long term self-medication for gastritis. His physical exam is normal except for slight tenderness in the RUQ. A CBC reveals macrocytic, megaloblastic anemia.

Which diagnostic test would be most helpful at this point?

a. ECG and electrolytes
b. Liver function, B_{12} and folic acid levels, and electrolytes
c. Chest radiograph and ultrasound of the gallbladder
d. Blood albumin levels and bone marrow studies

23. Ms. Z, a 35-year-old female, comes into the clinic demanding to be seen immediately. She is agitated and complaining loudly of police brutality. She states that she was unjustly jailed overnight because of a misunderstanding and that she was shackled for more than three hours causing bruises on her wrists and ankles. Upon further elaboration she states the police altered a blood test and said her blood alcohol level was 300.

This information alone indicates:

a. Paranoid ideation
b. Alcoholism
c. Need for legal services referral
d. The patient may have a drinking problem

24. Non-compliance with medication is a concern in outpatient treatment of patients with mental health problems. Which of the following would be least helpful in promoting medication regimen compliance?

a. Client involvement in treatment decision making
b. Providing the client with information about expected action and side effects of the medications
c. Arranging follow-up visits with whatever staff are available
d. Maintaining telephone communication with the patient to monitor effects and response to medication

25. One of the most effective treatments for alcoholism is:

a. Psychoanalysis
b. Active participation in A.A.
c. Aversion therapy with Antabuse
d. Active participation in Al-Anon

26. Ms. C is brought to the emergency room from a party by her friends. She is stuporous, confused, and has pinpoint pupils.

These signs are consistent with:

a. PCP intoxication
b. Heroin use
c. LSD
d. Amphetamine withdrawal

27. A 23-year-old male comes to the clinic to obtain treatment for a cut on his arm he received in a street fight. His face is badly bruised from a previous fight. He is unkempt and shows evidence of poor personal hygiene. He has a history of alcohol abuse. At present he is tachycardic and has an elevated blood pressure. His pupils are dilated and he is slightly diaphoretic. He complains of chest pain.

These signs are consistent with:

a. Acute alcohol intoxication
b. Chronic heroin use
c. Recent use of hallucinogenics
d. Recent use of cocaine

28. A young male adult is brought into the emergency room by the police. He is highly agitated and hostile and verbally abusive and threatening. He has several lacerations and bruises he sustained in a fight at a disco where he "tore the place apart."

    You should:

    a. Suspect police brutality
    b. Suspect LSD use
    c. Try to talk the patient down and keep him oriented
    d. Be prepared to administer Haldol

29. Which of the following IS NOT associated with physiologic dependance?

    a. Heroin
    b. Phenobarbital
    c. LSD
    d. Amphetamines

30. Mark is an 18-year-old brought to the student health clinic complaining of chest pain and palpitations. He is highly anxious and perspiring. His roommate states he thinks he took some kind of drug.

    In addition to myocardial infarction (MI) these symptoms could indicate intoxication or overdose of which of the following?

    a. Heroin
    b. Alcohol
    c. PCP
    d. Cocaine

31. Your first action in this case should be to:

    a. Arrange for emergency room transfer
    b. Prepare for cardiopulmonary support
    c. Draw blood gasses
    d. Do nothing until he is seen by a physician

32. To enhance the excretion of PCP from the body give:

    a. Haloperidol
    b. Ascorbic acid
    c. Valium
    d. A phenothiazine

33. Which pharmacologic agent is contraindicated in persons on PCP?

    a. Valium
    b. Phenothiazine
    c. Haloperidol
    d. Ascorbic acid

34. CNS rebound is seen in withdrawal of:

    a. Depressants
    b. Stimulants
    c. Hallucinogenics
    d. Alcohol

35. Aggressive behavior can be seen with abuse of which of the following?

    a. Amphetamines
    b. Depressants
    c. Hallucinogenics
    d. Any psychoactive substance

Answers

1. d	13. b	25. b
2. a	14. a	26. b
3. c	15. d	27. d
4. a	16. a	28. d
5. d	17. b	29. c
6. c	18. d	30. d
7. a	19. b	31. b
8. a	20. a	32. b
9. b	21. c	33. b
10. d	22. b	34. b
11. c	23. c	35. d
12. d	24. c	

25/35 70%

Bibliography

American Psychiatric Association. (1994). *Diagnostic and statistical manual of mental disorders* (4th ed.). Washington, DC: Author.

Bhatia. S. C., & Bhatia, S. K. (1997). Major depression: Selecting safe and effective treatment. *American Family Physician, 55,* 1683–1694.

Boswell, E. B., & Stoudemire, A. (1996). Major depression in the primary care setting. *The American Journal of Medicine, 101,* (supplement 6A), 3S–9S.

Buck, B., Shaw, S., Cleary, P., Delbanco, T. L., & Aronson, M. D. (1987). Screening for alcohol abuse using the CAGE questionnaire. *American Journal of Medicine, 82,* 231–235.

Buffum, M. D., & Buffum, J. C. (1997). The psychopharmacologic treatment of depression in elders. *Geriatric Nursing, 18,* 144–149.

Cole, S., & Raju, M. (1996). Making the diagnosis of depression in the primary care setting. *The American Journal of Medicine, 101,* (supplement 6A), 10S–17S.

Eisendrath, S. J. (1998). Psychiatric disorders. In L. M. Tierney, S. J. McPhee, & M. A. Papadakis (Eds.). *Current medical diagnosis and management (37th ed., pp. 973-1030).* Stamford, CT: Appleton & Lange.

Foreman, M. D., & Zane, D. (1996). Nursing strategies for acute confusion in elders. *American Journal of Nursing, 96*(4), 44–52.

Goldberg, J. R. (1996). The P-450 system: Definition and relevance to the use of antidepressants in medical practice. *Archives of Family Medicine, 5,* 406–412.

Lundquist, R. S., Bernens, A., & Olsen, C. G. (1997). Comorbid disease in geriatric patients: Dementia and depression. *American Family Physician, 55,* 2687–2694.

Pinkowish, M. D. (1997). Rational use of the newer antidepressants. *Patient Care,* March 30, 49–50, 55–57, 62, 67–77.

Pokorny, A., Miller, B. A., & Kaplan, H. B. (1972). The brief MAST: A shortened version of the Michigan alcoholism screening test. *American Journal of Psychiatry, 129,* 342–345.

Simon, L., Jewell, N., & Brokel, J. (1997). Management of acute delirium in hospitalized elderly: A process improvement project. *Geriatric Nursing, 18,* 151–154.

Sussman, N., & Stahl, S. (1996). Update in the pharmacology of depression. *The American Journal of Medicine, 101,* (Supplement 6A), 26S–36S.

Valente, S. M. (1996). Diagnosis and treatment of panic disorder and generalized anxiety in primary care. *The Nurse Practitioner*, *21*(8), 26–47.

Wichowski, H. C., & Benishek, D. (1996). An assessment tool to identify panic disorder. *The Nurse Practitioner*, *21*(8), 48, 53–55, 58–59.

Care of the Aging Adult

Debbie G. Kramer

Demographics of Older Adults

The elderly population in America is increasing rapidly. The rates are significantly higher than for other segments of the population. A greater number of aged persons are living longer and healthier due to improved health care and a healthier lifestyle. The average U.S. life span has increased appreciably since the beginning of the century. The average life expectancy at birth increased by almost two years during the past decade. The term "elderly" is generally accepted as referring to persons 65 years and older.

- Definitions of Late Adulthood:
    1. Age 65 to 74 years—the young-old
    2. Age 75 to 84 years—the middle-old
    3. Age 85 and over—the oldest-old

- Population Statistics (U.S. Census Bureau, 1995)
    1. In 1900, individuals aged 65 and over numbered 3.1 million persons—one in every 25 Americans
    2. By 1994, the elderly comprised one in eight (33.2 million); an 11-fold increase
    3. The Census Bureau projects the elderly population will more than double to 80 million, one in five persons, between now and 2050
    4. Fastest growing subgroup is the oldest-old, also referred to as the frail elderly—3 million persons and 10% of the elderly
    5. Greatest growth spurt will be seen when the "baby-boomers" enter the 65 and over group, between the years of 2010 and 2030
    6. The "baby-boomers" will number 19 million in 2050 when they become the oldest-old, making them 24% of elderly Americans and 5% of all Americans

- Gender Statistics
    1. Elderly women outnumber elderly men by three to two—20 million to 14 million (1994 data)
    2. In 1993, the life expectancy for women was 79 years and 72 years for men
    3. Men have higher death rates at each age

- Marital Status and Living Arrangements

1. In 1993, 75% of non-institutionalized elderly men were married and living with their spouses

2. 41% of their female counterparts were married and living with their spouses

3. Older women were three times more likely than men to be widowed—48% versus 14%; eight out of ten elderly persons living alone are women

4. The likelihood of living alone or in a residential care facility increases with age

5. Only 9% of non-institutionalized persons aged 65 to 69 years needed assistance with their activities of daily living (ADL), whereas 50% of the 85 and over age group required such assistance

- Income and Poverty

    1. Living below the government defined poverty level increases with age

    2. Older women (16%) have higher poverty rate than older men (9%)

    3. Elderly African-Americans (33%) and Hispanics (22%) outnumber Whites (11%) with low income levels

    4. Within each race/ethnic group, poverty is more prevalent for women than men; income varies with differences in age, gender, race, ethnicity, marital status, living arrangements, educational level, former occupation, and work history

- Educational Status

    1. Better education is correlated with a healthier, longer life

    2. In 1993, 60% of non-institutionalized elderly as compared to 85% of those under age 65 completed high school

    3. The oldest-old were more likely to have only an eighth grade education or less (24% versus 6%); the level of education decreases with age

    4. 12% of the elderly have college degrees versus 20% of those aged 55 to 59 and 27% of persons aged 45 to 49

- Racial/Ethnic Diversity

    1. In 1995, 85 out of 100 elderly were White

2. By 2050, 67 out of 100 persons will be non-White

3. Hispanics will rise from 4% to 16% of the older population

Theories of Aging (Spirduso, 1995)

Aging is a process that occurs to an organism with the passage of time, eventually resulting in death. Understanding by scientists of the mechanisms of the theories of aging may show an interaction and inter-relatedness among the theories in the future.

- Genetic Theories

    1. Gene—process of aging is dictated by preprogrammed genetic components influenced by biological markers such as puberty and menopause; one or more genes control cellular aging process and specific genes may influence longevity

    2. Error - catastrophe—an early theory suggesting errors occur through somatic mutations, chromosomal rearrangements or genetic material transcriptions

    3. DNA—mutations occur in the mitochondria of DNA and continually mount upwards throughout an individual's lifetime, causing aging

    4. Hayflick limit or cell aging—cells will multiply and divide only a finite number of times; genetically preprogrammed

- Damage Theories

    1. Chemical—chemical reactions occur naturally and result in irreversible molecular defects; may occur from air, food, smoking and the like; if insults and injuries outweigh the repairing process, the system fails

    2. Cross-linkage—atoms or molecules have chemical sites that may link to DNA in the cell; damaged DNA is repaired by body's defense mechanism; if cross-linkage impedes transport of nutrients and information, the damage cannot be repaired

    3. Free-radical—free radicals are oxygen metabolites produced by one-electron reduction of oxygen that can produce damage and lead to cell death

- Gradual Imbalance Theories

1. Autoimmune—immune system loses its ability to distinguish normal material from foreign antigens and begins to destroy its host

2. Gradual imbalance—brain, endocrine or immune system begins to fail, possibly at different rates, causing an imbalance and decreased effectiveness

3. Neuroendocrine regulatory system—enables body to adapt to real or perceived challenges such as changes in workload, temperature, or psychological threats

- Wear and Tear—mechanical and biological features of aging; irreversible damage occurs over time

- Social Theories

  1. Disengagement theory (not currently supported)—individuals inevitably become withdrawn from society as a function of aging; acceptable to both the individual and society

  2. Activity theory—maintenance of activity, social roles and social supports directly related to satisfaction with life and self-concept; quality of activities more important than quantity

- Developmental Theories

  1. Erik Erickson's resolution of psychological conflict—ego integrity vs. despair

  2. Robert Peck expanded upon Erickson's conflict of aging

     a. Ego differentiation vs. work role preoccupation

     b. Body transcendence vs. body preoccupation

     c. Ego transcendence vs. ego preoccupation

  3. Daniel Levinson's Seasons of Life—individual must ultimately come to terms with the inevitability of death; focus is on the relationship of physical changes to personality

  4. Developmental tasks theory

     a. Adjust to decreasing physical strength and health

     b. Adjust to retirement and reduced income

     c. Adjust to death of partner

     d. Establish affiliation with peers

      e.   Adapt to social rules

      f.   Establish satisfactory physical living arrangements

Interview and Health History

The goal of the interview is to obtain a complete and accurate health history. It is a subjective account of the individual's status. Much of the information obtained will be utilized to formulate diagnoses and a plan of care.

- Develop a Relationship
  1. Develop a climate of trust
  2. Establish a caring relationship
  3. Identify the chief complaint
  4. Maintain a goal-directed interview, as older adults may have long and complex histories
     a. Direct flow of conversation—avoid a "positive" review of systems-answering "yes" to all questions
     b. Ask specific questions, but allow individual to elaborate
     c. Design questions to address one issue at a time
- Communication
  1. Speak slowly; do not shout; lower octaves are generally heard more clearly
  2. Help interpret patient's feelings; ask for clarification
  3. Convey warmth and concern through listening, appropriate touch
  4. Observe for signs of anxiety, exhaustion, nervousness
  5. Understand social mores, cultural differences, language barriers, personal biases
- Environment
  1. Provide a quiet, private setting
  2. Set time limit, as the elderly may tire
  3. Sit face-to-face to ensure eye contact; exhibit a relaxed, but concerned atmosphere

4. Provide good lighting and ventilation; avoid light source shining from behind you as it creates shadows and glares

- Health History: Format

  1. Biographical data—important to obtain name and phone number of closest relative

  2. Family history

     a. Parents' health history; cause of death (if applicable)

     b. History of diabetes, heart and kidney disease, cancer, alcoholism, drug abuse, mental illness and other major medical problems in family

  3. Occupation—any environmental or occupational exposure to pulmonary toxins; adjustment to retirement; source of income

  4. Medications—prescriptions, over-the counter, nontraditional modalities, home remedies

  5. Smoking history, illegal drug use history

  6. Allergies, drug sensitivities, foods

  7. Mental health problems

  8. Nutrition evaluation

     a. General

        (1) Attitude towards eating—alone, with family or caregiver

        (2) Appetite

        (3) Consumption, special dietary restrictions

        (4) Meal preparation

        (5) Shopping

        (6) Alcohol use/abuse

     b. Significant weight loss (at least 5% of usual body weight)—sudden (days to weeks) vs. gradual weight loss

     c. Common causes of weight loss

        (1) Cancer (lung, GI, lymphoma, GU)—up to 36% of cases

        (2) Diabetes and hyperthyroidism

        (3) Depression, anxiety and dementia

   (4) AIDS—do not rule out high-risk behaviors in elderly such as homosexuality, IV drug abuse, history of blood transfusion or infected spouse

 9. Sleep

  a. Note patterns—hour of bedtime/sleep, daytime fatigue/naps, insomnia

  b. Sleep aids—pharmacological and non-pharmacological

  c. Normal changes of sleep patterns with aging

   (1) Longer stage 1, light sleep

   (2) Shorter stages 3 and 4, decreased 20%—deep sleep shorter, therefore less restful nights

   (3) Increased sleep apnea of 10 seconds or more without awakening

   (4) Increased time awake during night

 10. Exercise patterns, recreational profile

 11. Review of systems

  a. Systematic review of elderly individual

  b. Subjective data collected

  c. Diseases may present atypically

 12. Preventive health practices—check frequency of screening tests such as Papanicolaou smear, testicular and prostate exams, stool guaiac test, sigmoidoscopy, cholesterol level, mammograms

- Past Medical History

 1. Hospitalization and operations

 2. Vaccinations—influenza, pneumonia, hepatitis, tetanus

 3. Accidents, injuries, falls

 4. Childhood and adult illnesses

 5. Communicable disease history

  a. Tuberculosis

  b. Influenza

  c. HIV status

  d. Sexually transmitted diseases

  e. Streptococcal infections

  f. Hepatitis

- Health Practices, Religious Implications

  1. Blood transfusion acceptance/denial

  2. Dietary restrictions

  3. Fasting on certain holidays

  4. Sabbath restrictions for procedures, activities

- Safety Assessment

  1. Environment

      a. Home—stairs, scatter rugs, electrical wires, telephone cords, locks on doors and windows

      b. Neighborhood—sidewalks, location of stores, banks, post office, pharmacy

      c. Community services

      d. Crime

  2. Driving—loss of independence if taken away (difficult decision); must weigh the risks versus benefits of action

  3. Elder abuse—recent and increasingly common form of domestic violence

      a. Estimated to be approximately 1 million persons

      b. Abuser frequently is caregiver or family

      c. Physical or psychological abuse, neglect

- Patient Self-Determination Act (1990)—encourage patient to discuss this with family and health care provider and act upon wishes

  1. Advance directives—indicates intent of patient based on his/her wishes with right to refuse any or all interventions of medical care

  2. Living will—a contract specifying the patient's wishes concerning the end of his/her life; varies according to state in which he/she resides; a copy should be given to the health care provider and family member

    3. Durable power of attorney for health care—authorizes an agent to make medical decisions on behalf of the patient when the patient is unable

    4. Physician-assisted suicide may become an issue

Living Situations and Income Status

    1. Socialization

    2. Support systems in place such as family and friends

    3. Available resources in the community

    4. Effect of change in financial resources upon retirement or disability

    5. Assess role and status of caregiver; care of the caregiver

Functional Assessment

- Definition—method used to measure an individual's impairment and/or disability through physical, emotional, cognitive and social parameters

    1. Physical function identifies sensorimotor ability

    2. Emotional function focuses on coping mechanisms

    3. Cognitive function identifies intellectual and reasoning capabilities

    4. Social function evaluates ability to maintain social roles

- Certain deficits affect functional status

    1. Visual and auditory deficits may precipitate or worsen confusion

    2. Unfamiliar surroundings may cause confusion, sleep disturbances

    3. Musculoskeletal injury resulting in mobility impairment, dependence, loss of control and sleep disturbances

- Determine ability to perform activities of daily living (ADL) and self-care activities independently using the Index of Independence in Activities of Daily Living Scale (Katz, 1983)

    1. Elderly tend to overrate abilities; underrate disabilities

    2. Family members tend to underrate abilities

    3. Index ranks ability to perform basic functions such as bathing, dressing, feeding and continence

- Determine ability to perform Instrumental Activities of Daily Living (IADL) (Katz, 1983)

    1. More complex personal tasks such as cooking and shopping

    2. More complex independent functions such as taking care of finances, banking and managing medications

- Cognitive status assessments are used to detect causes of cognitive impairment

    1. Short Portable Mental Status Questionnaire (SPMSQ) is used to identify the presence and degree of intellectual impairment by testing orientation, memory concerning self-care, remote memory and math (Pfeiffer, 1975)

    2. The Mini-Mental State Exam (MMSE) is used to identify cognitive aspects of mental functions such as orientation, attention, recall and language (Folstein, Folstein & McHugh, 1975)

- Other functional issues may be assessed such as medical conditions, communication, senses, resources and behavior problems

Physical Assessment

An essential component of the evaluation from which valuable information can be obtained; an organized, systematic approach such as head-to-toe or major organ system should be utilized

- General Inspection

    1. Provide initial assessment of health status

    2. Identify specific characteristics—posture, gait, appearance

    3. Determine if exhibiting altered concentration due to pain, memory loss, agitation, and other signs of focusing deficits

    4. Identify strengths, disabilities and limitations

- Normal Aging Changes in the Elderly: General Appearance

    1. Fat increases by 30% and water decreases by 53% by age 70; fat distribution shifts from extremities to trunk

    2. Weight increases until about age 50 and then begins to fall; longevity favors individuals who are ''ideal'' weight or slightly above

    3. Anatomic size and height—elderly lose one to two inches due to

thinning of cartilage between vertebrae and poor posture; kyphosis; males and females lose approximately one-sixteenth of an inch each year beginning around age 30

- Integumentary System
    1. Anatomical and physiological changes
        a. Decreased elasticity—increased wrinkles, folds, sagging, dry skin resulting in poor turgor
        b. Decreased perspiration—increased heat tolerance, poor temperature regulation
        c. Body and facial hair grays, thins; increased facial hair on women
        d. Nail growth slows, thickens; hypertrophy common
        e. Eyebrows coarse, bristle-like
        f. Cell regeneration slower
        g. Thinning of epithelial cells and subcutaneous fat layers
    2. Clinical implications
        a. Increased risk of infection
        b. Decreased wound healing
        c. Pruritus
        d. Poorly supported blood vessels rupture easily causing purpura
        e. Common benign skin lesions
            (1) Seborrheic/senile keratosis—macular-papular, dark, warty areas seen on face, neck and trunk
            (2) Cherry angioma—small, round, red, domed papules seen on trunk and proximal extremities
            (3) Cutaneous skin tags—pedunculated papillomas seen on neck, chest and intertriginous sites
            (4) Common blue nevus—benign, firm, dark-blue/gray/black, well-defined papule, usually seen on hands and feet
        f. Sun exposure changes

        (1)   Solar lentigo—flat, brown, pigmented macule on exposed areas only

        (2)   Solar keratosis—single or multiple discreet, dry, rough, scaly lesions on face, neck and hands

3. Abnormal changes and disease

    a.   Infections—viral, bacterial, fungal

    b.   Skin ulcerations

    c.   Ingrown toenails

    d.   Bunions, corns, calluses

    e.   Onychomycosis—fungal infection of nails

    f.   Abnormal skin lesions

        (1)   Actinic keratosis—pre-cancerous macular, irregular, scaly lesions seen on hands, arms, neck and face

        (2)   Squamous cell carcinoma—malignant soft, red-brown lesion of skin and mucous membrane arises as result of exogenous carcinogens such as sunlight or x-rays; seen on exposed areas, especially face, ears, scalp and arms

        (3)   Basal cell carcinoma—most common type of skin cancer; hard pearly-gray or pink, round, oval lesion with depressed center; usually on forehead, eyelids, nose and lips

        (4)   Malignant melanoma—round, oval, brown or tan irregular macular lesions seen mostly on trunk, arms, legs; familial tendency, not as common in older population

- Cardiovascular System

1. Anatomical and physiological changes

    a.   Slight decrease in heart size

    b.   Decreased cardiac output and cardiac reserve; heart fills and expels blood less efficiently

    c.   Increased peripheral vascular resistance

    d.   Increased ectopic activity

    e.   Decreased resting heart rate; increased with exercise/stress, takes longer to return to baseline; decreased exercise tolerance

   f. Increased rigidity and thickness of valves

  2. Clinical implications

   a. Orthostatic hypotension

   b. Increased narrow or wide pulse pressure

   c. Unilateral or bilateral pain or swelling in lower extremities

   d. Varicosities—tortuous peripheral vessels

   e. Functional systolic murmurs increase with age

   f. S_4 commonly heard

   g. Heart rate < 60 or > 90 beats per minute may be diagnostically significant

   h. BP of 90/60 to 140/90 acceptable

  3. Abnormal changes and disease

   a. Hypertension or isolated systolic hypertension

   b. Coronary artery disease—may present with fatigue, confusion, dizziness, dyspnea, palpitations; may *not* present with pain

   c. Cerebrovascular disease—may present as confusion, headache

   d. Congestive heart failure—may present as confusion/delirium, anxiety, shortness of breath, cough and/or palpitations

   e. Arrhythmias—may present with restlessness, diaphoresis, syncope

   f. Peripheral vascular disease

    (1) Arterial—claudication

    (2) Venous—stasis

    (3) Trophic changes with decreased peripheral hair distribution

- Respiratory System

  1. Anatomical and physiological changes

   a. Decreased vital capacity, decreased tissue elasticity

   b. Increased residual volume, decrease in functional alveoli

   c. Increased diameter of the chest

    d. Decreased ability to clear lungs, less efficient cough

    e. Decreased diffusion of gases

    f. Decreased strength of expiratory muscles, more rigid intercostal muscles

    g. Decreased clearance of congestion

    h. Kyphosis may be present

2. Clinical implications

    a. Increased antero-posterior diameter

    b. Barrel chest, retraction

    c. Decreased ventilation at lung bases

    d. Pallor, cyanosis

    e. Nail clubbing

    f. Vesicular breath sounds, bilateral basilar crackles

    g. Decreased reserve

    h. Decreased response to exercise, stress and disease

3. Abnormal changes and disease

    a. Asthma, bronchitis, emphysema

    b. Tumor, lung cancer

    c. Pleural effusion

    d. Pneumonia—atypical presentation of tachypnea, confusion, chest pain, dyspnea and often no fever or low grade fever

    e. Tuberculosis

    f. Atelectasis

    g. Infection

    h. Adventitious sounds—rhonchi, crackles, wheezing, pleural friction rub

    i. Tachypnea, irregular breathing, labored breathing

    j. No breath sounds

- Breasts
  1. Anatomical and physiological changes
     a. Atrophy of fatty tissue and glands, pendulous breasts
     b. May appear nodular
     c. Increased sagging
     d. Nipples are lower
     e. Elderly men may have increased breast size
  2. Clinical implications
     a. Wide variation of size, symmetry, contour, texture, pigmentation
     b. Gynecomastia for men
  3. Abnormal changes and disease
     a. Unilateral mass, pain, tenderness, cancer
     b. Grossly unequal
     c. Redness, bloody discharge
     d. Dimpling
     e. Fixed inversion or retraction of nipple
- Gastrointestinal System
  1. Anatomical and physiological changes
     a. Decreased saliva
     b. Decreased mastication
     c. Decreased peristalsis
     d. Weakening of lower esophageal sphincter
     e. Lower esophageal sphincter often fails to relax
     f. Decreased gastric acid secretion
     g. Decreased hepatic metabolism
     h. Decreased pancreatic secretion
     i. Decreased insulin release
  2. Clinical implications

    a.   Constipation, fecal impaction

    b.   Indigestion

    c.   Increased sensitivity to medication in GI tract

    d.   Increased response to alcohol, nicotine, chocolate, peppermint and caffeine

    e.   Periodontal disease

    f.   Malnutrition

3.   Abnormal changes and disease

    a.   Diabetes

    b.   Nutritional deficiencies

    c.   Gastroesophageal reflux disease

    d.   Hiatal hernia

    e.   Intestinal obstruction, jaundice

    f.   Stool changes—black, tarry; blood; mucus; light tan or gray color

- Genitourinary and Reproductive Systems

   1.   Anatomical and physiological changes

    a.   Renal changes

       (1)   Decreased kidney function, number of nephrons and glomerular filtration rate (GFR)

       (2)   Decreased bladder capacity and muscle tone

       (3)   Decreased sphincter control

       (4)   Increased frequency, urgency, nocturia

    b.   Hormonal changes

       (1)   Decreased estrogen in females

       (2)   Decreased testosterone in males

       (3)   Atrophy of ovaries, uterus and vagina

       (4)   Development of firmer testes, may be smaller

       (5)   Sclerosis of penile arteries and veins

            (6)   Decreased seminal fluid, sperm number, motility

            (7)   Pubic hair thins and grays

            (8)   Prostate gland enlargement

            (9)   Decreased vaginal secretions

2. Clinical implications

    a. Asymptomatic urinary tract infections

    b. Urinary incontinence

    c. Atrophic vaginitis, foul-smelling vaginal discharge

    d. Pelvic prolapse

    e. Benign prostatic hypertrophy

    f. Drug toxicity

    g. Urinary retention

    h. Impotency

    i. Testicular enlargement, nodules

3. Abnormal changes and disease

    a. Cervical, ovarian cancer/disease/nodules

    b. Testicular, penile cancer/lesions/nodules

    c. Bladder, kidney cancer/disease/lesions

- Endocrine System

1. Anatomical and physiological changes

    a. Decreased size, number and activity of sweat glands

    b. Decline in body's cooling mechanism

    c. Decreased ability to perspire

    d. Decreased ability to metabolize glucose

    e. Reduced insulin secretion

    f. Delayed insulin response

2. Clinical implications

    a. Dehydration

    b. Hyperthermia

    c. Hypoglycemia

  3. Abnormal changes and disease

    a. Diabetes mellitus

    b. Tumors

    c. Thyroid disease

- Musculoskeletal System

  1. Anatomical and physiological changes

    a. Bone demineralization

    b. Decreased strength and endurance, range of motion

    c. Joint and cartilage erosion

    d. Loss of flexibility in the joints

    e. Bony growths at joints

    f. Decreased muscle mass

    g. Bony prominences develop

  2. Clinical implications

    a. Gait disturbances

    b. Falls

    c. Loss of height

    d. Hallus valgus—bunions

    e. Hammer toes

    f. Valgus, varus deformities

    g. Lordosis, scoliosis, kyphosis

    h. Stiffness and decreased range of motion of joints

  3. Abnormal changes and disease

    a. Osteoporosis

    b. Degenerative joint disease

    c. Fractures—vertebrae, hip, colles' (fracture of lower end of radius)

    d. Extra-articular pathologic changes—bursitis, fibrositis

      e.   Swelling, tenderness pain in joints

- Sensory System

   1. Vision

      a.   Anatomical and physiological changes

         (1)   Lens yellows and clouds

         (2)   Pupils smaller, but remain equal

         (3)   Decreased tear production

         (4)   Lens stiffen

         (5)   Decreased peripheral vision

         (6)   Difficulty in color discrimination

         (7)   Eyelids thinning, increased stretching, poor fit; entropion and ectropion

         (8)   Conjunctiva pale and less white

         (9)   Arcus senilis

      b.   Clinical implications

         (1)   Decreased visual acuity

         (2)   Decreased adaptation to darkness

         (3)   Corneal irritation

         (4)   Decreased peripheral vision

         (5)   Dry appearance

         (6)   Progressive eyelid relaxation

      c.   Abnormal changes and disease

         (1)   Macular degeneration

         (2)   Blindness

         (3)   Retinal detachment

         (4)   Glaucoma

         (5)   Cataracts

   2. Hearing

      a.   Anatomical and physiological changes

    (1) Decreased discrimination of pitch and acuity

    (2) Decreased sensitivity to higher frequency sounds

    (3) Excessive cerumen, hair growth in canal

    (4) Tympanic membranes may lose mobility

  b. Clinical implications

    (1) Vertigo, tinnitus

    (2) Diminished hearing

    (3) Auricle loses elasticity, lobe elongates

  c. Abnormal changes and disease

    (1) Tumors

    (2) Deafness

    (3) Presbycusis

    (4) Otosclerosis

    (5) Impacted cerumen

    (6) Tophi, pain

3. Head/throat/neck/nose

  a. Anatomical and physiological changes

    (1) Decreased sense of smell; difficulty distinguishing specific odors

    (2) Decreased size of thyroid gland

    (3) Atrophy of pharynx, larynx

    (4) Nose sags, appears longer

    (5) Lymph nodes may be noted—less than 1 cm in size, soft discrete and mobile considered normal variation

  b. Clinical implications

    (1) Marked asymmetry of face

    (2) Increased size of lymph nodes

    (3) Soft voice

    (4) Difficulty swallowing

        (5)   Postnasal drip

   c.   Abnormal changes and disease

        (1)   Loss of smell

        (2)   Allergic rhinitis

        (3)   Cracks, fissures of lips

        (4)   Head, neck, throat nodules/cancer

4.   Taste

   a.   Anatomical and physiological changes

        (1)   Decreased number of taste buds, papillary atrophy

        (2)   Difficulty distinguishing specific tastes

        (3)   Teeth yellow, increased space between teeth

        (4)   Decreased ability to chew

   b.   Clinical implications

        (1)   Loss of interest in eating

        (2)   Poor fitting dentures, loose or broken teeth

        (3)   Dehydration

   c.   Abnormal changes and disease

        (1)   Oral cancer

        (2)   Ulcerations

5.   Touch

   a.   Anatomical and physiological changes

        (1)   Decreased receptors

        (2)   Lower ability to distinguish temperature and pain

   b.   Clinical implications

        (1)   Decreased sensation

        (2)   Numbness, tingling

        (3)   Potential for burns, injury

   c.   Abnormal changes and disease

        (1)   Loss of feeling

(2)   Scalding, frostbite

- Neurological system
  1. Anatomical and physiological changes
     a. General decrease in cerebral blood flow
     b. Global brain atrophy
     c. Slowed response to heat and cold
     d. General slowing of reaction time
     e. Sluggish deep tendon reflexes
     f. Loss of vibratory sensation
  2. Clinical implications
     a. Benign senile tremors
     b. Decreased coordination and balance
     c. Wide-based gait
     d. Nystagmus
     e. Decreased response to pain
  3. Abnormal changes and disease
     a. Ataxia
     b. Dysphasia, aphasia
     c. Dysarthria
     d. Parkinson's disease
     e. Senile dementia/Alzheimer's disease
     f. Delirium
     g. Cerebrovascular accident (CVA)
     h. Vertigo

Common Selected Problems of the Older Adlut

For review of other common health problems that affect the elderly see "Gerontological Nursing Certification Review Guide," published by Health Leadership Associates

Common Neurological Disorders and Mental Health Issues

- Delirium—acute change of mental status with disturbance of attention and cognition due to an organic cause; common problem of hospitalized elderly

    1. Definitive diagnostic features

        a. Acute onset; may be worse at night; "sundowning"

        b. Varying course

        c. Psychotic symptoms

            (1) Often iatrogenic—related to medications or fluid and electrolyte imbalance

            (2) Initial presentation of many serious and treatable medical disorders

            (3) Initial presentation in many common disorders, for example:

                (a) Urinary tract infection

                (b) Long history of alcohol abuse combined with an anticholinergic or narcotic

        d. Visual and auditory hallucinations

        e. Frequent disorientation

    2. Common medications causing delirium

        a. Narcotics

        b. Benzodiazepines

        c. Anticholinergics

        d. Antidepressants

        e. Barbiturates

        f. Antihypertensives

        g. Digoxin

        h. Antibiotics such as cephalosporins, aminoglycosides and metronidazole

        i. H_2 blockers such as cimetidine

    3. Conditions predisposing the elderly to development of delirium

    a. Head injury

    b. Dementia

    c. History of significant substance abuse

    d. Advanced medical illness or organ failure

4. Effective treatment

    a. May be difficult; interventions that help orientation

    b. Keep out of bed during waking hours

    c. Presence of family members

    d. Bedroom lights kept on at night; use of clock and calendar

    e. Regular schedule

    f. Trial of low-dose neuroleptic medication or high-potency anti-psychotic

- Dementia—gradual regression and loss of intellectual functioning, such as thinking, remembering, and reasoning, of sufficient severity to interfere with daily functioning

  1. Definitive diagnostic features

    a. Impaired judgement

    b. Change in personality

    c. Mood swings

    d. Erratic behavior

    e. Significant short term memory impairment

    f. Impairment in abstract thinking

    g. Aphasia, apraxia, agnosia

  2. Major causes of dementia

    a. Alzheimer's disease (AD)

        (1) Affects 2.5 million Americans, increasing from 0.6% from age 65 to 70 to 8.4% over age 85

        (2) Most common type of dementia; 16% of women and 6% of men who survive to an average life expectancy will develop Alzheimer's disease

        (3)   Gradual onset

        (4)   Senile plaques and neurofibrillary tangles seen on autopsy

   b.   Multi-infarct dementia (MID)

        (1)   Onset may be sudden

        (2)   Generalized symptoms of disorientation, confusion, behavior change

        (3)   MID coexists in 15 to 20% of AD

        (4)   Risk factors include high blood pressure, vascular disease, diabetes, or previous stoke

   c.   Parkinson's disease (P.D.)

        (1)   Lack of dopamine which controls muscle activity

        (2)   Symptoms include tremors, stiffness, and slow speech

        (3)   Late in the course, some individuals develop dementia

   d.   Other related disorders include Huntington's disease, Creutzfeldt-Jakob disease, Pick's disease, and normal pressure hydrocephalus

   e.   Other causes of dementia are alcohol, drugs, nutritional and metabolic disorders; rarely a tumor

 3.   Effective treatment

   a.   Good preventive health practices may impact the risk of developing dementia

   b.   Use of lists to assist with memory impairment

   c.   Correct vision and hearing deficits

   d.   Use of day hospital and outpatient day care centers

   e.   Make little environmental changes to avoid confusion

   f.   Drug therapy shows limited success at present

- Depression—psychiatric condition which is an affective disorder characterized by physical, cognitive and emotional symptoms; frequently under diagnosed in the elderly and less likely to be treated than in younger adults; decrease in cognitive functioning may be falsely attributed to dementia when the underlying cause is actually depression

1. Definitive diagnostic features

   a. Regular markedly depressed mood

   b. Cognitive symptoms worsen; inability to concentrate

   c. Loss of interest in life, vegetative symptoms

   d. Lack of pleasure in almost all activities

   e. General feeling of worthlessness

   f. Significant unintentional weight loss or weight gain

   g. Insomnia or hypersomnia

   h. Improvement in mentation seen with treatment

   i. Past and family history more likely

2. Marked depressive symptoms noted with the following medical conditions

   a. Endocrine/metabolic disorders (thyroid disease, diabetes mellitus, hypokalemia, anemia)

   b. Brain tumors

   c. COPD

   d. Vitamin deficiencies

   e. Neurological disorders (Parkinson's disease, stroke, multiple sclerosis, seizure disorder)

   f. Drug therapy used to treat medical conditions

   g. Alcohol abuse

   h. Chronic pain

   i. Cancer

3. Complications in diagnosing in the elderly

   a. Behavioral and cognitive changes of the aging central nervous system (CNS) make the differential diagnosis of depression versus dementia challenging

   b. Presence of other major medical conditions

   c. Common complaints of insomnia, awakening during sleep or sleepy during day

4. Effective treatment

    a. Counseling, psychotherapy

    b. Exercise, diet, rest

    c. Cautious trial of pharmacologic interventions—in most cases, the dosage should be reduced 30 to 50%

- Suicide—increasing rates in this population, higher than at younger ages; multiple losses and decreased internal and external resources contribute to incidence; perceived intolerable psychological distress, frustration and unmet needs

1. Risk factors

    a. Sex (male-rate is seven times higher than for older women)

    b. Race (white)

    c. Marital status (divorced, separated or single)

    d. Economic status (low, unemployed)

    e. Mental illness (depression, schizophrenia and individuals in early stages of dementia who are aware of their deficits are at highest risk)

    f. Health, pain (cancer, AIDS, dialysis patients)

    g. Alcohol abuse, dependence

    h. Bereavement (especially within one year of a loss, retirement)

    i. Social isolation

    j. Previous attempts

2. Types

    a. Overt suicide—specific act which terminated life (weapon, hanging, poison, toxic fumes)

    b. Covert suicide—destructive behaviors that erode health and lead to death

        (1) Alcohol abuse, drug abuse

        (2) Medication misuse (overdosage or omission)

        (3) Smoking

        (4) Poor dietary habits, self-starvation

       (5) Ignoring disease symptoms

3.   Treatment—prevention depends on prompt recognition of signs; autonomy and confidentiality do not take priority over one's safety

    a. May be difficult

    b. Close observation during acute phase

    c. Identify and treat underlying depression

    d. Excellent listening skills and willingness to listen

    e. Ensure safe environment; determine if hospitalization is indicated

Pharmacotherapy and the Elderly

Age-related physiological changes result in elderly being at high risk for side effects and toxic effects; compounded when chronic diseases are present

- Important Issues

1.   Cost of prescription medications for elderly account for 30% of all prescription medications, and 40% to 50% of all non-prescription medications in United States

2.   More than $3 billion a year are spent by elderly on prescription and nonprescription drugs

3.   Majority of elderly have one or more chronic conditions such as arthritis, hypertension, heart disease and diabetes which are treated with multiple medications

4.   Increased number of adverse drug reactions (ADR); ADR have occurred in 30% of elderly outpatients and account for up to 10% of hospital admissions

    a. Reflective of number and type of medications taken

    b. Frequent use of over-the-counter, self-prescribed medication, home remedies

    c. Multiple health care providers with lack of coordination of care

    d. Multiple pharmacies used with lack of ability to identify potential drug interactions

    e. Do not assume that behavior change is age-related

5. Common ADR in the elderly include edema, nausea, vomiting, anorexia, dizziness, diarrhea, constipation, confusion, and urinary retention; should not be misinterpreted as signs and symptoms of illness or due to the aging process

- Physiological Changes—may lead to increased plasma concentrations of drugs

    1. Decreased tolerance of standard dosages; toxic reactions occur at lower doses

    2. Decreased metabolism—usually occurs in the liver which is decreased in sized with decreased blood flow

    3. Decreased absorption—decreased liver enzyme activity and gastric emptying time; gastric pH increased

    4. Variable distribution—lean muscle mass decreases and fat tissue increases; fat soluble drugs have longer duration; water soluble drugs have smaller volume of distribution and higher plasma concentrations; increased adipose tissue can cause increased storage of lipid-soluble drugs

    5. Decreased ability to excrete drugs due to decreased glomerular filtration rate (GFR); results in decreased excretion time for medication; GFR declines 50% between third and ninth decades of life

- Potential Side Effects of Commonly Prescribed Drugs

    1. Confusion—digoxin, cimetidine, dopamine agents, antihistamines, hypnotics, sedatives

    2. Anorexia—digoxin

    3. Fatigue/weakness—diuretics, antidepressants, antihypertensives

    4. Ataxia—sedatives, hypnotics, anticonvulsants, antipsychotics

    5. Forgetfulness—barbiturates

    6. Constipation—anticholinergics

    7. Diarrhea—oral antacids

    8. GI upset—iron, nonsteroidal anti-inflammatory drugs (NSAID), salicylates, corticosteroids, estrogens, alcohol

    9. Tinnitus—analgesics

    10. Urinary retention—anticholinergics

11. Orthostatic hypotension—antihypertensives, sedatives, diuretics, antidepressants

12. Depression—benzodiazepines

13. Delirium—corticosteroids, sedatives, antihistamines

14. Dizziness—sedatives, antihypertensives, anticonvulsants, diuretics

- Problems With Use of Medication

  1. Overuse—elderly feel when they seek care from a health care provider, they should receive a prescription

  2. Misuse—self-prescribing habits, changing dosages, use of old prescriptions, use of friend's medication, poor history given to provider, out-dated prescriptions

  3. Knowledge deficit—difficulty understanding due to educational level *or* misunderstanding due to hearing deficits, *or* inadequate information provided by health care professional

  4. Memory deficit—forget purpose, dosage, frequency of taking medication, may accidentally repeat dosage

  5. Cost—may not purchase medication due to limited financial resources

  6. Visual deficit—inability to properly read label, may take wrong medication

  7. Mobility problems—difficulty opening bottles, small tablets hard to handle, splitting pills in half is sometimes necessary, difficulty manipulating inhalers

  8. Multiple providers/multiple pharmacies—conflicting/duplicate medications prescribed by various health care practitioners; generic and brand name prescriptions being taken concurrently

- Recommendations for drug use in the elderly—identify factors that predispose the elderly to ADR, e.g., multisystem disease, greater severity of disease, female gender, small body size, hepatic or renal disease, previous drug reactions; proceed cautiously with the following:

  1. Clear indication for use

  2. Reliably effective drug

  3. Shortest duration appropriate

4. Lowest dosage, "start low, go slow"

5. Cost effective

6. Will it enhance quality of life

7. Avoid adverse outcomes

8. Evaluate patient compliance

9. Identify resource person to assist in administering if necessary

10. Use calenders, pill boxes, and large print to assist

11. Use of devices to aid administration such as spacers for inhalers

Preventive Health Care Recommendations (U.S. Preventive Services, 1996)

The focus is to prevent disease or injury and promote health. Life expectancy has improved, but chronic diseases remain the major causes of death. The elderly have a greater absolute risk of disease and respond positively to preventive measures. Implement the following by using a tracking system such as a checklist or flowsheet.

- History—annual review and recommendations for persons over age 65

    1. Dietary intake—protein-calorie malnutrition is common

    2. Functional status—identify issues

    3. Substance abuse

        a. Tobacco—directly and negatively affects both health and financial status

        b. Alcohol—heavy use is more than two drinks/day

        c. Illegal drug use

        d. Abuse of prescription medications

    4. Physical activity—exercise and physical fitness improve multiple physiological functions such as cardiorespiratory capacity, muscle strength, endurance, range of motion, sleep and cognitive function; reduces falls and injury

- Physical Examination

    1. Height and weight, blood pressure

    2. Clinical breast exam

3. Complete skin exam

4. Thyroid nodules (if history of irradiation), auscultation for carotid bruits (if risk factors for cerebrovascular, cardiovascular, or neurological disease)

5. Oral cavity examination

- ***Recommended*** screening tests by U.S. Preventive Services

    1. Fasting glucose if marginally obese, or family history of diabetes

    2. Papanicolaou smear—perform if no previously documented screen is consistently negative or hysterectomy was performed because of cervical cancer or its precursors; otherwise there is insufficient evidence for routine Pap testing over age 65

    3. Dipstick urinalysis

    4. Mammography—every one to two years

    5. PPD—if at high risk for close/personal contact with disease

    6. Fecal occult blood/sigmoidoscopy—annual fecal occult blood and flexible sigmoidoscopy every three to five years

    7. Electrocardiogram with two or more risk factors (high blood cholesterol, hypertension, smoking, diabetes mellitus, family history of coronary artery disease)

    8. Thyroid function tests

    9. Glaucoma and visual acuity testing

    10. Hearing impairment testing

    11. Total cholesterol in older persons with major coronary heart disease risk factors (smoking, hypertension, diabetes)

- Immunizations

    1. Influenza vaccine—annually

    2. Pneumococcal vaccine once

    3. Tetanus - diphtheria toxoids (Td) should be completed for adults who have not received the primary series; periodic Td boosters

- Routine screening—data does **not** yet indicate *for or against* routine screening for the following:

    1. Depression in asymptomatic patients

2. Dementia in asymptomatic patients

3. Osteoporosis with bone densitometry in postmenopausal women, but women should be counseled about hormone prophylaxis

4. Controversy over whom and how to screen for colon and prostate cancers; digital rectal exams and serum tumor markers such as PSA are not routinely recommended for prostate cancer screening; should be limited to males with a greater than 10 years life expectancy

5. Total cholesterol in asymptomatic patient

Questions
Select the best answer

1. Since the turn of the 20th century, the population over age 65 has increased by:

   a. 3-fold
   b. 5-fold
   c. 11-fold
   d. 20-fold

2. By the year 2050, the elderly population will:

   a. Begin to decrease
   b. Level off at 50 million persons
   c. Include those persons 55 and over
   d. More than double to 80 million

3. Elderly women outnumber elderly men:

   a. Three to two
   b. Twenty million to ten million
   c. Five to two
   d. Two to one

4. Which of the following elderly groups have lower income levels:

   a. African-American males over age 65
   b. Elderly African-Americans and Hispanics
   c. Middle and oldest-old Asians
   d. Oldest-old Whites

5. Better education has proven to improve one's life. The following statement is true:

   a. Half of the elderly have completed high school
   b. The elderly are as likely to have only completed 8th grade as persons under 75 years old
   c. Middle-old have the highest percentage of college degrees
   d. Lack of education increases with age

6. Racial and ethnic differences in the aging population exist. It is predicted that:

   a. The African-American population will double

b. The Asian population will triple
c. The Hispanic population will quadruple
d. The White population will decrease by 20%

7. When performing a health history on the elderly, which of the following should the nurse practitioner avoid?

a. Standing near the window so the patient can see the interviewer more clearly
b. Implications of cultural differences and social mores
c. Asking open-ended questions, but keeping conversation focused
d. Observing for signs of fatigue

8. A common cause of weight loss in the elderly is:

a. Hypothyroidism
b. Hyperthyroidism
c. Delirium
d. Hemophilia

9. Which statement is most accurate about the sleep patterns of older persons?

a. Sleep apnea of 10 seconds or more may occur awakening the elderly
b. The elderly fall asleep quickly but awaken frequently during the night
c. The elderly have difficulty falling asleep, but then sleep soundly
d. There are shorter stages 3 and 4 and longer stage 1 sleep cycles

10. Elder abuse is presently a problem in the United States. Which of the following statements regarding elder abuse is not true?

a. The most common abusers are the family or caregivers
b. Physical abuse is four times more common than psychological abuse
c. It is a common form of domestic violence
d. Up to 10% of the elderly may be subjected to one type of abuse

11. Which of the following is not included in the Patient Self Determination Act of 1990?

a. Durable power of attorney for health care
b. Living will
c. Organ donation
d. Indication of patient's intent for medical care

12. In performing activities of daily living:

    a. The elderly overrate their own abilities
    b. The family members overrate their loved one's ability
    c. The elderly cannot manage their finances well
    d. The elderly frequently pay for services such as cooking and cleaning

13. When observing general physical findings, the nurse practitioner is aware that:

    a. The elderly lose one to two inches in height due to the thickening of the cartilage
    b. The fat distribution shifts from the trunk to the extremities
    c. Weight is constant
    d. Fat increases as water decreases

14. Anatomical and physiological changes of the integument system include:

    a. Decreased heat tolerance
    b. Increased wrinkles, folds and sagging
    c. Coarse body and facial hair
    d. Rapid nail growth with easy breaking of nails

15. Which of the following clinical implications related to the skin do not occur in the elderly?

    a. Risk of infection decreases
    b. Decreased wound healing
    c. Sun exposure changes
    d. Pruritus

16. Which of the following is a normal age-related change of the cardiovascular system?

    a. Slightly increased heart size
    b. Decreased exercise tolerance
    c. Decreased peripheral vascular resistance
    d. Presence of S_3 heart sound

17. Coronary artery disease may present with the following abnormal changes and/or disease?

    a. Dyspnea and palpitations
    b. Isolated systolic hypertension
    c. Congestive heart failure

    d. Arrhythmias

18. Which of the following aging changes of the respiratory system is not found in the elderly?

    a. Decreased vital capacity and tissue elasticity
    b. Increased residual volume
    c. Decreased anterior-posterior diameter of the chest
    d. Less efficient cough and clearance of congestion

19. Normal age-related changes frequently result in atypical presentation of illness in the elderly client. Which of the following signs and symptoms of pneumonia is frequently not found in the elderly?

    a. High fever
    b. Tachypnea
    c. Confusion
    d. Chest pain

20. The elderly have breast-related variations. Which statement is true?

    a. Elderly men have a decrease in breast size
    b. There is atrophy of the fatty tissue and a nodular appearance
    c. Significantly unequal breast size is a normal variation
    d. Dimpling and bloody discharge are often seen

21. Which of the following is not a normal age related change of the GI tract?

    a. Decreased gastric acid secretions
    b. Decreased response to alcohol, caffeine and nicotine
    c. Constipation and indigestion
    d. Weakening of the esophageal sphincter

22. Which of the following is a result of normal age-related changes of the GU system?

    a. Asymptomatic urinary tract infections
    b. Urinary incontinence
    c. Urinary retention
    d. Urgency, frequency and nocturia

23. Which of the following is not a result of endocrine changes?

    a. Decreased sweat gland activity

  b. Decreased glucose metabolism
  c. Increased ability to perspire
  d. Response to insulin is delayed

24. Abnormal disease processes of the musculoskeletal system include:

  a. Osteoporosis, degenerative joint disease
  b. Bony growths at joints
  c. Decreased strength and endurance
  d. Decreased muscle mass

25. Which of the following is not a normal physiological change of the eyes?

  a. Decreased visual acuity
  b. Poor color discrimination
  c. Yellowing, clouding and stiffening of the lens
  d. Degeneration of the macula

26. Aging results in a variety of normal, non-pathological changes in the body. Which of the following is a normal, age-related change in the structure or function of the ear?

  a. Decreased discrimination of pitch and acuity
  b. Increased sensitivity to low-pitched sounds
  c. Decreased hair growth in the canals
  d. Increased mobility of the tympanic membrane

27. Variations in the elderly's ability to taste are related to:

  a. Decreased taste buds
  b. Increased ability to distinguish specific tastes
  c. Development of new taste buds
  d. Difficulty swallowing

28. Mrs G. is an 86-year-old female who lives alone. She has been functionally independent until two days ago when her daughter found her to be disheveled, incontinent of urine, and "talking nonsense." When evaluating Mrs. G. to rule out causes of delirium, the nurse practitioner knows that which of the following is not typically a cause?

  a. Infection
  b. Polypharmacy
  c. Hyponatremia
  d. Depression

29. Alzheimer's disease is characterized by:

    a. Long-term memory loss more dramatic than short term
    b. Acute onset
    c. Plaques and tangles
    d. Affects elderly men and women equally

30. Which of the following is not a diagnostic feature of depression?

    a. Inability to concentrate
    b. Short-term memory impairment
    c. Mood swings
    d. Unintentional weight loss or gain

31. Risk factors for suicide in the elderly include:

    a. Elderly, married females
    b. Dementia, depression
    c. Limited educational background
    d. Minority ethnic groups

32. It is important to remember that physiological changes in the elderly affect drug therapy. Which of the following statements is true?

    a. Metabolism of drugs usually occurs in the kidneys
    b. The liver increases in size in relation to the number and types of drugs used
    c. Gastric pH is decreased
    d. Decreased ability to excrete drugs is due to the decreased GFR

33. The U.S. Preventive Services Task Force made the following recommendation for routine screening of all individuals over 65 years old:

    a. Total cholesterol annually
    b. Prostatic specific antigen annually
    c. Complete skin exam annually
    d. Papanicolaou smear annually on all females

34. Controversy exists for routine screening. The following is not recommended for screening of the elderly?

    a. PPD if at high risk
    b. Bone densitometry for osteoporosis
    c. Td boosters periodically
    d. Fasting glucose with a positive family history

Answers

1. c	12. a	23. c
2. d	13. d	24. a
3. a	14. b	25. d
4. b	15. a	26. a
5. d	16. b	27. a
6. c	17. a	28. d
7. a	18. c	29. c
8. b	19. a	30. c
9. d	20. b	31. b
10. b	21. b	32. d
11. c	22. d	33. c
		34. b

Bibliography

Bates, B. (1995). *A guide to physical examination and history taking* (6th ed.). Philadelphia: J. B. Lippincott.

Bennett, J. C., & Plum, F. (Eds.). (1996). *Cecil textbook of medicine* (20th ed). Philadelphia: W. B. Saunders.

Cassel, C. K., Cohen, H. J., Larson, E. B., Meier, D. E., Resnick, N. M., & Rubenstein, L. Z. (Eds.). (1997). *Geriatric medicine.* New York: Springer.

Cassidy, K. (1996). Health assessment of the elderly. In C. Kopac & V. Millonig (Eds.), *Gerontological nursing certification review guide for the generalist, clinical specialist, and nurse practitioner* (pp. 42-67). Potomac, MD. Health Leadership Associates.

Fitzpatrick, T. B., Johnson, R. A., Polano, M. K., Suurmon, D., & Wolff, K. (1997). *Color atlas of synopsis of clinical dermatology* (3rd ed.). New York: McGraw-Hill.

Folstein, M. F., Folstein, S. E., & McHugh, P. R. (1975). Mini-mental state: A practical method for grading the cognitive state of patients for the clinician. *Journal of Psychiatric Research, 12,* 189-198.

Forciea, M. A., & Lavizzo-Mourey, R. J. (1996). *Geriatric secrets.* Philadelphia: Hanley & Belfus.

Guide to clinical preventive services. U.S. preventive services task force (2nd ed.). (1996). Baltimore: Williams & Wilkins.

Katz, S. (1983). Assessing self-maintenance: Activities of daily living, mobility, and instrumental activities of daily living. *Journal of the American Geriatric Society, 31,* 721-727.

Lueckenotte, A. G. (1994). *Pocket guide to gerontological assessment* (2nd ed.). St. Louis: Mosby.

Pfeiffer, E. (1975). A short portable mental status questionnaire for the assessment of organic brain deficit in elderly patients. *Journal of The American Geriatric Society, 23,* 433-441.

Spirduso, W. W. (1995). *Physical dimensions of aging.* Human Kinetics. Champaign, IL: Human Kinetics.

U.S. Census Bureau (1995). (Revised May 13, 1997). *Statistical briefs.* Economics and Statistical Administration, U.S. Department of Commerce.

Advanced Practice Trends/Issues and Health Policy

Leanne C. Busby

Introduction

Advanced practice registered nurses (APRN) must be alert to the rapidity of changes in health policy and trends that impact their practice and their patients. This chapter will review the advanced practice role, advanced practice trends and issues, and the impact of health policy on advanced practice nursing. Although current information is presented, the reader is encouraged to contact local and State regulatory bodies for particular practice requirements.

Advanced Practice Nursing

- Definition of Advanced Practice Registered Nursing
    1. National Council of State Boards of Nursing (NCSBN)—"practice based on the knowledge and skills acquired in a basic nursing education, through licensure as a registered nurse, and in graduate education and experience, including advanced nursing theory, physical and psychosocial assessment, and treatment of illness" (NCSBN, 1992, p. 6).
    2. American Nurses Association (ANA)—"professional nurses who have successfully completed a graduate program of study in a nursing specialty or related field that provides specialized knowledge and skills that form the foundation for expanded practice roles in health care" (ANA, 1996).

- Role Development
    1. Pediatric nurse practitioner (PNP) provided model for other emerging nurse practitioner (NP) specialties
    2. Original role was seen as an opportunity to improve access to care, and as one solution to physician shortage
        a. Originally there was both support and resistance for new role
        b. Early research focused on quality, cost effectiveness, productivity, clinical decision making skills and job satisfaction
        c. Policy makers originally saw NP as physician extenders
        d. In 1973 PNPs organized National Association of Pediatric Nurse Associates and Practitioners (NAPNAP) to establish guidelines for PNP practice

    e.   During 1980 to 1989—more physicians resulted in less need for NP

    f.   During 1990 to 1998—increased emphasis on primary care resulted in decreased need for specialty care; NP seen as viable, cost effective member of health care delivery team

- Educational Preparation

    1.   In 1964, Dr. Loretta C. Ford and Dr. Henry K. Silver started first PNP program at University of Colorado Health Sciences Center in Denver, Colorado.

        a.   1960's studies suggested children were receiving less than adequate care due to physician shortage

        b.   American Academy of Pediatrics (AAP) surveyed physicians and found that most physicians were willing to delegate certain health care delivery tasks to nurses in new expanded role

        c.   Length of first program was four months of study and 18 months of clinical practice

        d.   Most early programs were certificate programs and were located both within and outside academic medical centers

    2.   By 1989, 85% of federally funded NP programs were at Master's degree level

    3.   Typical programs today are one to two years of full time study or two to four years of part time study (Harper, 1996)

    4.   Curriculum

        a.   Core graduate nursing content includes: Nursing theory, organizational/leadership theory, ethical/legal issues, multicultural care, economics, community based care, managed care, and health care delivery systems

        b.   Advanced practice core content includes: Advanced health assessment, pharmacology, physiology, advanced pathophysiology or other related sciences depending on the APRN specialty; clinical decision making process, advanced nursing interventions/therapeutics, health promotion/disease prevention, community based practice, role differentiation, and interpersonal and family theory

        c.   APRN specialty content includes information that is unique to type of APRN role, information that is unique to health care needs of respective specialty population, information that supports standards and competencies established by professional specialty organizations, clinical decision making applied to specialty practice, and faculty supervised clinical practice experience (Harper, 1996)

Advanced Practice Trends and Issues

- Components of Advanced Practice Registered Nursing Role
    1. Coordinator of care
    2. Patient advocate
    3. Accountable for patient outcomes and cost effectiveness
    4. Direct care giver
    5. Educator
    6. Administrator
    7. Researcher
    8. Consultant
    9. Case manager
    10. Change agent
- Scope and Standards of Advanced Practice
    1. Standards of practice
        a. Described by ANA (1996) as authoritative statements by which to measure quality of practice, service or education
        b. Establishes minimum levels of acceptable performance
        c. Provides consumer with means to measure quality of care received (Hawkins & Thibodeau, 1996)
        d. Both generic and specific specialty standards exist
        e. Specialty groups have also developed standards, some of which are: National Association of Pediatric Nurse Associates and Practitioners (NAPNAP), American Academy of Nurse Practitioners (AANP), Association for Women's Health, Obstetric, and Neonatal Nurses (AWHONN) (formerly NAACOG)
        f. Can be used to provide legal expectations of practice but were

not designed to define standards of practice for clinical or legal purposes

2. Scope of practice

   a. Based on what is legally allowable in each State under its Nurse Practice Act

   b. Provides guidelines for nursing practice

   c. Is not mandated

   d. Varies widely from State to State (Hawkins & Tibodeau, 1996)

   e. Fluid and evolving (Hanson, 1996)

   f. Often based on legal requirements within State and national standards

3. Nurse practice acts

   a. Authorizes Boards of Nursing in each state to establish statutory authority for licensure of registered nurses (RN)

   b. Authority includes use of title, authorization for scope of practice, and disciplinary grounds (Bosna, 1997)

   c. Evolves from statutory law which, after interpretation, becomes regulatory language

- Credentialing

   1. Mandates accountability/responsibility for competent practice

   2. Validation of required education, licensure, and certification

   3. Necessary to assure public of safe health-care provided by qualified individuals

   4. Necessary to assure compliance with federal and State laws related to nursing practice

   5. Acknowledges APRN advanced scope of practice

   6. Should provide appropriate avenues for public or individual practice complaints

   7. Allows profession to be accountable to public and its members by enforcing professional standards for practice (Hickey, Ouimette, & Venegoni, 1996)

- Certification
    1. Definition: Process by which nongovernmental agency or association confirms that an individual licensed professional has met certain predetermined standards as specified by that profession for specialty practice
    2. Purpose: To assure the public that an individual has mastered a body of knowledge and acquired skills in a particular specialty
    3. May be required for State licensure and reimbursement
    4. Required for APRN practice in some States (Hickey, Ouimette, & Venegoni, 1996)

- Prescriptive Authority
    1. Ensures educational preparation in therapeutic regimens
    2. Addressed State by State with varying degrees of authority
    3. Over 49 States provide some degree of prescriptive authority at present
    4. Depending on full scope of state law, an APRN may obtain a federal Drug Enforcement Agency (DEA) registration number
    5. Requires pharmacology education within graduate programs and continuing education to maintain authority

- Hospital staff admitting privileges: Possibility of hospital staff membership opened to nonphysician providers by Joint Commission on Accreditation of Health Care Organizations (JCAHO) in 1983

- Practice Issues
    1. Collaborative practice
        a. Purpose: To enhance quality of care and improve patient outcomes
        b. Definition: ANA's *Nursing: A Social Policy Statement* (1995) describes collaboration as "true partnership" in which all players have and value power, recognize and accept separate and combined areas of responsibility and activity, and share common goals
        c. Interdisciplinary teams are form of collaborative practice

    d. Provides for ongoing continuity and coordination of care (Hickey, Ouimette, & Venegoni, 1996)

2. Case management

    a. Purpose: To mobilize, monitor and control resources that patient uses over course of an illness while maintaining a balance between quality and cost (Hickey, Ouimette, & Venegoni, 1996)

    b. Definition: Comprehensive and systematic approach to providing quality community-based health care

    c. Components of role

        (1) Planning care for cost effectiveness and optimal outcomes

        (2) Procuring and coordinating care

        (3) Monitoring and evaluating outcomes

        (4) Performing physical assessments

        (5) Selecting lab oratory and other tests

        (6) Prescribing medications (Hawkins & Thibodeau, 1996)

        (7) Requires that provider have strong communication skills and clinical expertise

        (8) Provides care along continuum, decreases fragmentation of services, enhances patient and family quality of life, and contains costs

    d. Key features associated with models of case management:

        (1) Standardized appropriate use of resources aimed at identified outcomes within appropriate time frames

        (2) Promotes collaborative practice among disciplines

        (3) Promotes coordinated continuity of care over course of illness

        (4) Promotes job satisfaction for providers

        (5) Promotes patient and provider satisfaction with care delivery while minimizing cost to institution (Hickey, Ouimette, Venegoni, 1996)

    e. Populations that would benefit from case management

        (1)   Those for whom course of treatment is costly and unpredictable

        (2)   Those who experience frequent or chronic readmissions to hospital

        (3)   Those involved with multiple providers or multiple disciplines (Hickey, Ouimette, & Venegoni, 1996)

3.   Quality improvement

    a.   Definition: ''The organized creation of beneficial change... the attainment of unprecedented levels of performance.'' (Juran, 1989, p. 28)

    b.   Program directed toward assuring and defining excellence and accountability for quality of care provided

    c.   Alternative terms—Total Quality Management (TQM); Continuous Quality Improvement (CQI); differs from Quality Assurance (QA) in being a continuous rather than episodic process

    d.   Provides norms, criteria, and standards by which to evaluate and measure program or process (Hawkins & Tribodeau, 1996)

    e.   Provides framework for systematic, continuous evaluation of practice through identification of norms, criteria, and standards that measure program effectiveness and minimize liability

    f.   Can decrease exposure to liability

    g.   Mechanisms of quality improvement

        (1)   Peer review

            (a)   Recognize and reward nursing practice

            (b)   Leads to higher standards of practice

            (c)   Discourages practice beyond scope of legal authority

            (d)   Improves quality of care (Bodenheimer & Grumbach, 1996)

            (e)   Provides for accountability and responsibility

        (2)   Other methods of evaluation

            (a)   Audit—retrospective measurement of quality

        (b)   Interviews and questionnaires

        (c)   Patient satisfaction surveys or interviews

4.   Risk management

   a.   Systems and activities designed to recognize and intervene to decrease risk of injury to patients and subsequent claims against health care providers; based on assumption that many injuries to patients are preventable

   b.   Evaluates sources of legal liability in practice such as:

        (1)   Patients

        (2)   Procedures

        (3)   Quality of record keeping

   c.   Includes educational activities that decrease risk in identified areas

5.   Malpractice

   a.   Professional misconduct, unreasonable lack of skill, infidelity in professional or fiduciary duties, or illegal or immoral conduct that results in harm to the patient

   b.   Alleged failure on the part of professional to render services with the degree of care, diligence and precaution that another member of same profession in similar circumstances would render to prevent injury to someone else

   c.   Malpractice insurance

        (1)   Does not protect APRN from charges of practicing medicine without a license if APRN is practicing outside legal scope of practice for that State

        (2)   National Practitioner Data Bank collects information on adverse actions against health care practitioners, including nurses; once clinical privileges are granted by hospitals, bank can be queried every two years

        (3)   Types of coverage

            (a)   Occurrence coverage—covers event of malpractice which occurred during policy period, regardless of date of discovery or when claim filed

        (b) Claims made coverage—covers only claims filed during policy coverage period, regardless of when event occurred; optional tail coverage contract extends the coverage of a claims made policy into the future to cover all claims filed after the basic claims made coverage period

6. Negligence—failure of individual to do what a reasonable person would do that results in injury to another

7. Reimbursement

   Whether working independently, sharing a joint practice with a physician, or employed in a hospital or within a managed care system, APRN must be reimbursed appropriately. Standards that determine private pay insurance mechanisms are often modeled after federal policies such as Medicaid and Medicare. However, even when the federal government establishes mandates that encourage direct payment of nonphysician healthcare providers, barriers to reimbursement are often encountered in State level rules and regulations (Hanson, 1996).

   a. Medicaid

       (1) Authorized in 1965 as Title XIX of Social Security Act

       (2) Federal/State matching program with federal oversight

       (3) Financed through federal and State taxes, with between 50% and 83% of total Medicaid costs covered by federal government

       (4) Does not cover all people below federal poverty level, but State Medicaid programs are required by federal government to cover certain categories such as:

           (a) Recipients of Aid to Families with Dependent Children (AFDC)—(States set own eligibility requirements for AFDC)

           (b) People over 65, blind, or totally disabled who are eligible for cash assistance under federal Supplemental Security Income (SSI) program

           (c) Pregnant women (for pregnancy-related services only) and children under six with family incomes up to 133% of federal poverty level

        (d)   Children born after September 1983 in families whose income is at or below federal poverty level

  (5) States can choose to cover "medically needy"

  (6) Coverage required for certain services

        (a)   Hospital and physician services

        (b)   Laboratory and radiographic services

        (c)   Nursing home and home health care services

        (d)   Prenatal and preventive services

        (e)   Medically necessary transportation

  (7) States can add services to list and can place certain limitations on federally mandated services

  (8) Although Medicaid recipients cannot be billed for services, States can impose nominal co-payments or deductibles for certain services (Bodenheimer & Grumbach, 1996)

  (9) Other insurance or third party payment must be exhausted before Medicaid will pay for services

b. Medicare

  (1) Federally mandated program, established in 1965, provides health insurance for aged and disabled individuals

  (2) Eligibility covers hospital service, physician services, and other medical services

  (3) Income level does not impact eligibility

  (4) Medicare Part A

        (a)   Those 65 years of age and older who are eligible for Social Security are automatically enrolled, whether or not they are retired—persons are eligible for Social Security when they (or their spouses) have paid into Social Security system through employment for 40 quarters or more

        (b)   Those who have paid into system for less than 40 quarters can enroll in Medicare Part A by paying monthly premium

(c) Those who are under age 65 and are totally and permanently disabled may enroll in Medicare Part A after receiving Social Security disability benefits for 24 months

(d) Those with chronic renal disease requiring dialysis or transplant may also be eligible for Part A without a two year waiting period

(e) Services covered include some hospitalization costs; some skilled nursing facility costs, although custodial care is not covered; home health care–100% for skilled care; 80% of approved amount for medical equipment; and hospice care–100% for most services

(f) Payment for hospitization is based on projected costs of caring for patient with a given problem—each Medicare patient admitted to a hospital is classified according to a diagnosis-related group (DRG); the hospital is then paid a predetermined amount for each patient admitted with the given DRG, if hospital costs are above payment rate, the hospital must absorb loss; if costs are below payment rate, hospital allowed to keep a percentage of excess

(g) APRN not paid directly for services delivered in a hospital

(5) Medicare Part B—Supplementary Medical Insurance (SMI)

(a) Monthly premium is charged

(b) Some-low income people are eligible to have monthly premium paid by Medicaid

(c) Financed by general federal revenues and by Part B monthly premiums

(d) Covers all medically necessary services—80% of an approved amount after annual deductible; includes physician services, physical, occupational, and speech therapy; medical equipment and diagnostic tests, and some preventive care such as Pap tests, mammograms, hepatitis B, pneumococcal and influenza vaccines can be included in medical expenses

c. APRN—Medicaid/Medicare coverage

    (1) Omnibus Budget Reconciliation Act (OBRA) 1989— mandated Medicaid reimbursement for certified pediatric and family nurse practitioners began July 1, 1990; providers required to practice within the scope of State law and do not have to be under supervision or associated with a physician or other provider

    (2) Level of payment determined by States—reimbursement rates range from 70% to 100% of fee-for-service physician Medicaid rate (Pearson, 1998)

    (3) Pediatric and family nurse practitioners may bill Medicaid directly after attaining provider number from State Medicaid agency

    (4) States can elect to pass laws allowing them to extend Medicaid payment to other types of NP not identified in federal statutes

    (5) As of August 5, 1997, new legislation has expanded direct Medicare reimbursement for APRN in all geographic locations

    (6) Self-employed APRN can now be reimbursed at 85% of physician fee schedule without direct physician supervision

    (7) When APRN is employed by physician, the physician practice may receive 100% of customary physician charge, according to "Incident to" rules (Buppert, 1998)

    (8) APRN must be RN currently licensed to practice in the State in which services are rendered; must meet requirements for NP practice in State in which services are rendered; must be currently certified as a primary care NP; must have successfully completed a formal advanced practice educational program of at least one academic year that includes at least four months of classroom instruction and awards a degree, diploma, or certificate

OR, have successfully completed a formal advanced practice educational program and have been performing in that expanded role for at least 12 months during the 18-month period immediately preceding February 8, 1978, the effective date for the provision of services of NP as reflected in the conditions for certification for rural health clinics

(9) NP covered services are limited to services an NP is legally authorized to perform under the State law in which the NP practices and must meet training, educational and experience requirements prescribed by the Secretary of Health and Human Services

(10) NP services covered under Part B if service would be considered physician's services if furnished by MD or Doctor of Osteopathy (DO); if NP is legally authorized to perform services in the state in which they are performed; if services are performed in collaboration with MD/DO (collaboration specified as a process whereby NP works with physician to deliver health care within scope of NP expertise with medical direction and appropriate supervision as provided for in jointly developed guidelines or other mechanisms defined by federal regulations and law of the state in which services are performed); and services are otherwise precluded from coverage because of one of the statutory exclusions

(11) "Incident to" refers to services provided as an integral, yet incidental, part of the physician's personal, professional services in the course of diagnosis or treatment of injury or illness—these services must occur under direct personal supervision of a physician, and the APRN must be an employee of the physician or physician group; services must occur during the course of treatment where the physician performs an initial service and subsequent services in a manner that reflects the physician's active participation and management of the course of treatment—direct personal supervision does not mean that the physician must be in the same room as the APRN, however, the physician must be present in the office

suite and available for assistance and direction while the APRN provides patient care (Buppert, 1998)

(12) When APRN performs "incident to" service in physician's office, billing must be submitted to Medicare by employing physician, under the physician's name, provider number and CPT code—payment is made at full physician rate and is paid to physician or physician practice

(13) When APRN provides service in skilled nursing facility, or nursing facility located in urban area as defined by law, Medicare payment can be obtained—medicare reimbursement is also available for APRN services in skilled nursing facilities (SNF) in nonrural areas on a reasonable charge basis; this amount may not exceed physician fee schedule amount for service and payment is made to the APRN's employer

d. APRN coverage—other third party payors

(1) Reimbursement from private insurers varies according to State insurance commission and is contract specific

(2) Civilian Health and Medical Program of the United States (CHAMPUS)

(a) Federal health plan which covers health care for military personnel and their families

(b) Applies to surviving dependents of service personnel and retirees

(c) APRN reimbursed for services

(3) Federal Employees Health Benefit Program (FEHBP)

(a) One of largest employer sponsored group health insurance programs

(b) APRN recognized as designated health care provider

e. Methods of payment for advanced practice nurses

(1) Fee-for-service model

(a) Unit of payment is visit or procedure

        (b) Can occur with utilization review in which case payor has right to authorize or deny payment of expensive medical interventions such as hospital admission, extra hospital days, and surgery

    (2) Episodic model

        (a) One sum is paid for all services delivered during a given illness

        (b) DRG fee payment

    (3) Capitation model, PPO, and HMO are covered in section on Managed Care in this chapter

- Professional Organizations
  1. Purpose and benefit
     a. Collective voice to promote nursing and quality care
     b. Monitor/influence laws and regulations
     c. Disseminate information
     d. Study practice issues
     e. Establish practice standards
  2. Examples
     a. American Academy of Nurse Practitioners (AANP)
     b. Association for Womens Health, Obstetrics & Neonatal Nurses (AWHONN)
     c. American College of Nurse Practitioners (ACNP)
     d. National Association of Nurse Practitioners in Reproductive Health (NANPRH)
     e. National Association of Pediatric Nurse Associates and Practitioners (NAPNAP)
     f. National Association of School Nurses (NASN)
     g. American Nurses Association (ANA)
     h. National Conference of Gerontological Nurse Practitioners (NCGNP)
     i. Nurse Practitioner Associates for Continuing Education (NPACE)

- Research in Advanced Practice
    1. Major trend is outcome studies
    2. Funding sources—Agency for Health Care Policy and Research (AHCPR), National Institutes of Health (NIH), National Institute for Nursing Research (NINR)
    3. Sources of research findings
        a. Conferences
        b. Scholarly publications
        c. Distribution of summaries of research studies (Hawkins & Thibodeau, 1996)
    4. Use of research in practice setting
        a. Develop research-based clinical pathways
        b. Track clinical outcomes and variances
        c. Demonstrate quality and cost effectiveness of care
        d. Give structure to demonstration projects
        e. Persuade lawmakers of NP value and contriburions in today's health care system
        f. Improve quality and patient outcomes
    5. Benefit of research for patients
        a. Provides thorough understanding of patient situation
        b. Provides more accurate assessment of situations
        c. Increases effectiveness of interventions
        d. Increases provider sensitivity to patient situations
        e. Assists providers to more accurately determine need for and effectiveness of interventions (Hickey, Ouimette, & Venegoni, 1996)
    6. Barriers to research utilization
        a. Time and cost of conducting research studies
        b. Resistance to change in work setting
        c. Lack of rewards for using research findings

    d. Lack of understanding or uncertainty regarding research outcomes (Hickey, Ouimette, & Venegoni, 1996)

  7. Strategies to overcome barriers to research utilization

    a. Creation of organizational culture that values and uses research

    b. Creation of environment where questions are encouraged, critical thinking is appreciated, and nursing care is evaluated

    c. Support for research through time allocation and financial commitment (Hickey, Ouimette & Venegoni, 1996)

Health Policy

- Policy Influences

  1. Healthy People 2000

    a. Published in 1990 by U.S. Department of Health and Human Services

    b. Purpose—commit nation to obtain three broad goals

      (1) Increase span of healthy life for all Americans

      (2) Reduce health disparities among Americans

      (3) Achieve access to preventive services for all Americans (DHHS, 1990, p.6)

    c. Contains 300 specific objectives based on 22 priority areas leading to socially and economically productive lives

    d. Objectives focus on equal access, acceptability, availability, continuity, cost and quality of care

    e. Objectives organized within broad categories of health promotion, health protection, and preventive services

    f. Identifies priority of systematic collection, analysis, interpretation, dissemination, and use of data to understand national health status and plan effective prevention programs

    g. Individuals, communities and organizations are responsible for determining how they will achieve the goals by the year 2000 (Hickey, Ouimette & Venegoni, 1996)

  2. Prevention guidelines

    a. ''Put Prevention Into Practice''—campaign established by U.S.

Public Health Service to enhance delivery of preventive care in primary care practice

b. *Clinicians Handbook of Preventive Services: Put Prevention Into Practice,* published by American Nurses Association (ANA) in 1996 to disseminate practical and comprehensive reference on preventive services to primary care clinicians; document includes:

    (1) Health screening schedules for early disease detection and immunization

    (2) Disease prophylaxis issues

    (3) Risk factor counselling techniques

    (4) Educational resources on preventive care (Hickey, Ouimette & Venegoni, 1996)

c. *Guide to Clinical Preventive Services* (U.S. Preventive Services Task Force, 1989) presents national clinical preventive services guidelines for practice and educational settings

    (1) Age and gender specific

    (2) Suggests targeted examinations, immunizations and health counseling that should be part of periodic health visits

3. Nursing's Agenda for Health Care Reform

a. Published in 1991 by ANA

b. Supports creation of a health care system that assures access, quality, and services at affordable costs

c. Supports ongoing primary care

d. Calls for basic core of essential health services to be available to all and for restructured health care system focusing on consumers and their health and health care delivery in familiar, convenient sites

e. Proposes shift from focus on illness and cure to orientation toward wellness and care

f. Supports provisions for long-term care and insurance reforms that assure improved access to coverage

      g.   Calls for establishment of public/private sector review of resource allocations, cost reduction plans, and fair and consistent reimbursement for all providers

- Utilization of Health Policy

    1.   Shifting trend toward primary care and early preventive measures supports need for APRN

    2.   Four major factors influence health care delivery services

        a.   Payors—individual health care consumers, businesses that pay for health insurance for employees, and government through public programs and entitlement programs such as Medicare and Medicaid

        b.   Insurers—take money from payors, assume risks, and pay providers

        c.   Providers—includes hospitals, physicians, nurses, APRN, physician assistants, pharmacies, home health agencies, and long term care facilities

        d.   Suppliers—pharmaceutical and medical supply industries

    3.   Legislative strategies and political involvement

        a.   APRN must be aware and informed of political process

        b.   APRN must be unified and must closely monitor policy issues

        c.   APRN must create local networks to remove barriers and develop practice guidelines (Hanson, 1996)

- Types of Health Care Delivery Systems

    1.   Primary health care

        a.   Institute of Medicine (IOM) definition—''primary care is the provision of integrated, accessible health care services by clinicians who are accountable for addressing a large majority of personal health care needs, developing a sustained partnership with patients, and practicing in the context of family and community (Committee on Future of Primary Care, 1994)''

        b.   Activities and/or functions define boundaries of primary care, such as curing or alleviating common illnesses and disabilities

        c.   Entry point to a system that includes access to secondary care and tertiary care

    d. Attributes include care that is accessible, comprehensive, coordinated, continuous, and accountable

    e. Strategy for organizing health care system as a whole; gives priority and allocates resources to community-based care rather than hospital-based acute care

    f. Providers of primary care:

        (1) Medical specialties such as family medicine, general internal medicine, general pediatrics, obstetrics and gynecology as specified in the Clinton administration's Health Security Act

        (2) Other experts have included NP and physician assistants (PA) as primary care providers (PCP)

    g. Many definitions stress self-responsibility for health (Hickey, Ouimette, & Venegoni, 1996)

2. Managed care

    a. Definition: Delivery system designed to manage health care through variety of relationships that connect consumers, sponsors, providers and third party payors

    b. System has existed for many years in this country beginning in 1938 with the creation of Kaiser Health Plan (Bodenheimer & Grumbach, (1996)

    c. Objectives

        (1) Manage use and price of health care delivery system

        (2) Control type, level and frequency of treatment

        (3) Restrict level of reimbursement for services

    d. Designed to control costs while assuring quality care

    e. Suggests obligation to manage is shared among providers, consumers and payers

        (1) Providers can no longer dictate price of care delivery— assume more financial risk for population assigned to them for care

        (2) Consumers have fewer choices of coverage and providers, and more financial responsibility

      (3)   Payors manage healthcare dollars through benefit design, selective contracting, and shifting financial risk to providers (Hickey, Ouimette, & Venegoni, 1996)

  f. Types of managed care plans

     (1) Health Maintenance Organizations (HMO)

        (a) Most common type

        (b) By 1994, enrollment at 52 million (20.3% of population)

        (c) Offer pre-established benefit package which includes preventive, inpatient and outpatient care

        (d) HMO contracts with providers to provide care to enrollees

        (e) Providers at financial risk resulting in incentive to provide high quality, cost effective care

        (f) Enrollees select a primary care provider (PCP) who manages total care by authorizing specialty visits, hospitalization, and other services

        (g) PCP referred to as "gatekeeper" and is typically MD, PA or APRN

     (2) Preferred Provider Organizations (PPO)

        (a) Compromised managed care option that is alternative between indemnity and HMO insurance

        (b) Uses financial incentives to influence consumer and provider behaviors

        (c) Refers to variety of arrangements between insurers, providers, and third-party payers rather than standard plan

        (d) Many owned by large insurance companies such as Prudential, Travelers and Aetna

        (e) Available primarily to employed commercial population

     (3) Point of Service Plans (POS)

        (a) Plan that enables consumers to decide at the point

at which they require service, whether or not to use a provider inside or outside the network

    (b)   If variation of HMO plan, PCP coordinates care for enrollees—if variation of PPO plan, enrollees may choose lower cost options outside of provider network

    (c)   Most rapidly growing type of managed care

  (4) Integrated delivery systems

    (a)   Vertical integration of services refers to different levels of care that are combined into a seamless system in which patients move smoothly among all components of delivery system

    (b)   Consists of capitated payment scheme in which the financial risk is shifted from payor to provider; unit of value is cost per member per month (PMPM); provider is responsible for specific target population for which they receive age and gender adjusted budget; in order to remain financially sound, providers must keep target population healthy

    (c)   Low cost, high quality service is the goal of an integrated delivery system and adds value to what consumers and payors purchase

    (d)   Rationing of resources emphasizes the provision of appropriate but not unlimited care in which the PCP assumes responsibility for provision and management of care

g. Reimbursement under managed care

  (1) Providers accept financial risk for care provided to specific population of enrollees

  (2) Payment is capitated

    (a)   Provider receives payment in advance

    (b)   Payment level reflects expected utilization by enrolled population for which provider is responsible

      (3) Provider must control volume and cost

      (4) Efficiency usually rewarded through bonus payments for operating within budget and meeting goals for quality and efficiency

  h. Impact of managed care on APRN

      (1) APRN must be able to demonstrate organization, professionalism, and strong interpersonal skills

      (2) APRN must understand what managed care is and how it is evolving

      (3) APRN must have strong clinical and financial skills

      (4) APRN must be able to adjust to evolving system

      (5) APRN must be able to facilitate internal and external linkages

      (6) APRN must be able to provide and manage care at different levels including:

         (a) Primary care

         (b) Case management

         (c) Utilization management

         (d) Patient advocacy

         (e) Education

         (f) Quality assurance

         (g) Resource management (Hickey, Ouimette, & Venegoni, 1996)

  i. Response of APRN to managed care

      (1) Determine ways to become more efficient without sacrificing interactions with patients

      (2) Engage in lobby activities to facilitate placement on provider panels

      (3) Study and document effectiveness of APRN care delivery

         (a) Collect data on time spent in preventive care delivery

(b) Critically evaluate conceptual approach to care delivery

(c) Investigate and document quality of care delivered by APRN (Hardy Havens, 1996)

Questions
Select the best answer

1. If the three broad goals of *Healthy People 2000* are met, the nation will:

    a. Increase healthy life span, reduce health disparities and increase access to health care for all Americans

    b. Increase healthy life span, increase access and improve economics related to health for all Americans

    c. Increase healthy life span, reduce health disparities, and improve economics related to the health of all Americans

    d. Reduce health disparities, increase access to health care services and make life more socially acceptable for all Americans

2. The achievement of the *Healthy People 2000* goals is the primary responsibility of:

    a. The federal government

    b. Local governments

    c. Individuals, communities and organizations

    d. The Department of Health and Human Services (DHHS)

3. Preventive health guidelines include references to:

    a. Immunizations, health screening, disease prophylaxis, education and infection control

    b. Immunizations, counselling, health screening, disease prophylaxis and education

    c. Health screening, disease prophylaxis, counselling and CPR

    d. Health screening, disease prophylaxis, education, immunizations and CPR

4. Nursing's Agenda for Health Care Reform:

    a. Is supportive of equal access, high quality, cost effective care

    b. Is a mandate to all nurses in the U.S.

    c. Is a summary of nursing research related to health care reform

    d. Is a report of the status of nursing in the 1990s

5. Originally, the nurse practitioner role was established to:

    a. Improve access to care and partially solve physician shortage

    b. Improve the nursing shortage and improve access to care

    c. Improve working conditions of nurses while improving access to care

    d. Improve nursing's image through expansion of the role

6. Early nursing research focused on:

    a. The response of policy makers to the nursing shortage
    b. The effectiveness of the NP as a primary care giver
    c. An effort to demonstate quality and cost effectiveness of NP
    d. The role of the NP as a physician extender

7. Which of the following is not a major factor influencing health care delivery services?

    a. Providers
    b. Payors
    c. Insurers
    d. Legislators

8. All definitions of primary health care include:

    a. The concept of universal access and accountability
    b. The concept of universal access and AIDS prevention
    c. The concept of universal access and a focus on self-responsibility for health
    d. The concept of universal access and a focus on reimbursement for services rendered

9. Standards of practice are:

    a. Authoritative statements used to measure quality
    b. Used to measure outcome but are not authoritative
    c. Designed for legal purposes
    d. Not designed for legal purposes and cannot be used to measure quality

10. Quality improvement activities include:

    a. Defining excellence and legal accountability
    b. Peer review, Quality Assurance plans, and patient satisfaction surveys
    c. Defining four practice domains
    d. Systems to decrease risk of injury to patients

11. Most risk management programs are based on the assumption that:

    a. Many injuries to patients are preventable
    b. Most legal liability is a result of poor documentation
    c. Most injuries to patients are not preventable
    d. Malpractice insurance is generally unnecessary

12. If an APRN practices beyond his/her scope:

    a. Malpractice insurance will protect him/her from a charge of practicing medicine without a license
    b. Malpractice insurance will not protect him/her from a charge of practicing medicine without a license
    c. He or she is legally accountable to the certifying agency
    d. The collaborating physician is legally accountable to the certifying agency

13. Standards of practice may be used to:

    a. Establish minimal levels of performance
    b. Establish reimbursement schemes for APRN
    c. Mandate nursing practice across the nation
    d. Mandate nursing practice in certain states

14. Scope of practice:

    a. Is identical across the States
    b. Is determined by the federal government
    c. Is mandated by the federal government
    d. Varies from State to State

15. Medicaid provides health insurance coverage to:

    a. Certain categories of people whose personal income falls below the federal poverty level
    b. Anyone whose personal income falls below the federal poverty level
    c. Newborns, pregnant women and those over 65 whose personal income falls below the federal poverty level
    d. Those who are elderly

16. Medicaid reimbursement is available to an APRN:

    a. Practicing in federally designated areas
    b. At a rate that is between 80% and 100% of the physician rate
    c. Only if the APRN is in collaborative practice with a physician
    d. Who practice in nursing homes only

17. Medicare reimbursement for services:

    a. Is not dependent on the patient's income level
    b. Depends on the patient's income level
    c. Is not available to APRN under any circumstances

d. Is only available to APRN who is in collaborative practice with a physician

18. Medicare Part A covers:

   a. Hospital, skilled nursing facility, and hospice care
   b. All medically necessary services
   c. Skilled nursing facility care only
   d. Hospice care only

19. Medicare Part B covers:

   a. All medically necessary services
   b. Inpatient hospital care
   c. Outpatient physician services only
   d. Skilled nursing facility and hospice care

20. To receive Medicare reimbursement, APRN must:

   a. Be nationally certified and maintain prescriptive privileges
   b. Maintain a current license in the state in which they are practicing
   c. Practice in a designated medically underserved area
   d. Practice with a physician

21. The term "incident to" refers to:

   a. The occasions when an APRN practices independently but occasionally consults with a physician
   b. The notion that the physician must be present in the office suite and immediately available to provide assistance in order for the APRN to bill for services rendered
   c. The notion that a physician must examine the patient along with the APRN if Medicare is to be billed for services rendered
   d. Medicaid only and is not pertinent to Medicare billing

22. "Incident to" billing is specific to:

   a. Medicare
   b. Medicaid
   c. Medicare and Medicaid
   d. Private insurance companies.

23. The Civilian Health and Medical Program of the United States (CHAMPUS):

    a. Is a federal health plan which covers health care for military personnel and their families and recognizes APRN as reimbursable provider
    b. Is a federal health plan which covers health care for military personnel and recognizes APRN as reimbursable providers
    c. Is a federal health plan which covers health care for military personnel and their families but does not recognize APRN as reimbursable providers
    d. Only covers hospital expenses of military personnel and their families

24. The knowledge base of the APRN is based on:

    a. Medical content
    b. Theoretical content only
    c. Scientific content and theory
    d. Theory and research

25. The role of the APRN has traditionally focused on:

    a. The delivery of primary health care to all people
    b. The delivery of acute health care to all peopl.
    c. Chronic care
    d. The medical model

26. The nurse practitioner role began:

    a. With the establishment of a pediatric nurse practitioner program in an effort to expand the role of the registered nurse in order to meet the needs of the children of the nation
    b. As a result of the new entitlement programs, Medicare and Medicaid
    c. When it was evident that the medical schools across the U.S. could not prepare enough family practitioners to meet the nation's need
    d. As an experimental program at Duke University Medical Center

27. Legal authority for APRN practice is granted by:

    a. Federal law
    b. Regulations from the Department of Health and Human Services
    c. State law and regulations
    d. The Board of Medicine in most States

28. Direct reimbursement to APRN has resulted in:

    a. Increased access to cost-effective, quality primary care

b. Increased malpractice claims against APRN
c. Decreased consumer choice of health care provider
d. Proliferation of APRN in independent practice

29. Malpractice insurance:

    a. Protects an APRN from charges of practicing medicine without a license when they are practicing outside the legal scope of practice
    b. Does not protect an APRN from charges of practicing medicine without a license when they are practicing outside the legal scope of practice
    c. Does not pay for legal defense if the APRN is practicing beyond the legal scope of practice
    d. Is important, but should not be purchased if the facility in which the APRN is employed carries good coverage

30. Collaborative practice:

    a. Limits autonomy and not reasonable in current managed care environment
    b. Will enhance quality of care and improve patient outcomes
    c. Will limit consumer choice of providers
    d. Excludes the concept of interdisciplinary teams

31. Case management:

    a. Balances quality and cost of patient care
    b. Has not been found to be cost effective
    c. Decreases the autonomy of the APRN
    d. Is rarely used today

32. The major trend in health policy research today is:

    a. Outcome studies
    b. Primary care studies
    c. Studies that compare practice strategies of MD and NP
    d. Studies that compare patient satisfaction with the care delivered by MD versus NP

33. Current prescriptive authority for APRN:

    a. Varies among the States
    b. Is fairly consistent among the States
    c. Provides DEA numbers for APRN
    d. Allows APRN to move freely from State to State

34. Managed care is a term that describes:

    a. An established system of health care delivery that is mandated by the federal government
    b. A network of providers who contract to provide services for a specific group of enrollees
    c. A system that does not recognize APRN as primary provider
    d. A network of hospitals and nursing homes that provide care to chronically ill people

35. Certification is:

    a. A procedure through which the government appraises and grants certification to an APRN
    b. Granted by the individual States
    c. Governed by each State's Board of Nursing
    d. A process in which a non-governmental agency or group verifies that an APRN has met certain predetermined standards for specialty practice

36. Licensure:

    a. Is a federal process that is used to standardize health care facilities
    b. Is granted by a State government agency and grants permission to engage in the practice of a given profession
    c. Cannot be used to prohibit anyone from practicing a given profession
    d. Is a federal process that is used to standardize educational programs

37. Reimbursement under managed care:

    a. Requires that the provider accept the financial risk for the care provided to a specific population of enrolled patients
    b. Requires that the managed care organization accept the financial risk for the care provided to a specific population of enrolled patients
    c. Does not reward efficient care delivery
    d. Is not available to APRN

38. An integrated delivery system:

    a. Is one that delivers high quality care but is often not cost effective
    b. Delivers a vertical integration of services with a capitated payment scheme
    c. Does not include rationing of resources
    d. Does not include a capitated payment scheme

Answers

1. a	14. d	27. c
2. c	15. a	28. a
3. b	16. b	29. b
4. a	17. a	30. b
5. a	18. a	31. a
6. c	19. a	32. a
7. d	20. b	33. a
8. a	21. b	34. b
9. a	22. a	35. d
10. b	23. a	36. b
11. a	24. c	37. a
12. b	25. a	38. b
13. a	26. a	

Bibliography

American Nurses Association. (1996). *Clinician's handbook of preventive services: Put prevention into practice.* Washington, DC: Author.

Bodenheimer, T. S. & Grumbach, K. (1996). *Understanding health policy: A clinical approach.* Norwalk, CT: Appleton & Lange.

Bosna, J. (1997). Using nurse practitioner certification for state nursing regulation: An update. *The Nurse Practitioner: The American Journal of Primary Health Care, 22*(6), 213–216.

Buppert, C. (1998). Reimbursement for nurse practitioner services. *The Nurse Practitioner: The American Journal of Primary Health Care, 23*(1), 67–81.

Hanson, C. M. (1996). Health policy issues: Dealing with the realities and constraints of advanced nursing practice. In A. B. Hamric, J. A. Spross, & C. M. Hanson (Eds.) *Advanced practice nursing: An integrative approach* (pp. 496–515). Philadelphia: W. B. Saunders.

Hardy Havens, D. M., Ronan, J. P., & Hannan, C. (1996). Maintaining the nurse practitioner identity in a world of managed care. *Journal of Pediatric Health Care, 10,* 86–88.

Harper, D. (1996). Education for advanced nursing practice. In A. B. Hamric, J. A. Spross, & C. M. Hanson (Eds.) *Advanced practice nursing: An integrative approach* (pp. 57–80). Philadelphia: W. B. Saunders.

Hawkins, J. W., & Thibodeau, J. A. (1996). *The advanced practice nurse: Current issues* (4th ed.). NY: Tiresias Press.

Hickey, J. V., Ouimette, R. M., & Venegoni, S. L. (1996). *Advanced practice nursing: Changing roles and clinical applications.* Philadelphia: Lippincott.

Juran, M. (1989). *Juran on leadership for quality: An executive handbook.* NY: The Free Press.

National Council of State Boards of Nursing. (1992). *Position paper on the licensure of advanced practice nursing.* Chicago: Author.

Pearson, L. (1998). Annual update of how each state stands on legislative issues affecting advanced nursing practice: A survey of legal authority, reimbursement status, and prescriptive authority. *The Nurse Practitioner: The American Journal of Primary Health Care, 23*(1), 14–66.

U.S. Department of Health and Human Services, (1990). *Healthy people 2000: National health promotion and disease prevention objectives* (DHHS Publication No. PHS 91-50213). Washington, DC: Agency for Health Care Policy and Research.

U.S. Preventive Services Task Force. (1996). *Guide to clinical preventive services.* (2nd ed.) Baltimore, MD: Williams & Wilkins.

INDEX

Health Leadership Associates
Nurse Practitioner Continuing Education
Programs

Analysis of the 12-lead ECG

This course is designed for advanced practice nurses. During this 8 hour course you will review cardiac electrophysiology, the cardiac cycle and cardiac muscle function as a basis for 12-lead ECG interpretation; analysis of dysrhythmia, conduction abnormalities, atrial abnormalities, ventricular hypertrophy, axis deviation, myocardial ischemia and myocardial infarction. A one hour practice workshop completes the program. A comprehensive course syllabus is included.

Pharmacology for Nurse Practitioners: A Comprehensive Review and Update

This 30 hour course is designed as a comprehensive presentation and review of pharmacology from the physiologic perspective. In addition to presenting the pharmacokinetics and pharmacodynamics of drugs (indications, contraindications, mechanisms of action, excretion and side effects profile) the corresponding body system physiology will be presented in a format that makes the pharmacology easy to understand and apply in clinical practice. A comprehensive course syllabus is included.

Suturing Review and Practice

This $2\frac{1}{2}$ hour course is designed for nurse practitioners who do not have significant suturing experience. Whether you have been taught but haven't practiced, or have never been taught at all, this program will introduce and reinforce skills that you have not had the opportunity to develop. A brief didactic session on wound assessment and preparation is followed by hands-on instruction and practice of the simple interrupted and vertical mattress techniques.

For information on these and other programs contact:
Health Leadership Associates, Inc.
P.O. Box 59153
Potomac, MD 20859
1-800-435-4775

For information on Certification Review Courses, Home Study Programs and Review Books contact:

Health Leadership Associates, Inc.
Post Office Box 59153
Potomac, Maryland 20859

1-800-435-4775

REVIEW BOOK/AUDIO CASSETTE ORDER FORM
HEALTH LEADERSHIP ASSOCIATES, INC.

PLEASE PRINT OR TYPE

NAME: _____

ADDRESS: Street _____ Apt. # _____ City _____ State _____ Zip Code _____

TELEPHONE: _____ (HOME) _____ (WORK)

Section 1: AUDIO CASSETTES

Professional "live" audio recordings of Review Courses are approximately 15 hours in length unless otherwise noted and include detailed course handouts. Continuing Education contact hours are available for these audio cassette Home Study Programs.

QTY	REVIEW COURSE TITLE	PRICE	
___	Acute Care Nurse Practitioner	$150.00	___
___	Adult Nurse Practitioner	$150.00	___
___	Analysis of the 12-Lead ECG (Available 6/99)	$75.00	___
___ **	Childbearing Management	$45.00	___
___	Clinical Specialist in Adult Psychiatric and Mental Health Nursing	$150.00	___
___	Family Nurse Practitioner (Consists of ANP, PNP & Childbearing Management Courses)	$330.00	___
___ *	Gerontological Nurse	$75.00	___
___	Gerontological Nurse Practitioner	$150.00	___
___	Home Health Nurse	$150.00	___
___	Inpatient Obstetric/Maternal Newborn/ Low Risk Neonatal/Perinatal Nurse	$150.00	___
___	Medical-Surgical Nurse	$150.00	___
___ **	Menopause Lecture	$30.00	___
___	Midwifery Review	$150.00	___
___ *	Pediatric Nurse	$75.00	___
___	Pediatric Nurse Practitioner	$150.00	___
___	Pharmacology Review and Update (Available 4/99)	$300.00	___
___ *	Psychiatric and Mental Health Nurse	$75.00	___
___ **	Test Taking Strategies and Techniques	$20.00	___
___	Women's Health Care Nurse Practitioner	$150.00	___

*8 Hour Course, ** 2-4 Hour Course*

SUB TOTAL: _____

Maryland Residents add 5% sales tax: _____

CEU FEE ($25/course, except FNP course $35): *OPTIONAL*

Shipping: 2-4 Hour Course $5.00 _____

All other Courses $10.00 _____

TOTAL: _____

PAYMENT DUE METHOD OF PAYMENT

☐ Check or money order (US funds, payable to Health Leadership Associates, Inc.) A $25 fee will be charged on returned checks.

☐ Purchase Order is attached. P.O. # _____

☐ Please charge my: ☐ MasterCard ☐ Visa ☐ AMEX ☐ Discover

Credit Card# _____ Exp. date _____

Signature _____

Print Name _____

REVIEW GUIDES & AUDIO CASSETTES

1) Section 1 Total $ _____

2) Section 2 Total $ _____

3) Section 3 Total $ _____   *(All prices subject to change without notice)*

TOTAL PAYMENT DUE $ _____

Section 2: REVIEW BOOKS

QTY	BOOK TITLE	PRICE	
___	Adult Nurse Practitioner Certification Review Guide (third edition)	$47.75	___
___	Family Nurse Practitioner Certification Review Guide Set (Includes ANP, PNP, and Women's Health Care NP Guides)	$123.25	___
___	Gerontological Nursing Certification Review Guide for the Generalist, Clinical Specialist, and Nurse Practitioner (revised edition)	$47.75	___
___	Pediatric Nurse Practitioner Certification Review Guide (third edition)	$47.75	___
___	Psychiatric Certification Review Guide for the Generalist and Clinical Specialist in Adult, Child, and Adolescent Psychiatric and Mental Health Nursing (second edition)	$47.75	___
___	Women's Health Care Nurse Practitioner Certification Review Guide	$47.75	___
___	TODAY and TOMORROW'S WOMAN – MENOPAUSE: BEFORE AND AFTER (Girls of 16 to Women of 99)	$19.95	___

STUDY QUESTION BOOKS

QTY		PRICE	
___	Acute Care Nurse Practitioner Certification Study Question Book	$30.00	___
___	Adult Nurse Practitioner Certification Study Question Book	$30.00	___
___	Family Nurse Practitioner Certification Study Question Book Set (Includes ANP, PNP and WHCNP Study Question Books)	$60.00	___
___	Pediatric Nurse Practitioner Certification Study Question Book	$30.00	___
___	Women's Health Care Nurse Practitioner Certification Study Question Book	$30.00	___

SUB TOTAL: _____

Maryland Residents add 5% sales tax: _____

CEU FEE ($20 per book, except FNP Set $35): *OPTIONAL*

Shipping: $9.00 FNP Set: _____

$5.00 for one book: _____

$2.00 for each additional book: _____
(Except $1.00 for each add'l. *Today and Tomorrow's Woman*)

TOTAL: _____

For orders of 10 or greater call 1-800-435-4775.

Section 3: REVIEW BOOK/AUDIO CASSETTE DISCOUNT PACKAGES

A discounted rate is available when purchasing Review Book(s) and Audio Cassettes together. When purchasing packages, indicate Book/Audio Cassette selections in sections 1 and 2. *Does not apply to Study Question Books.* Calculate amount due in this section.

QTY	PACKAGE SELECTION	PRICE	
_____	8 Hour Course / 1 Review Guide	$120.00	___
_____	15 Hour Course / 1 Review Guide	$190.00	___
_____	FNP Package	$415.00	___

FNP Package consists of Adult NP, Pediatric NP, Women's Health Care NP Guides & Audio Cassettes of the ANP, PNP, and Childbearing Management Courses.

SUB TOTAL: _____

Maryland Residents add 5% sales tax: _____

CEU Fee ($35 per package, except FNP Package $45) *OPTIONAL*

TOTAL: (Shipping charge included in package rate) _____

RETURN POLICY

Due to the nature of the material contained in the review books and audio cassettes, returns on books ONLY will be accepted one week post delivery. No returns on audio cassettes except for defective audio cassettes which will be replaced.

MAIL TO:	Health Leadership Associates, Inc. P.O. Box 59153 Potomac, MD 20859
OR PHONE:	(800) 435-4775; (301) 983-2405
OR FAX:	(301) 983-2693